P9-BHS-809

Aging

Nineteenth Edition

06/07

EDITOR

Harold Cox

Indiana State University

Harold Cox, professor of sociology at Indiana State University, has published several articles in the field of gerontology. He is the author of *Later Life: The Realities of Aging* (Prentice Hall, 2000). He is a member of the Gerontological Society of America and the American Sociological Association's Occupation and Professions Section and Youth Aging Section.

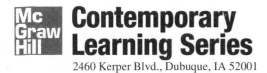

Contemporary Learning Series

2460 Kerper Blvd., Dubuque, IA 52001

Visit us on the Internet
http://www.mhcls.com

Credits

1. **The Phenomenon of Aging**
   Unit photo—© Getty Images/Scott T. Baxter
2. **The Quality of Later Life**
   Unit photo—© Ryan McVay/Getty Images
3. **Societal Attitudes Toward Old Age**
   Unit photo—© Getty Images/Skip Nall
4. **Problems and Potentials of Aging**
   Unit photo—© Ryan McVay/Getty Images
5. **Retirement: American Dream or Dilemma**
   Unit photo—© The McGraw-Hill Companies, Inc./Christopher Kerrigan
6. **The Experience of Dying**
   Unit photo—© Royalty Free/CORBIS
7. **Living Environment in Later Life**
   Unit photo—© Getty Images/Skip Nall
8. **Social Policies, Programs, and Services for Older Americans**
   Unit photo—Kerry Edwards 2004, Inc./Dave Scull, photographer

Copyright

Cataloging in Publication Data
Main entry under title: Annual Editions: Aging. 2006/2007.
1. Aging—Periodicals. I. Cox, Harold, *comp.* II. Title: Aging.
ISBN-13: 978–0–07–351614–1   ISBN-10: 0–07–351614–7   658'.05   ISSN 2072–3808

Nineteenth Edition

Cover image © Scott T. Baxter/Getty Images, Oliver Ribardiere/Getty Images, Martial Colomb/Getty Images, Andersen Ross/Getty Images, Corbis/
Royalty Free, Digital Vision/Punchstock and Photos.com
Printed in the United States of America   1234567890QPDQPD9876   Printed on Recycled Paper

Editors/Advisory Board

Members of the Advisory Board are instrumental in the final selection of articles for each edition of ANNUAL EDITIONS. Their review of articles for content, level, currentness, and appropriateness provides critical direction to the editor and staff. We think that you will find their careful consideration well reflected in this volume.

Preface

In publishing ANNUAL EDITIONS we recognize the enormous role played by the magazines, newspapers, and journals of the public press in providing current, first-rate educational information in a broad spectrum of interest areas. Many of these articles are appropriate for students, researchers, and professionals seeking accurate, current material to help bridge the gap between principles and theories and the real world. These articles, however, become more useful for study when those of lasting value are carefully collected, organized, indexed, and reproduced in a low-cost format, which provides easy and permanent access when the material is needed. That is the role played by ANNUAL EDITIONS.

The decline of the crude birth rate in the United States and other industrialized nations combined with improving food supplies, sanitation, and medical technology has resulted in an ever increasing number and percentage of people remaining alive and healthy well into their retirement years. The result is a shifting age composition of the populations in these nations—a population composed of fewer people under age 20 and more people 65 and older. In 1990, approximately 3 million Americans were 65 years old and older, and they composed 4 percent of the population. In 2000, there were 36 million persons 65 years old and older, and they represented 13 percent of the total population. The most rapid increase in the number of older persons is expected between 2010 and 2030 when the "baby boom" generation reaches the age of 65. Demographers predict that by 2030 there will be 66 million older persons representing approximately 22 percent of the total population. The growing number of older people in the population has made many of the problems of aging immediately visible to the average American. These problems have become widespread topics of concern for political leaders, government planners, and average citizens.

Moreover, the aging of the population has become a phenomenon of the United States and the industrialized countries of Western Europe—it is also occurring in the underdeveloped countries of the world as well. An increasing percentage of the world's population is now defined as aged.

Today almost all middle-aged people expect to live to retirement age and beyond. Both the middle-aged and the elderly have pushed for solutions to the problems confronting older Americans. Everyone seems to agree that granting the elderly a secure and comfortable status is desirable. Voluntary associations, communities, and state and federal governments have committed themselves to improving the lives of older persons. Many programs for senior citizens, both public and private, have emerged in the last 15 years.

The change in the age composition of the population has not gone unnoticed by the media or the academic community. The number of articles appearing in the popular press and professional journals has increased dramatically over the last several years. While scientists have been concerned with the aging process for some time, in the last two decades there has been an expanding volume of research and writing on this subject. This growing interest has resulted in this nineteenth edition of *Annual Editions: Aging 06/07*.

This volume is representative of the field of gerontology in that it is interdisciplinary in its approach, including articles from the biological sciences, medicine, nursing, psychology, sociology, and social work. The articles are taken from the popular press, government publications, and scientific journals. They represent a wide cross section of authors, perspectives, and issues related to the aging process. They were chosen because they address the most relevant and current problems in the field of aging and present a variety of divergent views on the appropriate solutions to these problems. The topics covered include demographic trends, the aging process, longevity, social attitudes toward old age, problems and potentials of aging, retirement, death, living environments in later life, and social policies, programs, and services for older Americans. The articles are organized into an anthology that is useful for both the student and the teacher.

The goal of *Annual Editions: Aging 06/07* is to choose articles that are pertinent, well written, and helpful to those concerned with the field of gerontology. Comments, suggestions, or constructive criticism are welcomed to help improve future editions of this book. Please complete and return the postage-paid article rating form on the last page of this volume. Any anthology can be improved. This one will continue to be improved—annually.

Harold Cox

Harold Cox
Editor

Contents

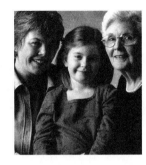

UNIT 1
The Phenomenon of Aging

The concepts in bold italics are developed in the article. For further expansion, please refer to the Topic Guide and the Index.

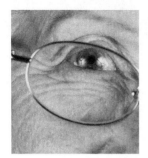

UNIT 2
The Quality of Later Life

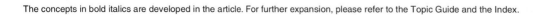

UNIT 3
Societal Attitudes Toward Old Age

The concepts in bold italics are developed in the article. For further expansion, please refer to the Topic Guide and the Index.

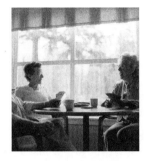

UNIT 4
Problems and Potentials of Aging

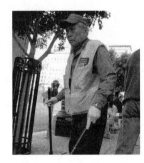

UNIT 5
Retirement: American Dream or Dilemma?

The concepts in bold italics are developed in the article. For further expansion, please refer to the Topic Guide and the Index.

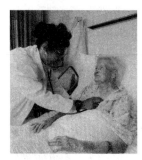

UNIT 6
The Experience of Dying

The concepts in bold italics are developed in the article. For further expansion, please refer to the Topic Guide and the Index.

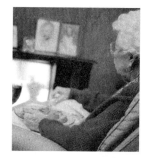

UNIT 7
Living Environment in Later Life

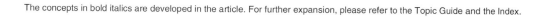

UNIT 8
Social Policies, Programs, and Services for Older Americans

The concepts in bold italics are developed in the article. For further expansion, please refer to the Topic Guide and the Index.

The concepts in bold italics are developed in the article. For further expansion, please refer to the Topic Guide and the Index.

Topic Guide

This topic guide suggests how the selections in this book relate to the subjects covered in your course. You may want to use the topics listed on these pages to search the Web more easily.

On the following pages a number of Web sites have been gathered specifically for this book. They are arranged to reflect the units of this *Annual Edition*. You can link to these sites by going to the student online support site at *http://www.mhcls.com/online/*.

ALL THE ARTICLES THAT RELATE TO EACH TOPIC ARE LISTED BELOW THE BOLD-FACED TERM.

Adulthood, late
2. The Economic Conundrum of an Aging Population
9. Successful Aging
10. The Do or Die Decade
18. Will You Still Need Me When I'm…84? More Couples Divorce After Decades

Aging
2. The Economic Conundrum of an Aging Population
3. A Study for the Ages
4. Puzzle of the Century
5. The Demographic Drivers of Aging
7. The Coming Death Shortage: Why the Longevity Boom Will Make Us Sorry To Be Alive
9. Successful Aging
10. The Do or Die Decade
12. Society Fears the Aging Process
13. Ageism in America

Alternative lifestyles
11. We Can Control How We Age

Alzheimer's disease
19. The Disappearing Mind
20. Alzheimer's Disease as a "Trip Back in Time"

Assisted living
30. (Not) the Same Old Story
31. A Home for the Rest of Your Life
32. Assisted Living: How Much Assistance Can You Really Count On?
35. Long-Term Care: The Ticking Bomb

Attitudes toward aging
12. Society Fears the Aging Process
13. Ageism in America
14. The Activation of Aging Stereotypes in Younger and Older Adults
15. The Under-Reported Impact of Age Discrimination and Its Threat to Business Vitality

Baby boomers
22. Reshaping Retirement: Scenarios and Options

Biology of aging
1. Elderly Americans
3. A Study for the Ages
4. Puzzle of the Century
9. Successful Aging
11. We Can Control How We Age
29. Trends in Causes of Death Among the Elderly

Brain
9. Successful Aging
10. The Do or Die Decade
19. The Disappearing Mind
20. Alzheimer's Disease as a "Trip Back in Time"

Centenarians
4. Puzzle of the Century
6. Will You Live to Be 100?
11. We Can Control How We Age

Cognition
9. Successful Aging
19. The Disappearing Mind
20. Alzheimer's Disease as a "Trip Back in Time"

Death
7. The Coming Death Shortage: Why the Longevity Boom Will Make Us Sorry To Be Alive
26. More Hospice Patients Forgoing Sustenance
27. Expectancy of Spousal Death and Adjustment to Conjugal Bereavement
28. Start the Conversation
29. Trends in Causes of Death Among the Elderly

Demography
1. Elderly Americans
2. The Economic Conundrum of an Aging Population
5. The Demographic Drivers of Aging

Diet
3. A Study for the Ages
6. Will You Live to Be 100?

Drugs
34. Have Seniors Been Dealt a Bad Hand? Medicare's Drug Discount Cards
37. Prescription for Change

Economic status
7. The Coming Death Shortage: Why the Longevity Boom Will Make Us Sorry To Be Alive
15. The Under-Reported Impact of Age Discrimination and Its Threat to Business Vitality
17. Breakthrough
22. Reshaping Retirement: Scenarios and Options
23. Old. Smart. Productive.
24. Work, Retirement, and Well-Being
36. Universalism Without the Targeting: Privatizing the Old-Age Welfare State
37. Prescription for Change
38. Riding Into the Sunset

Education
11. We Can Control How We Age
13. Ageism in America

Elder care
31. A Home for the Rest of Your Life
32. Assisted Living: How Much Assistance Can You Really Count On?
35. Long-Term Care: The Ticking Bomb

Internet References

The following internet sites have been carefully researched and selected to support the articles found in this reader. The easiest way to access these selected sites is to go to our student online support site at *http://www.mhcls.com/online/*.

AE: Aging 06/07

The following sites were available at the time of publication. Visit our Web site—we update our student online support site regularly to reflect any changes.

General Sources

Alliance for Aging Research
http://www.agingresearch.org/

The nation's leading non-profit organization dedicated to improving the health and independence of Americans as they age through public and private funding of medical research and geriatric education.

ElderCare Online
http://www.ec-online.net/

This site provides numerous links to eldercare resources. Information on health, living, aging, finance, and social issues can be found here.

FirstGov
http://www.firstgov.gov/

Whatever you want or need from the U.S. government, it's here on FirstGov.gov. You'll find a rich treasure of online information, services and resources.

UNIT 1: The Phenomenon of Aging

The Aging Research Centre
http://www.arclab.org/

The Aging Research Centre is dedicated to providing a service that allows researchers to find information that is related to the study of the aging process.

Centenarians
http://www.hcoa.org/centenarians/centenarians.htm

There are approximately 70,000 centenarians in the United States. This site provides resources and information for and about centenarians.

National Center for Health Statistics
http://www.cdc.gov/nchs/agingact.htm

NCHS is the Federal Government's principal vital and health statistics agency. NCHS is a part of the Centers for Disease Control and Prevention, U.S. Department of Health and Human Services.

UNIT 2: The Quality of Later Life

Aging with Dignity
http://www.agingwithdignity.org/

The non-profit Aging With Dignity was established to provide people with the practical information, advice and legal tools needed to help their loved ones get proper care.

The Gerontological Society of America
http://www.geron.org

The Gerontological Society of America promotes the scientific study of aging, and it fosters growth and diffusion of knowledge relating to problems of aging and of the sciences contributing to their understanding.

The National Council on the Aging
http://www.ncoa.org

The National Council on the Aging, Inc., is a center of leadership and nationwide expertise in the issues of aging. This private, nonprofit association is committed to enhancing the field of aging through leadership, service, education, and advocacy.

UNIT 3: Societal Attitudes Toward Old Age

Adult Development and Aging: Division 20 of the American Psychological Association
http://www.iog.wayne.edu/APADIV20/APADIV20.HTM

This group is dedicated to studying the psychology of adult development and aging.

American Society on Aging
http://www.asaging.org/index.cfm

The American Society on Aging is the largest and most dynamic network of professionals in the field of aging.

Canadian Psychological Association
http://www.cpa.ca/contents.html

This is the contents page of the Canadian Psychological Association. Material on aging and human development can be found at this site.

UNIT 4: Problems and Potentials of Aging

Alzheimer's Association
http://www.alz.org

The Alzheimer's Association is dedicated to researching the prevention, cures, and treatments of Alzheimer's disease and related disorders, and providing support and assistance to afflicted patients and their families.

A.P.T.A. Section on Geriatrics
http://geriatricspt.org

This is a component of the American Physical Therapy Association. At this site, information regarding consumer and health information for older adults can be found.

Caregiver's Handbook
http://www.acsu.buffalo.edu/~drstall/hndbk0.html

This site is an online handbook for caregivers. Topics include nutrition, medical aspects of caregiving, and liabilities of caregiving.

Caregiver Survival Resources
http://www.caregiver.com

Information on books, seminars, and information for caregivers can be found at this site.

AARP Health Information
http://www.aarp.org/bulletin

Information on a BMI calculator, the USDA food pyramid, healthy recipes and health related articles can be found at this site.

International Food Information Council

http://www.ific.org/

At this site, you can find information regarding nutritional needs for aging adults. This site focuses on information for educators and students, publications, and nutritional information.

University of California at Irvine: Institute for Brain Aging and Dementia

http://www.alz.uci.edu/

The Institute for Brain Aging and Dementia is dedicated to the study of Alzheimer's and the causes of mental disabilities for the elderly.

UNIT 5: Retirement: American Dream or Dilemma?

American Association of Retired People

http://www.aarp.org

The AARP is the nation's leading organization for people 50 and older. AARP serves their needs through information, education, advocacy, and community service.

Health and Retirement Study (HRS)

http://www.umich.edu/~hrswww/

The University of Michigan Health and Retirement Study surveys more than 22,000 Americans over the age of 50 every two years. Supported by the National Institute on Aging, the study paints an emerging portrait of an aging America's physical and mental health, insurance coverage, financial status, family support systems, labor market status, and retirement planning.

UNIT 6: The Experience of Dying

Agency for Health Care Policy and Research

http://www.ahcpr.gov

Information on the dying process in the context of U.S. health policy is provided here, along with a search mechanism. The agency is part of the Department of Health and Human Services.

Growth House, Inc.

http://www.growthhouse.org/

This award-winning web site is an international gateway to resources for life-threatening illness and end of life care.

Hospice Foundation of America

http://www.HospiceFoundation.org

On this page, you can learn about hospice care, how to select a hospice, and how to find a hospice near you.

Hospice HotLinks

http://www.hospiceweb.com/links.htm

Links with information about all aspects of hospice care can be found at this site.

UNIT 7: Living Environment in Later Life

American Association of Homes and Services for the Aging

http://www.aahsa.org

The American Association of Homes and Services for the Aging represents a not-for-profit organization dedicated to providing high-quality health care, housing, and services to the nation's elderly.

Center for Demographic Studies

http://cds.duke.edu

The Center for Demographic Studies is located in the heart of the Duke campus. The primary focus of their research is long-term care for elderly populations, specifically those 65 years of age and older.

Guide to Retirement Living Online

http://www.retirement-living.com

An online version of a free publication, this site provides information about nursing homes, continuous care communities, independent living, home health care, and adult day care centers.

The United States Department of Housing and Urban Development

http://www.hud.gov

News regarding housing for aging adults can be found at this site sponsored by the U.S. federal government.

UNIT 8: Social Policies, Programs, and Services for Older Americans

Administration on Aging

http://www.aoa.dhhs.gov

This site, housed on the Department of Health and Human Services Web site, provides information for older persons and their families. There is also information for educators and students regarding the elderly.

American Federation for Aging Research

http://www.afar.org/

Since 1981, the American Federation for Aging Research (AFAR) has helped scientists begin and further careers in aging research and geriatric medicine.

American Geriatrics Society

http://www.americangeriatrics.org

This organization addresses the needs of our rapidly aging population. At this site, you can find information on health care and other social issues facing the elderly.

Community Transportation Association of America

http://www.ctaa.org

C.T.A.A. is a nonprofit organization dedicated to mobility for all people, regardless of wealth, disability, age, or accessibility.

Consumer Reports State Inspection Surveys

http://www.ConsumerReports.org

To learn how to get state inspection surveys and to contact the ombudsman's office, click on "Personal Finance," then select "Assisted Living."

Medicare Consumer Information From the Health Care Finance Association

http://cms.hhs.gov/default.asp?fromhcfadotgov=true

This site is devoted to explaining Medicare and Medicaid costs to consumers.

National Institutes of Health

http://www.nih.gov

Information on health issues can be found at this government site. There is quite a bit of information relating to health issues and the aging population in the United States.

The United States Senate: Special Committee on Aging

http://www.senate.gov/~aging/

This committee, chaired by Senator Gordon Smith, Oregon, deals with the issues surrounding the elderly in America. At this site, you can download committee hearing information, news, and committee publications.

We highly recommend that you review our Web site for expanded information and our other product lines. We are continually updating and adding links to our Web site in order to offer you the most usable and useful information that will support and expand the value of your Annual Editions. You can reach us at: *http://www.mhcls.com/annualeditions/.*

UNIT 1

The Phenomenon of Aging

Unit Selections

1. **Elderly Americans**, Christine L. Himes
2. **The Economic Conundrum of an Aging Population**, Robert Ayres
3. **A Study for the Ages**, Nancy Shute
4. **Puzzle of the Century**, Mary Duenwald
5. **The Demographic Drivers of Aging**, Kevin Kinsella and David R. Phillips
6. **Will You Live to Be 100?**, Thomas Perls and Margery Hutter Silver
7. **The Coming Death Shortage: Why the Longevity Boom Will Make Us Sorry To Be Alive**, Charles C. Mann

Key Points to Consider

- What factors contribute to the increasing life expectancy of the American people? What challenges do aging Americans face?

- Why are older Americans healthier than ever before?

- Will it ever be possible to slow down the aging process? Would this be desirable? Why or why not?

- What are the problems and advantages that society must consider in facing the increased aging population? Give examples.

Student Website

www.mhcls.com/online

Internet References

Further information regarding these websites may be found in this book's preface or online.

The Aging Research Centre
http://www.arclab.org/

Centenarians
http://www.hcoa.org/centenarians/centenarians.htm

National Center for Health Statistics
http://www.cdc.gov/nchs/agingact.htm

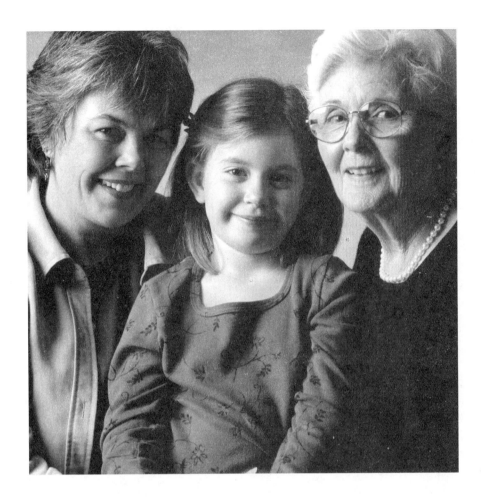

The process of aging is complex and includes biological, psychological, sociological, and behavioral changes. Biologically, the body gradually loses the ability to renew itself. Various body functions begin to slow down, and the vital senses become less acute. Psychologically, aging persons experience changing sensory processes; perception, motor skills, problem-solving ability, and drives and emotions are frequently altered. Sociologically, they must cope with the changing roles and definitions of self that society imposes on the individual. For instance, the role expectations and the status of grandparents is different from those of parents, and the roles of the retired are quite different from those of the employed. Being defined as "old" may be desirable or undesirable, depending on the particular culture and its values. Behaviorally, aging individuals may move slower and with less dexterity. Because they are assuming new roles and are viewed differently by others, their attitudes about themselves, their emotions, and, ultimately, their behavior can be expected to change.

Those studying the process of aging often use developmental theories of the life cycle—a sequence of predictable phases that begins with birth and ends with death—to explain individuals' behavior at various stages of their lives. An individual's age, therefore, is important because it provides clues about his or her behavior at a particular phase of the life cycle, be it childhood,

adolescence, adulthood, middle age, or old age. There is, however, the greatest variation in terms of health and human development among older people than among any other age group. While every 3-year-old child can be predicted to have certain developmental experiences, there is a wide variation in the behavior of 65-year-old people. By age 65, we find that some people are in good health, employed, and performing important work tasks. Others of this cohort are retired but in good health. Still others are retired and in poor health. Others have died prior to the age of 65. The articles in this section are written from biological, psychological, and sociological perspectives. These disciplines attempt to explain the effects of aging and the resulting choices in lifestyle, as well as the wider cultural implications of an older population.

In the article "Elderly Americans," Christine Himes delineates the increases in life expectancy and the aging of the American population that has occurred during the last century. Robert Ayres in "The Economic Conundrum of an Aging Population" examines the effect of a smaller labor force and a larger, older population on industrialized countries throughout the world. In "A Study For the Ages," Nancy Shute reports on the results of a longitudinal study that followed the lifestyle of a sample of volunteers whose ages ranged from 20 to 90. Many of the losses formerly associated with aging were found to be treatable and versible. In "The Demographic Drivers of Aging," Kinsella and Phillips explain how a declining death rate, a declining crude birth rate, and an increase in life expectancy can lead to significant changes in the age composition of a population.

Thomas Perls and Margery Hutter Silver conducted a study at Harvard Medical School of long-living individuals. Following their research, they came up with a quiz that included dietary and lifestyle choices, as well as family histories to help the individual determine what his or her probabilities are of living to a very old age. In "The Coming Death Shortage," Charles Mann discusses the possible changes that could occur in the United States and other countries as a result of the projected increases in both life expectancy and life span. He perceives a shift in the power base of the country from the young to old and wonders if a gerontocracy will emerge.

Elderly Americans

by Christine L. Himes

The United States is in the midst of a profound demographic change: the rapid aging of its population. The 2000 Census counted nearly 35 million people in the United States 65 years of age or older, about one of every eight Americans. By 2030, demographers estimate that one in five Americans will be age 65 or older, which is nearly four times the proportion of elderly 100 years earlier, in 1930. The effects of this older age profile will reverberate throughout the American economy and society in the next 50 years. Preparing for these changes involves more than the study of demographic trends; it also requires an understanding of the growing diversity within the older population.

The lives and well-being of older Americans attract increasing attention as the elderly share of the U.S. population rises: One-fifth will be 65 or older in 2030.

The aging of the U.S. population in the next 20 years is being propelled by one of the most powerful demographic forces in the United States in the last century: the "baby boom" cohort, born between 1946 and 1964. This group of 76 million children grabbed media attention as it moved toward adulthood—changing school systems, colleges, and the workplace. And, this same group of people will change the profile and expectations of old age in the United States over the next 30 years as it moves past age 65. The potential effects of the baby boom on the systems of old-age assistance already are being evaluated. This cohort's consumption patterns, demand for leisure, and use of health care, for example, will leave an indelible mark on U.S. society in the 21st century. Understanding their characteristics as they near older ages will help us anticipate baby-boomers' future needs and their effects on the population.

Until the last 50 years, most gains in life expectancy came as the result of improved child mortality. The survival of larger proportions of infants and children to adulthood radically increased average life expectancy in the United States and many other countries over the past

century. Now, gains are coming at the end of life as greater proportions of 65-year-olds are living until age 85, and more 85-year-olds are living into their 90s. These changes raise a multitude of questions: How will these years of added life be spent? Will increased longevity lead to a greater role for the elderly in our society? What are the limits of life expectancy?

Increasing life expectancy, especially accompanied by low fertility, changes the structure of families. Families are becoming more "vertical," with fewer members in each generation, but more generations alive at any one time. Historically, families have played a prominent role in the lives of elderly people. Is this likely to change?

As much as any stage of the life course, old age is a time of growth, diversity, and change. Elderly Americans are among the wealthiest and among the poorest in our nation. They come from a variety of racial and ethnic backgrounds. Some are employed full-time, while others require full-time care. While general health has improved, many elderly suffer from poor health.

The older population in the 21st century will come to later life with different experiences than did older Americans in the last century—more women will have been divorced, more will have worked in the labor force, more will be childless. How will these experiences shape their later years?

The answers to these questions are complex. In some cases, we are confident in our predictions of the future. But for many aspects of life for the elderly, we are entering new territory. This report explores the characteristics of the current older population and speculates how older Americans may differ in the future. It also looks at the impact of aging on the U.S. society and economy.

Increasing Numbers

The United States has seen its elderly population—defined at those age 65 or older—grow more than tenfold during the 20th century. There were just over 3 million Americans age 65 or older in 1900, and nearly 35 million in 2000.

At the dawn of the 20th century, three demographic trends—high fertility, declining infant and child mortality, and high rates of international immigration—were acting in concert in the United States and were keeping

Table 1
U.S. Total Population and Population Age 65 or Older, 1900-2060

Year	Population (in thousands)		Percent 65+	Percent increase from preceding decade	
	Total	Age 65+		Total	Age 65+
Actual					
1900	75,995	3,080	4.1		
1910	91,972	3,950	4.3	21.0	28.2
1920	105,711	4,933	4.7	14.9	24.9
1930	122,755	6,634	5.4	16.1	34.5
1940	131,669	9,019	6.8	7.2	36.0
1950	150,697	12,270	8.1	14.5	36.0
1960	179,323	16,560	9.2	19.0	35.0
1970	203,212	20,066	9.9	13.4	21.2
1980	226,546	25,549	11.3	11.5	27.3
1990	248,710	31,242	12.6	9.8	22.3
2000	281,422	34,992	12.4	13.2	12.0
Projections					
2020	324,927	53,733	16.5	8.4	35.3
2040	377,350	77,177	20.5	7.5	9.8
2060	432,011	89,840	20.8	7.0	9.6

Note: Data from 1900 to 1950 exclude Alaska and Hawaii. All data refer to the resident U.S. population.

Sources: U.S. Census Bureau publications: *Historical Statistics of the United States: Colonial Times to 1970* (1975); *1980 Census of Population: General Population Characteristics* (PC80-1-B1); *1990 Census of Populations: General Population Characteristics* (1990-CP1); *Census 2000 Demographic Profile*, (www.census.gov/Press-Release/www/2001/tables/dp_us_2000.xls, accessed Sept. 19, 2001); and *Population Projections of the United States by Age, Sex, Race, Hispanic Origin, and Nativity: 1999 to 2100* (www.census.gov/population/projections/nation/summary/np-t4-a.txt, accessed Sept. 25, 2001).

the population young. The age distribution of the U.S. population was heavily skewed toward younger ages in 1900, as illustrated by the broad base of the population age-sex pyramid for that year in Figure 1. The pyramid, which shows the proportion of each age and sex group in the population, also reveals that the elderly made up a tiny share of the U.S. population in 1900. Only 4 percent of Americans were age 65 of older, while more than one-half (54 percent) were under age 25.

But adult health improved and fertility fell during the first half of the century. The inflow of international immigrants slowed considerably after 1920. These trends caused an aging of the U.S. population, but they were interrupted after World War II by the baby boom. In the post-war years, Americans were marrying and starting families at younger ages and in greater percentages than they had during the Great Depression. The surge in births between 1946 and 1964 resulted from a decline in childlessness (more women had at least one child) combined with larger family sizes (more women had three or more children). The sustained increase in birth rates during their 19-year period fueled a rapid increase in the child population. By 1970, these baby boomers had moved into their teen and young adult years, creating a bulge in that year's age-sex pyramid shown in Figure 1.

The baby boom was followed by a precipitous decline in fertility: the "baby bust." Young American women reaching adulthood in the late 1960s and 1970s were slower to marry and start families than their older counterparts, and they had fewer children when they did start families. U.S. fertility sank to an all-time low. The average age of the population started to climb as the large baby boom generation moved into adulthood, and was replaced by the much smaller baby-bust cohort. By 2000, the baby-boom bulge had moved up to the middle adult ages. The population's age structure at younger and older ages became more evenly distributed as fluctuations in fertility diminished and survival at the oldest ages in-

4

Figure 1

U.S. Population by Age and Sex, 1900, 1970, 2000, and 2030

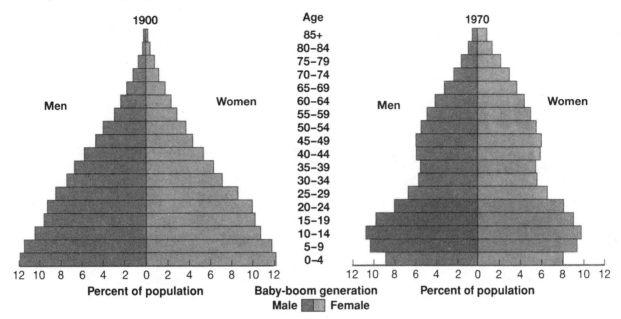

Note: U.S. population in 1900 does not include Alaska or Hawaii. The baby-boom generation includes persons born between 1946 and 1964.

Sources: U.S. Census Bureau Publications: *Historical Statistics of the United States: Colonial times to 1970* (1975); *Census 2000 Summary File* (SFI) (http://factfinder.census.gov, accessed Sept. 5, 2001); and "Population Projections of the United States by Age, Sex, Race, Hispanic Origin, and Nativity: 1999 to 2100" (www.census.gov/population/projections/nation/summary/np-t4-a.txt, accessed Sept. 25, 2001).

creased. By 2030, the large baby-boom cohorts will be age 65 and older, and U.S. Census Bureau projections show that the American population will be relatively evenly distributed across age groups, as Figure 1 shows.

The radical shift in the U.S. population age structure over the last 100 years provides only one part of the story of the U.S. elderly population. Another remarkable aspect is the rapid growth in the number of elderly, and the increasing numbers of Americans at the oldest ages, above ages 85 or 90. The most rapid growth in the 65-or-older age group occurred between the 1920s and the 1950s (see Table 1). During each of these decades, the older population increased by at least 34 percent, reaching 16.6 million in 1960. The percentage increase slowed after 1960, and between 1990 and 2000, the population age 65 or older increased by just 12 percent. Since the growth of the older population largely reflects past patterns of fertility, and U.S. fertility rates plummeted in the 1930s, the first decade of the 21st century will also see relatively slow growth of the elderly population. Fewer people will be turning 65 and entering the ranks of "the elderly." Not until the first of the baby-boom generation reaches age 65 between 2010 and 2020 will we see the same rates of increase as those experienced in the mid-20th century.

In the 1940s and 1950s, the rapid growth at the top of the pyramid was matched by growth in the younger ages—the total U.S. population was growing rapidly, and the general profile was still fairly young. That was not the case in the second half of the 20th century, as the share of

the population age 65 or older increased to around 12 percent. The elderly share will increase much faster in the first half of the 21st century. This growth in the percentage age 65 or older constitutes population aging.

Many policymakers and health care providers are more concerned about the sheer size of the aging baby-boom generation than the baby boom's share of the total population. The oldest members of this group will reach age 65 in 2011, and by 2029, the youngest baby boomers will have reached age 65. This large group will continue to move into old age at a time of slow growth among younger age groups. The Census Bureau projects that 54 million Americans will be age 65 or older in 2020; by 2060, the number is projected to approach 90 million. The size of this group, and the general aging of the population, are important in planning for the future. Older Americans increasingly are healthy and active and able to take on new roles. At the same time, increasing numbers of older people will need assistance with housing, health care, and other services.

The Oldest-Old

The older population is also aging as more people are surviving into their 80s and 90s. In the 2000 Census, nearly one-half of Americans age 65 or older were above age 74, compared with less than one-third in 1950; one in eight were age 85 or older in 2000, compared with one in 20 in 1950 (see Figure 2).

(Figure 1-continued)

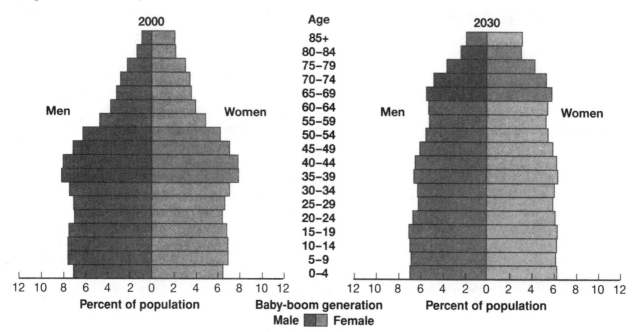

As the baby boomers enter their late 60s and early 70s around 2020, the U.S. elderly population will be younger: The percentage ages 65 to 74 will rise to 58 percent, as shown in Figure 2. By 2040, however, just 44 percent will be 65 to 74, and 56 percent of all elderly will be age 75 or older.

Those age 85 or older, the "oldest-old," are the fastest growing segment of the elderly population. While those 85 or older made up only about 1.5 percent of the total U.S. population in 2000, they constituted about 12 percent of all elderly. More than 4 million people in the United States were 85 or older in the 2000 Census, and by 2050, a projected 19 million will be age 85 or older. These oldest-old will make up nearly 5 percent of the total population, and more than 20 percent of all elderly Americans. This group is of special interest to planners because those 85 or older are more likely to require health services.

Gender Gap

Women outnumber men at every age among the elderly. In 2000, there were an estimated three women for every two men age 65 or older, and the sex ratio is even more skewed among the oldest-old.

The preponderance of women among the elderly reflects the higher death rates for men than women at every age. There are approximately 105 male babies born for every 100 female babies, but higher male death rates cause the sex ratio to decline as age increases, and around age 35, females outnumber males in the United States. At age 85 and older, the ratio is 41 men per 100 women.[1]

Changes in the leading causes and average ages of death affect a population's sex ratio. In 1900, the average sex ratio for the U.S. total population was 104 men

for every 100 women. But during the early 1900s, improvements in health care during and after pregnancy lowered maternal mortality, and a greater proportion of women survived to older ages. Adult male mortality improved much more slowly; death rates for adult men plateaued during the 1960s.

In recent years, however, male mortality improved faster than female mortality, primarily because of a marked decline in deaths from heart disease. The gender gap at the older ages has narrowed, and it is expected to narrow further. The U.S. Census Bureau projects the sex ratio for those age 65 or older to rise to 79 men for every 100 women by 2050. A sex ratio of 62 is anticipated for those age 85 or older.

Most elderly women today will outlive their spouses and face the challenges of later life alone: Older women who are widowed or divorced are less likely than older men to remarry. Older women are more likely than older men to be poor, to live alone, to enter nursing homes, and to depend on people other than their spouses for care. Many of the difficulties of growing older are compounded by past discrimination that disadvantaged women in the workplace and now threatens their economic security.

As the sex differential in mortality diminishes, these differences may lessen, but changes in marriage and work patterns, family structures, and fertility may mean that a greater proportion of older women will not have children or a living spouse. High divorce rates and declining rates of marriage, for instance, mean that many older women will not have spousal benefits available to them through pensions or Social Security.

Figure 2

Age Distribution of Older Americans, 1900–2000, and Projection to 2050

Percent of 65+ population

■ Age 65–74   ■ Age 75–84   ■ Age 85+

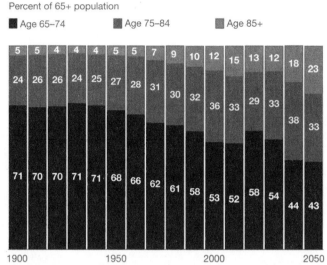

Sources: U.S. Census Bureau publications: *Historical Statistics of the United States: Colonial Times to 1970* (1975); *1980 Census of Population: General Population Characteristics* (PC80-1-B1); *1990 Census of Populations: General Population Characteristics* (1990-CP1); *Census 2000 Demographic Profile*, (www.census.gov/2001/tables/dp_us_2000.xls, accessed Sept. 19, 2001); and "Projections of the Resident Population by Age, Sex, Race, Hispanic Origin, 1990 to 2100" (www.census. gov/population/www/projections/natdet-D1A.html, accessed July 6, 2001).

Ethnic Diversity

The U.S. elderly population is becoming more racially and ethnically diverse, although not as rapidly as is the total U.S. population. In 2000, about 84 percent of the elderly population were non-Hispanic white, compared with 69 percent of the total U.S. population. By 2050, the proportion of elderly who are non-Hispanic white is projected to drop to 64 percent as the growing minority populations move into old age (see Figure 3). Although Hispanics made up only about 5 percent of the elderly population in 2000, 16 percent of the elderly population of 2050 is likely to be Hispanic. Similarly, blacks accounted for 8 percent of the elderly population in 2000, but are expected to make up 12 percent of elderly Americans in 2050.

The major racial and ethnic groups are aging at different rates, depending upon fertility, mortality, and immigration among these groups. Immigration has a growing influence on the age structure of racial and ethnic minority groups. Although most immigrants tend to be in their young adult ages, when people are most likely and willing to assume the risks of moving to a new country, U.S.

Figure 3

Elderly Americans by Race and Ethnicity, 2000 and 2050

Percent of population age 65+

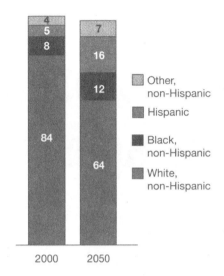

■ Other, non-Hispanic

■ Hispanic

■ Black, non-Hispanic

■ White, non-Hispanic

Note: The 2000 figures refer to residents who identified with one race. About 2% of Americans identified with more than one race in the 2000 census.

Sources: U.S. Census Bureau, *Census 2000 Demographic Profile* (2001); and U.S. Census Bureau, "Projections of the Resident Population by Age, Sex, Race and Hispanic Origin, 1999-2100" (www.census.gov/population/www/projections/natdet-D1A.html, accessed Sept. 19, 2001).

immigration policy also favors the entry of parents and other family members of these young immigrants. The number of immigrants age 65 or older is rapidly increasing as more foreign-born elderly move to the United States from Latin America, Asia, or Africa to join their children.[2] These older immigrants, plus the aging of immigrants who entered as young adults, are altering the ethnic makeup of elderly Americans.

References

1. U.S. Census Bureau, *Population Projections of the United States by Age, Sex, Race, Hispanic Origin, and Nativity: 1999 to 2100* (2000), accessed online at: www.census.gov/population/projections/nation/summary/np-t3-a.txt, on Sept. 19, 2001.
2. Janet M. Wilmoth, Gordon F. DeJong, and Christine L. Himes, "Immigrant and Non-Immigrant Living Arrangements in Later Life," *International Journal of Sociology and Social Policy* 17 (1997): 57–82.

The Economic Conundrum of an Aging Population

By Robert Ayres

In a large part of the world, old age is an incentive to have many children. That may seem puzzling to Europeans or Americans, for whom old age can be a welcome escape from the burdens of buying kids' clothes or paying for college tuition. Retired people in affluent countries usually have savings or pensions, as well as government-provided retirement income. But in poor countries, where hundreds of millions of people have no such income after they stop working, adult male children are the equivalent of social security. For this reason, there are strong cultural imperatives for children to provide support for their elderly parents, in preference (if a choice is necessary) to their own young. The result is a combination of too many children and too little care for those children—a potent formula for yet another generation of poorly educated and impoverished young people, including more young men whose frustrations make them prime prospects for militias and terrorists, and young women who have few prospects other than to have more children. It's a self-perpetuating cycle, which ironically becomes harder to break as life expectancies increase and the number of old people in poor countries continues to increase.

Aging Populations Have Fewer Children, But...

The incentives for having fewer children in rich industrialized countries are the mirror image of the reasons for having large families in poor countries. In poor countries, most people live on subsistence farms where child labor is valuable. In rich countries, most people live in cities where children are required by law to go to school. Children are an expensive luxury for people who live in cities and who have jobs outside the home. They must be housed, fed, and schooled. They add nothing to family income. If the mother has a job, she must find (and pay for) a baby-sitter or nanny to look after young children. Urban teenagers are often neglected by working parents, and too many of them—lacking adult guidance—engage in high-risk or costly

behavior, from profligate consumption of video games or TV shows exhibiting extreme violence, to unsafe sex, drug-taking, or even crime. If unemployed, children may be an economic burden on parents into their thirties. In Italy, especially, unmarried children have become notoriously inclined to continue to live with their aging parents and enjoy mama's cooking. For that reason, among others, Italy now has one of the lowest birth rates in the world. Some Italians would like to see that trend reversed.

The shift to a stable population will increase the "dependency ratio" of old to young. While that may stem environmental decline, it could bring economic hardship to the countries that first achieve it. The only real chance of escaping this dilemma is to eliminate the huge economic inequities that now prevail in the world.

Last fall, *The Economist* magazine published a story, "Work Longer, Have More Babies." The illustration showed a horrified young woman—presumably in shock over the news that she is expected to stop having fun and start reproducing, for the good of western society. The underlying message, of course, was that as the populations of rich countries get older, with smaller percentages of them of child-bearing age—and as fewer of them care to bear the expense of having kids in any case—the populations of those countries will shrink and their cultures will risk being overrun by others, whose populations are rapidly expanding.

It is true that all of the industrialized countries, including the United States, are aging. The number of old people supported by social security, compared to the number of younger employed people paying into the retirement system, is growing. This "dependency ratio"—the number of people over 65 as a percentage of the number in the 20-24 age group—is a good indicator of the fundamental demographic problem. This ratio is now just over 20 percent for the United States, about 27 percent for the Euro zone, and 28 percent for Japan. However, by 2050, according to the World Bank, the dependency ratio will be close to 46 percent for the United States, 60 percent for Europe, and 70 percent for Japan.

The number of workers supporting each German pensioner today, via the main government "pay-as-you-go" (PAYG) system, is about three. By 2030, if current trends continue, the number of active workers per pensioner will be only 1.5. If each of the active workers earned 100 Euros before the transfer, he (or she) would get to keep 60, and the retiree would also get 60 Euros (1.5 X 100 = 2.5 X 60 = 150). The other costs of government would be taken (via taxation) out of the 60 Euros of income each person has. Costs of government, net of pensions, are at least 25 percent of GDP for industrialized countries, so taxes would take at least 15 Euros from each worker and retiree. The original 100 Euros is therefore down to 45, or less. From that, the future worker must think about saving for his own future retirement when the over-stressed PAYG system collapses, as many people now expect.

A Demographic Dilemma

To an environmentalist, an aging population might seem a good thing—proof that birthrates have fallen and that overall population will stabilize or decline. But a small aging population like that of Italy, in a world of huge younger populations like those of China or Brazil, may not be sustainable. First, there's that pressure from those who don't want their traditional culture (of Italy, or Spain, or France) to be overrun, and who want to encourage their young families to have more children. But even if that weren't a factor, there'd be the economic pressure on a country with a high dependency ratio to alleviate the imbalance, by delaying retirements or reducing retirement benefits. There's also the kind of pressure created by the Bush administration in the United States, to allow active workers to divert part of their social security taxes into privately controlled savings or investment accounts. It's a tempting idea because share prices have increased in value faster than government bonds (in which social security funds are invested), but it would take money away from the PAYG funds available to support current retirees, thus imposing either a very large near-term tax burden or additional government debt to make up the difference.

All things considered, an aging population of non-workers will necessitate an increased tax burden or increased public sector debt, or both. In the past, a few countries have lived with taxes in the 50-percent range, especially in wartime, but not happily. However, this is no longer plausible. In a globalized world with no restrictions on capital flows, where nations compete for investment and where multinational firms can—and do—move money around at the touch of a button, high taxes are a major barrier to investment. In the world of 2030, the United States will be somewhat better off than Europe or Japan, thanks to its lower dependency ratio. On the other hand, China and India will have much lower dependency ratios than the United States, in addition to having lower wages. Even if they had to pay much higher wages, as they must do eventually, those countries would, and will, continue to absorb most of the capital available for investment, including whatever savings the workers of the (formerly) rich countries can manage to divert from current needs.

When environmentalists began to worry about population in the 1970s, the idea that having a *declining* population could spell trouble for a country might have seemed unimaginable. After all, wasn't that the ultimate goal? But in a globalized economy, a declining national population means a nation with a high percentage of elderly, non-working people will compete against nations of young, productive (often low-wage) people—and lose. The change of perspective since the 1970s can be attributed to three factors.

• First, *retirement ages have gotten younger*, putting greater burdens on the social security system. According to the European Commission, the average age of retirement in Western Europe was 65 in 1960, but is 60 today. Civil servants and some unionized workers, such as truck drivers, are able to retire considerably earlier. In the United States, the average age of retirement was 66 in 1960, but is down to under 63 today. Moreover, when firms "downsize," which happens with alarming frequency these days, they often do so by offering early retirement schemes to older workers without replacing them with younger ones. This cuts payroll costs and shifts some or all of the burden to the government. Employees who were previously paying into the social security system are suddenly withdrawing funds from the system.

• Meanwhile, *birth rates in the industrialized countries have declined*, just as environmentalists hoped they would—but with some unforeseen consequences. In 1950, the average overall birth rate in the European union was still above replacement (2 children per woman), at 2.7. Today it is 1.5 and falling. Similar rates are now observed in Japan, China, and Russia. In the United States, the birth rate is just above 2, in part because many of the country's Latino immigrants still prefer large families. If current trends continue, the working-age population of Europe will fall by 18 percent (40 million people) by 2050, while the corresponding U.S. group will increase by a similar amount. In that period the average age of the German population will increase to 54, while the average American will still be only 35. This discrepancy is very disturbing to most European economists, and politicians, who are concerned about economic competition with the United States, not to mention China and India.

• Finally, *life expectancies have been increasing* since the beginning of the 18th century, and especially fast since the early 19th century. When Thomas Malthus warned of explosive population growth, in 1798, the average life expectancy was probably no more than 35. When Otto von Bismarck introduced the first state pension in Germany in 1889, the average life expectancy was 48, whereas the retirement age was set at 70. No wonder the German PAYG system was fiscally sound when it was introduced. There were a lot of active workers and very few retirees. The ratio was probably more than 100 to 1. Now, of course, the life expectancy of Europeans, Japanese, and Americans alike is around 77 (slightly more for women, slightly less for men) and still rising.

An older population requires more health and other services, and produces less wealth, than a younger population. At least that is the conventional wisdom. What is certain is that existing pension plans and social security programs are in deep trouble, even in the United States, and more so in Europe and Japan.

What Would an Aging Society Be Like?

Imagine a society ruled by the old. College professors, army generals, CEOs, doctors, judges, and legislators would hang on to their jobs into their seventies or eighties, or even longer. Promotion in big corporations, civil service, colleges and universities, and the military officer corps would slow almost to a halt, as vacancies due to retirement become rare. Even poorly paid jobs like teaching children in primary or secondary schools, or nursing, or processing forms in government agencies, would most likely require advanced degrees. Computers already do much of the work formerly done by clerks and middle managers. Computers are learning to talk to each other. The need for human interfaces will continue to decline.

Highly skilled construction, repair, and maintenance jobs, such as heavy machine operation, auto repair, plumbing, masonry, plastering, plumbing, electrical work, and electronics repair, would continue to be important and well-paid. However, many such jobs tend to be passed on from father to son. Union membership would be essentially closed to outsiders. Without an expanding economy to absorb them, young people on the lower rungs of the education ladder would be chronically unemployed—or forced to take jobs that most people are unwilling to do, such as collecting and separating trash or cleaning fish.

It is unlikely that there would be enough such jobs for all. But unemployment, especially among the young, is socially destabilizing. Moreover, it discriminates against ethnic minorities of all kinds. It is not at all unlikely that half or more of the present U.S. prison population—disproportionately black and Hispanic, and the largest in the industrialized world—would never have got into trouble with the law if there had been enough decent job opportunities for the less privileged.

Of course there is nothing new about this situation. It has been with us for a long time. The children of the rich are less likely to steal or commit crimes for money, since they don't need to. If they are caught driving while drunk, or accused of date rape, they will be defended by high-priced lawyers or released on a convenient technicality to avert the expense of a trial without an assured outcome, or worse, the loss of a wealthy campaign contributor. When the rich commit financial crimes that cause vast losses for customers or shareholders, they can afford to hire even more expensive lawyers skilled in the black arts of confusion, obstruction, obfuscation, and delay. Very few millionaire malefactors are convicted, still fewer punished. In the future, as the rich get richer—and older people become more demographically dominant—this sort of inequity will almost surely get worse before it gets better.

One way it's likely to get worse is in access to medical services. The rich can afford services that the poor can only dream of. No matter what the Christian and/or Islamic fundamentalists and their moral police think, and no matter whether it is legal in the United States and other major Christian or Islamic countries, cloning of stem cells from human embryos for therapeutic purposes is on the way. Clinics will soon—probably within a decade—be available in China, Russia, the Ukraine, Armenia, or other countries, where custom-grown livers, kidneys, hearts, lungs, or even legs and arms can be had for a suitably high price. The technology is already well along in development. Demand will surely follow. The more effective the gene therapies and stem cell technologies become, the longer their lucky recipients will live—and block the promotion prospects for younger people.

Given these trends, there is growing risk that the aging society of a mature industrial nation will be an increasingly inequitable society, ruled by the rich (and the old) for their own benefit and perpetuation in power. It will be controlled by means of hired guardians who will perform the same duties as today's police and military, but with added civil powers. Having high unemployment or underemployment, and no real power, the rest of our urban society will inevitably revert to a form of existence analogous to that of the Romans who were kept satisfied and entertained by bread and circuses. Its bread will be junk food and its circuses will be our 200 TV channels and omnipresent movieplexes, as well as our sports stadiums and NASCAR race tracks. But just as Rome was overrun, this self-indulgent senior culture (more toys for 65-year-old boys, with fewer actual children) could well be overrun by needier and more aggressive outsiders.

In a society thus dominated by the old, the young are doubly disadvantaged—by their subordinate positions in the major institutions of society and by their reduced capacity to pay the costs of social security. But the real killer is the fact that these overburdened young Europeans, Americans, or Japanese will be competing with nations that have both cheaper wages *and* lower dependency ratios—countries that will not only get the lion's share of investment but also will have to spend less of it on supporting their elders. To a policymaker in Brussels, Washington, or Tokyo, the advent of stable population will look worrisome indeed—unless the inequities between the enviable "old" and hungry or resentful "young" countries are bridged.

Supporting the Old Without Lots More Young?

The standard economist's formula for dealing with overpopulation is economic growth. The reasoning behind this formula is uncomfortable for environmentalists, but there is an inescapable logic: people with higher incomes, in countries that have social security for the elderly, want and need fewer babies; they do not need children to provide security. So, there's an enormous dilemma. Economic growth drives consumption, and waste, which is the reason population is a problem in the first place. But economic growth is also what's necessary to raise incomes to the point where population stabilizes.

It's here where the politics of economic development and the population stabilization that can follow become complicated. Environmentalists are not alone in their uneasiness about the full-throttle economic growth that increases incomes but also increases consumption of nonrenewable resources, degrades the environment, and may undermine social stability. They find some of their concerns echoed by their most fanatical adversaries—fundamental Islamists who regard Western modernization as decadent, but who have notoriously suppressed women's empowerment. The discomfort is made all the more excruciating by the fact that the anti-capitalist Muslims have become de facto bedfellows with some of *their* ideological enemies, the pro-capitalist Christian conservatives, in their mutual hatred of the "sexual revolution" of the past quarter-century. Experts on population virtually all agree that female empowerment, starting with education, is a necessary condition for reducing birthrates.

What's needed, to raise incomes and empower women while *also* mitigating concerns about profligate consumption, is an engine to drive economic growth without the kind of consumption that depends on the exploitation of remaining stocks of natural resources. How would this engine differ from the one that now drives global GDP yet leaves hundreds of millions of people in poverty and dependence on children—and vulnerable to social unrest?

To begin with, it would probably be a more "dematerialized" economy, in which economic productivity is not so rigidly tied to the extraction of ever more oil, minerals, wood, and other physical resources from the Earth as it is now. Aside from the costs of the ecological disruption and pollution that such industries impose, past experience shows that logging, mining, and drilling concessions tend to benefit mainly the very few (and often very corrupt) who have the power to make such deals. The natural wealth has never been widely distributed beyond this elite group. Governments in countries like Nigeria or Indonesia, which still have important natural resource stocks of oil or timber, also have vast populations of poor people for whom having children is a source of income. For this reason alone, it is essential that the global community address the inequity problem—and the closely related problem of corruption—far more quickly and seriously than it has. The rich Western countries have a big stake in the equitable development of the rest of the world, because equitable growth is the only effective tool for ameliorating international terrorism and its close cousin, uncontrollable immigration.

In the short run, though, *controlled* immigration is probably one of the most promising answers to the conundrum raised at the beginning of this article—the lack of enough new young workers (because of declining birthrates) to replace the retiring workers. Immigrants are demonstrably hardworking and willing to do the jobs our own pampered children scorn. Immigrants (being predominantly young adults) even tend to pay more in taxes than they get back in social services. They are a bargain, economically speaking. They also have fewer children than their age group in their home countries, as well as contributing enormously to the economic development of their home countries by sending back significant amounts of their earnings to parents or siblings.

That's only a short-term, partial solution, however. In the larger picture, the rich countries need to provide far more development aid, and to provide it with much tighter—and smarter—strings, to prevent misuse. Investment by the private sector can and will be the dominant source of capital, but that investment should not be going into exploitation of increasingly scarce natural resources. International lending agencies should stop encouraging this sort of investment, and in fact they should create barriers to discourage or prevent it. By the same token, international development agencies should concentrate much greater efforts on education and on creating the institutions needed to assure the rule of law.

As long as there are large economic disparities between nations, there will be unstoppable pressures both to have more children in the poor countries and to endure uncontrolled immigration of the poor into richer countries. When incomes are more equitable worldwide, the problem of smaller working populations supporting their elders will continue to be a problem as birthrates decline, *but* with all nations then sharing common constraints, the present incentives to have more babies and/or migrate to richer countries will disappear. Instead of being shackled by the destabilizing effects of poor people having large families to produce free labor and/or illegally migrating into rich countries in search of jobs, all governments can then focus on finding ways to build economic productivity through an increasingly non-extractive economy, enough to allow people everywhere to support their elders while living comfortably in their home countries.

Robert Ayres *is professor emeritus of management and environment at the European business school INSEAD and King Gustav XVIth professor of environmental science in Sweden.*

A STUDY FOR THE AGES

Generations of volunteers are helping scientists to comprehend time's toll

By Nancy Shute

JOHN FREDERICK KIRBY IS 87, but the retired engineer still treks the quarter mile to his Scientists Cliffs, Md., mailbox twice a day to get the newspaper and the mail. His 60-year-old daughter, Rosemary Hill, moved nearby last year in case her dad needs help. And her nephew, 30-year-old Sean Kirby, still makes the three-hour drive from his home in Frederick, Md., down to his grandfather's, where he can walk the beach and hunt for fossilized shark teeth, as he did as a child. It's just an average family—but one that by being so very ordinary is helping to decipher a mystery of consuming interest to everyone: What happens as we age?

The Kirby-Hills, along with more than 1,100 other volunteers from their 20s to their 90s, are guinea pigs for the Baltimore Longitudinal Study of Aging. The 39-year-old federal effort has become one of the world's great medical studies—and the first to illuminate in detail how healthy people grow old. By tracking physical and mental changes in a total of 2,438 study participants over the decades, the BLSA has made medical history. BLSA researchers, to cite one noteworthy example, discovered in 1992 that a rise in the blood of a substance called prostate-specific antigen (PSA) might warn of prostate cancer five years before traditional exams detect it.

On a larger scale, the BLSA's mountain of data confirms the great good news about aging: It may be inevitable, but it's not immutable. Many losses of function once thought to be age related, such as decreased mobility or memory lapses, can be stopped or slowed. And many supposed indignities of aging turn out to be pure misconception. A few examples:
• Only 20 to 30 percent of people over 70 have symptoms of heart disease; an addi-

tional 25 percent have heart disease but no symptoms. "If you're in the other 50 percent, you're not going to die of your aging heart" says Jerome Fleg, a BLSA cardiologist. "You're going to be able to function essentially like a healthy 20- or 25-year-old for the activities of daily living."
• People don't get crankier as they age; personality is a constant after age 30. A peevish 80-year-old was a peevish 40-year-old.

On average, Americans say middle age ends and old age starts at age 64.

• Even into very old age, high blood cholesterol significantly raises the risk of cardiovascular disease. Thus, preventive measures like a low-cholesterol diet may well be worthwhile after age 70, particularly for people with heart disease.
• Senility is not inevitable. Only 10 percent of people over 65 ever develop dementia, and much of the cognitive decline that we associate with old age is due to treatable medical conditions and diseases such as depression, diabetes, and hypertension. The small decline in memory and reaction time that many people experience with age doesn't impair their intellectual ability. "Aging is not a disease," says Paul Costa, chief of the BLSA's Laboratory on Personality and Cognition. "The ravages of aging are somewhat of a myth."

The youthful old. If you don't believe that, check out the nearest octogenarian. John Frederick Kirby's generation is living proof that old age has already moved beyond doddering fogyhood. George Bush is 72. Lena Horne is 79. So is Mike Wallace.

George Burns was still cracking vaudeville jokes when he turned 100.

"What was old in the last century is not old anymore," says Robert Butler, chair of New York's International Longevity Center of the Mount Sinai School of Medicine and founding director of the National Institute on Aging (and 70 years old). "Even in my own career I've seen it. In the 1950s, the people coming into the nursing homes were age 65. Now they're in their 80s."

Only relatively recently have enough people lived long enough to warrant nursing homes. In 1900, the average life span was 47. It has zoomed to 79 now, largely because of improved sanitation and nutrition and better medical care, which have effectively eliminated two major causes of death: childbirth and infectious diseases like smallpox and polio. Social Security and Medicare have contributed, too, by granting people over 65 an unprecedented degree of financial security. (Poverty is not a healthful lifestyle.)

But with people living longer and baby boomers streaming into middle age, the nature of old age has become an economic issue as well as a physiological one. By 2040, 21 percent of the U.S. population will be over 65, up from 13 percent now. That fifth of the population is projected to consume half the nation's health care resources, compared with about a third today. In an era of limited government funding, health and independence may be the best insurance a senior citizen can have.

Birth of a notion. In 1958, when the BLSA was launched, researchers trying to grasp the biological factors of aging were frustrated by the paucity of good data. Aging studies then were largely cross-sectional, meaning that they compared people living at the same time: 80-year-olds in a nursing home with college students, say. Differences in experience, education, and affluence between the generations tainted the results.

So in February 1958, when noted National Institutes of Health gerontologist Nathan Shock got a call from William Peter, a physician and retired medical missionary, asking how he could donate his body for medical research after he died, Shock told him he'd be more useful alive than dead. The two men decided to start a longitudinal study that would track the same people over time. They recruited themselves, their families, and their friends. Shock and Peter prodded the NIH to fund the research; longitudinal studies take years before there's any payoff. Today, the BLSA receives $6 million a year in federal funds as its total budget—surely one of Uncle Sam's better investments. "It's one of the most influential long-term studies in the world," says Caleb Finch, a professor of gerontology at the University of Southern California. "It was the first serious investigation of healthy people from middle age into later life."

41% of Americans ages 30 to 64 say they will exercise regularly when they are old. 95% of those 65 and older say they do now.

The BLSA was more like a men's club at first, and an all-white one at that; women weren't included until 1978. Their numbers now equal the men's, and thanks to extensive recruiting, 13 percent of the participants are African American. These days, volunteers in their 20s and 80s and minorities are most sought after, says James Fozard, chief of the NIA's longitudinal studies branch. (To volunteer, contact the NIA Information Center at 800-222-2225, department 1.)

Since volunteers are self-selected, they tend to be better educated and better off than the average American. No one is paid, and participants make their own way to Baltimore once every two years for a 2½-day visit. Sixty percent live in the Baltimore-Washington region, but others come from Australia, Hawaii, and California. Almost nobody drops out.

John Frederick Kirby was one of the first volunteers; he was recruited by neighbors in Scientists Cliffs, a summer community on the Chesapeake Bay built by researchers in the 1930s. He then signed up his father and, later, his two daughters, two sons, and two grandsons. "The first time I went, I was really nervous," says grandson Michael Hill, 35, like his cousin Sean Kirby the fourth generation of Kirbys in the BLSA. "But I don't feel like a guinea pig. It's more like part of the team." Hill, in turn, recruited his wife. They go to Baltimore's Little Italy neighborhood for dinner after a day of CT scans. "It's kind of a nice romantic time for us" Hill says.

But hardly plush. Study subjects stay at Johns Hopkins Bayview Medical Center, across the street from BLSA headquarters, in a hospital wing so old that the gritty TV series *Homicide* once filmed there. After settling in, volunteers get a thorough physical exam and are steered through a gantlet of physical and psychological tests from simple hearing exams to the Guilford-Zimmerman Temperament Survey, a personality test. "It's not the typical physical," says Georgia Burnette, a 68-year-old retired nurse from Buffalo who has been a volunteer since 1991. "You don't have a thallium scan routinely. You don't have Dopplers of your carotids."

Rosemary Hill loathes the treadmill test, in which subjects are run until they're about to drop. "They have you all hooked up to tubes, with a clothespin on your nose." Other volunteers find the psychological tests unnerving. Fred Litwin, the 73-year-old owner of a Washington, D.C., used-furniture store, quit taking a memory test in which words are flashed on a screen; it unearthed a deeply buried fear, he says, of being labeled a "dummy." (Volunteers can refuse any test without being banished.) Despite infirmities that the examination might reveal, Litwin says the rigorous probing also bestows confidence. "Knowing that I'm being studied and that there are no surprises makes me feel good."

Oh, by the way… Sometimes there *are* surprises. "The physician assistant was palpating my belly, and while they do that you secretly wonder what they're looking for," Litwin says of his last visit. "She said, 'You have an aortal aneurysm.'" Such weak spots in the wall of the aorta, the body's major artery, can balloon and burst; Litwin's mother had died of an aneurysm 12 years before. The BLSA reported the finding to Litwin's personal physician (study doctors do not treat participants),

and Litwin had surgery that successfully repaired the artery. "That was really a lifesaver for me," Lutwin says.

Many volunteers cite the world-class medical work-up as reason enough to put up with the inconvenience—and the expense. (They get room and board but are not otherwise compensated.) Just as many participants say they like contributing to the research. "I really believe in what they're doing," says Jamie Netschert, a 46-year-old veterinarian from Northern Virginia who has been in the study for 23 years, following in the footsteps of his father. "I saw how much it meant to my dad."

Such devotion yields a rich investigative harvest. In the case of the prostate-cancer research, for instance, researchers pulled blood samples taken as long as 25 years ago, then drew fresh samples from the same participants. BLSA data—thousands of blood and tissue samples stashed in 22 freezers and results stored in a mainframe computer and dozens of file cabinets stacked to the ceiling—are open to scientists around the world, awaiting questions not yet posed.

71% of Americans expect to be in good health when they are old. But 28% say they won't be able to drive.

From the outset, the study's mission was to see if aging follows a predictable pattern. As results have built up, the BLSA researchers realized that while most people associate aging with gray hair, Medicare, and early-bird specials, it really starts in the mid-30s. Muscles begin to shrivel. Bones lose mass. Hearing and vision become less acute. The immune system loses some of its punch. Hormone levels drop. Lung capacity contracts. And the body gets a bit shorter every year.

Wrinkled but running. But these insults aren't meted out monolithically. Different people age at very different rates, and the variation expands with age. Even within the same person, organ systems seem to have individual internal clocks. While one person feels her age in an aching, arthritic back, another develops shortness of breath due to heart disease. A third may be balding and wrinkled but still running marathons. Aging is infinite in its variety. There is no single pattern.

How time takes its toll

Even if you're already 40 or 50, it could be decades before you fully realize you're aging. The loss of 40 percent of lung capacity by age 80, say, is so gradual that most people never sense the difference. Besides, the signposts on this page are population averages. As car people say, your mileage may vary.

Your 40s

- At 40, the body burns 120 fewer calories a day than at age 30, making weight control harder.
- The body is 5/8 of an inch shorter at 40 than at 30 and will continue to shrink by about 1/16 of an inch a year because of changes in posture, bone loss, and compression of the spongy disks that separate the vertebrae.
- Changes in the inner ear erode the ability to hear higher frequencies for men, who lose hearing more than twice as fast as women do.
- The eyes begin to have trouble focusing on magazines and other close objects as the lenses become thicker.

Your 50s

- With menopause, fertility ends, and lower estrogen speeds bone loss and raises the risk of heart disease.
- As the eye's sensitivity to contrast declines, the ability to see in dim light or under conditions of glare, or to catch sight of moving objects, diminishes.
- Loss of strength becomes measurable as muscle mass diminishes.
- Vulnerability to infections and cancer increases; the thymus, a gland that plays a key role in the immune system, has shrunk by 90 to 95 percent.

Your 60s

- Making out conversations becomes harder, especially for men, as high-frequency hearing deteriorates further. (Consonants, which carry most of the meaning of speech, largely consist of higher frequencies.)
- The pancreas, which processes glucose, works less efficiently. Blood-sugar levels rise and more people are diagnosed with adult-onset diabetes.
- Joints are stiff in the morning, particularly the knees, hips, and spine, because of wear and tear on the cartilage that cushions them.
- Men's sexual daydreams all but vanish after age 65. Researchers don't know why.

Your 70s

- Blood pressure is 20 to 25 percent higher than in the 20s; the thicker, stiffer artery walls can't flex as much with each heartbeat.
- Reaction to loud noises and other stimuli is delayed as the brain's ability to send messages to the extremities slows.
- Short-term memory and the ability to learn spoken material, like a new language, decline with changes in brain function.
- More than half of men show signs of coronary-artery disease.
- Sweat glands shrink or stop working in both men and women, raising the risk of heat stroke (but reducing the need for deodorant).

Your 80s

- Women become particularly susceptible to falling and to disabling hip fractures. They are generally weaker than men and by now have lost over half the bone mass in the hips and upper legs.
- Almost half of those over 85 show signs of Alzheimer's disease.
- The heart beats, at maximum exertion, about 25 percent slower than it did at age 20—but compensates by expanding and pumping more blood per beat.
- The stereotype notwithstanding, personality *doesn't* change with age. A cranky 80-year-old was a cranky 30-year-old.

The *why* of the aging process remains one of science's great unresolved questions. Theories fall into two camps: the "program" camp, in which genes, hormones, or the immune system is thought to be programmed to follow a biological clock to self-destruction to make room for the next generation, and the "error" camp, in which cells and organs are thought to wear out or to suffer environmental damage. Most gerontologists now think that we age because of complex interactions that involve all of these. And they do know one thing for sure: So far, no one has figured out how to push the human life span beyond 120 years or so. Most of us will barely make it two thirds of the way, and we want to make it as far as we can, eking out every last day.

Realizing that aging varies widely from person to person prompted BLSA researchers to search out characteristics that lead to a healthy, satisfying, successful old age. Reubin Andres, an expert in obesity and diabetes who has spent most of his career at the BLSA, determined that it's healthier to gain some weight, as much as a pound a year from about age 40 on, and that those famous Metropolitan Life height/weight charts were set too low for older people. "We published that, and that led to a controversy that continues," Andres says, smiling. Indeed: In other studies, rats fed an extremely low-calorie diet lived up to twice as long as their well fed peers. Studies are underway with monkeys to see if a low-calorie diet will have the same life-extending effect on primates. In the meantime, Andres stresses that he's not advocating obesity, a major risk factor for heart disease and diabetes. "But for such a large fraction of the American population, and women more than men, to be concerned about losing 5 pounds, even 10 pounds, is trivial. All they're doing is removing some of the pleasure of living."

Disbelief. The BLSA finding that personality doesn't change after age 30 challenged such a deeply held stereotype of old age that even the researchers didn't believe it at first. So they ran five different personality tests. And they extended the study over 18 years. And they polled friends and spouses of participants, in case people were deluding themselves. "Quite amazingly, we got the same picture of stability from spouses and peers," says Costa, chief of the BLSA's personality laboratory. "When we do see significant change, it's often a sign of disease, like Alzheimer's disease."

Of late the BLSA has put more resources into Alzheimer's, for many people the most terrifying curse of age. In March, BLSA researchers reported that participants who took ibuprofen for as little as two years had half the risk of contracting Alzheimer's as did those who took aspirin or acetaminophen. Many researchers believe inflammation plays a key role in Alzheimer's ability to damage brain tissue; if so, ibuprofen, a nonsteroidal anti-inflammatory, may reduce or prevent the damage. At this point no one knows what dose works best, so the BLSA isn't telling people to start downing ibuprofen, says Jeffrey Metter, a physician and the study's medical director. But if you're already taking ibuprofen for arthritis or another reason, he says, "reap the wealth of the benefits."

By looking at decades' worth of results of tests that measure mental acuity, Costa's laboratory found that BLSA participants who developed Alzheimer's showed subtle changes, particularly in memory, 10 to 20 years before the debilitating symptoms came to light. The researchers are now performing MRI (magnetic resonance imaging) and PET (positron emission tomography) scans of participants' brains to try to detect signs of early changes in the hippocampus and other structures, and are investigating suspected links between Alzheimer's and changes over the years in the way the body metabolizes glucose. By attacking the same question from different angles within the same population, the investigators hope to find early markers for Alzheimer's and, eventually, a way to treat people before the disease irrevocably damages the brain.

Balanced information

These reliable resources deliver the latest word on aging and health.

- **"How and Why We Age"** (1994, Ballantine Books, $24). Written by cell biologist Leonard Hayflick, this book is often cited by gerontologists as the best guide to aging for nonscientists. It is an engaging read and includes a chapter on the Baltimore Longitudinal Study of Aging.
- **National Institute on Aging.** Publications from the federal agency include "In Search of the Secrets of Aging" and a national guide to resources on aging. Call (800) 222-2225, department 1, or visit the World Wide Web *(www.nih.gov/nia/).* For updates on Alzheimer's disease, including free publications, contact the NIA's Alzheimer's Disease Education and Referral Canter by calling (800) 438-4380 or on the Web *(www.alzheimers.org/adear).*
- **Alliance for Aging Research.** This consumer group has free pamphlets like "Improving Health With Antioxidants." Write the group at 2021 K Street, N. W., Suite 305, Washington, DC 20006. *-N.S.*

BLSA researchers also are continuing their landmark research on prostate-specific antigen and prostate cancer, which is newly diagnosed in 334,500 men a year. Just this spring, they reported that the ratio of two forms of PSA in a man's blood can reveal cancer up to 10 years before a manual exam would. The sophisticated test also identifies the cancer as aggressive or slow growing, making it possible to determine a man's level of risk, eliminate unnecessary PSA tests, and more reliably decide when surgery is necessary.

No more roast. While it can take years for researchers to sift through the BLSA data and reach conclusions, the individuals studied have more immediate—and personal—reasons to be interested in the results. Burnette, the retired Buffalo nurse,

learned she had extremely high cholesterol and slightly elevated blood sugar. So she took up mall walking with a friend. "Walking six or seven days a week, 3 miles in an hour, has lowered my cholesterol by half," she says. The 16 pounds she lost didn't hurt, either. Sister Mary Pauline Hogan, a 57-year-old participant from Boston, likes a nice piece of roast beef. But she's a little overweight and has a family history of heart problems; her mother died at age 54. So Sister Pauline is eating more chicken, fish, and vegetables. That can be a challenge because as administrator of a convent for retired nuns of the Sisters of Charity of St. Elizabeth, she cooks supper for 20 people. "I'm doing a lot of stir-fry," she says. "We have a grill, and I'm getting really fancy with it."

Of course, heredity has a lot to do with how we age, and nobody has figured out how to pick his or her parents. But as a result of efforts like Burnette's and Sister Pauline's, over the years BLSA participants have markedly improved the group's overall cholesterol levels, blood pressure, and smoking rates. They're also eating less fat and more fiber. "On the negative side, we have more obesity [among participants], and there's not a lot of exercising," Metter says. "But we do see more people walking."

It would be easy to dismiss these behavior changes, arguing that BLSA participants are unnaturally dutiful when it comes to healthy behavior. But the BLSA participants aren't the only ones changing. Nationally, the death rate from heart disease, the No. 1 cause of death in the United States, dropped 50 percent between 1950 and 1990, and it wasn't just due to better medical care. Diet and lifestyle have changed, too.

The point is not that lifestyle changes can affect the aging process—no one has yet devised an antiaging elixir, despite claims touted in tabloids and in health-food stores—but that they can fend off or slow age-related diseases such as arthritis, diabetes, heart disease, and stroke. BLSA researchers and others agree that moderate, regular physical activity, whether it's walking, gardening, bicycling, or golf, lowers blood pressure, cholesterol, and glucose; helps relieve the pain and stiffness of arthritis; and recently was shown to be a powerful antidepressant in the elderly. Weight training is proving remarkably useful in combating age-related loss of strength, even in women in their 90s.

And older people are indeed more active than their counterparts were just 10 years ago. Fitness participation by people over 55 rose 73 percent from 1987 to 1995, according to a study commissioned by the Sporting Goods Manufacturers Association. If this trend continues, increasing numbers of old people will avoid the invalidism that many people still presume to be the penalty of old age.

Before joining the BLSA research team 10 years ago, Metter worked as a neurologist at a Veterans Administration hospital, where "you had the impression that getting old was really bad for your health." The patients were infirm, impaired by strokes and other ailments. Coming to the BLSA was an awakening. "You saw those people who were really aging for the most part successfully or were managing their illnesses" well. The BLSA participants' ability to negotiate the aging process, Metter says, "has major implications in terms of how we can live into our older age more healthy and productive."

Pushing the limits. And many BLSA participants are healthy and productive well past 65. Fred Litwin, at 73, rides his Honda 450 motorcycle to work every day, where he hauls furniture up four stories in a hand-hoisted elevator. His wife, Evelyn, 74, also a BLSA volunteer, is the director of an outdoor nursery school where she has worked for 35 years. "I've been outdoors more than indoors," Evelyn Litwin says. "I feel like quite a vigorous person." Lee Canfield, an 83-year-old retired national security analyst, spends hours chopping wood and tilling his 1-acre Falls Church, Va., garden. "I like to push myself fairly close to the limits," Canfield says. "I'm not as young as I was, so my limits are closing. But I get a heck of a lot done, and in the process I enjoy it immensely."

None of these people feels like a teenager. Litwin concedes a loss of strength and short term memory, and Canfield's back is so stiff he can hardly bend over. But they adjust and move on. "I didn't think I was aging until last week," says Maurine Mulliner, a Washington, D.C. resident who was one of the first women to join the BLSA and, at 92, is among its oldest volunteers. (A few others are also in their 90s.) "It's a great surprise."

Mulliner was in bed with painful spinal arthritis at the time. The flare-up was playing havoc with her calendar, usually thickly penciled with meetings to alleviate the District of Columbia's financial crisis, lunches at the tony Cosmos Club (she was the third female member), church events, and her daily hatha yoga session (she danced with the Chicago Opera ballet in the 1930s, until the Depression did it in). A Mormon childhood taught her good values and a healthy diet, Mulliner says. Sturdy stock helped, too; a grandmother who was a frontier doctor and a mother who was a politician taught her that women could do whatever they wanted. Mulliner did, including a long career as an official with the Social Security Administration, political activism (she helped found the Americans for Democratic Action), and a World War II posting to the U.S. Embassy in London.

"If we learn to accept change, that's key," Mulliner says of growing old. "The people who can accept what comes along and know that they're not going to be able to change much of it and make a reasonable adjustment are the ones who can do it best.

PUZZLE OF THE CENTURY

Is it the fresh air, the seafood, or genes? Why do so many hardy 100-year-olds live in, yes, Nova Scotia?

BY MARY DUENWALD

MAYBE IT'S THAT HER FACE is so smooth and pink or the way she aims her green eyes right into yours, talking fast and crisply articulating each word. Her gestures are as nimble as a hatmaker's. You would be tempted to say Betty Cooper isn't a day over 70. She's 101. "If I couldn't read, I'd go crazy," she says, lifting the magazine on her lap. "I like historical novels—you know, Henry VIII and Anne Boleyn and all that kind of stuff. I get a big batch from the Books for Shut-ins every three weeks, and I read them all."

Betty wears bifocals, and it's no small thing to see as clearly as she does after watching a century go by. Though her hearing is not what it used to be, a hearing aid makes up for that. Complications from a knee operation more than 30 years ago keep her from walking easily. But she continues to live in her own apartment, in Halifax, Nova Scotia, with assistance from women who drop by to cook meals, run errands and help her get around.

Cooper's health and independence confound the notion that living a very long life entails more pain and suffering than it's worth. "I do have a problem remembering," she allows. "I go to say someone's name and it escapes me. Then five minutes later, I remember it." Of course, lots of people half her age have that complaint.

BETTY COOPER is a diamond-quality centenarian, whose body and brain appear to be made of a special material that has scarcely worn down. But just being a Nova Scotian may have something to do with it. At least that's the suspicion of medical researchers who plan to study Cooper and others in Nova Scotia to learn more about the reasons for their very long—and hardy—lives. In parts of Nova Scotia, centenarians are up to 3 times more common than they are in the United States as a whole, and up to 16 times more common than they are in the world population.

Why? Nova Scotians have their own theories. "We're by the sea, and we get a lot of fresh air," says Grace Mead, 98, of Halifax. "I've always been one for fresh air."

"I was a very careful young girl," says Hildred Shupe, 102, of Lunenburg. "I never went around with men."

"I mind my own business," says Cora Romans, 100, of Halifax.

"The Lord just expanded my life, I guess," says Elizabeth Slauenwhite, 99, of Lunenburg. "I'm in His hands, and He looked after me."

Delima Rose d'Entremont, a tiny, brown-eyed woman of 103, of Yarmouth, says the piano helped keep her going. "I won two medals in music when I was younger, and I taught piano all my life," she says, sitting straight in her wheelchair and mimicking herself at the keys. She occasionally performs for friends at her nursing home, Villa St. Joseph-du-Lac.

Cooper grew up on a farm in Indian Harbor Lake, on the province's eastern shore, and remembers meals that few followers of today's nonfat regimens would dare contemplate. "I ate the right stuff when I was growing up," she explains. "Lots of buttermilk and curds. And cream—in moderation. And when I think of the homemade bread and butter, and the toast with cups of cocoa," she says, trailing off in a high-calorie rhapsody. Then she adds: "I never smoked. And I never drank to excess. But I don't know if that made the difference."

In some ways, Nova Scotia is an unlikely longevity hot spot; a healthful lifestyle is hardly the provincial norm. Physicians say that despite abundances of brisk sea air, fresh fish and lobster and locally grown vegetables and fruits, Nova Scotians as a group do not take exceptionally good care of themselves. "The traditional diet is not that nutritious," says Dr. Chris MacKnight, a geriatrician at Dalhousie University in Halifax who is studying the centenarians. "It's a lot of fried food." Studies show that obesity and smoking levels are high and exercise levels low. Also, the two historically most important industries—fishing and logging—are dangerous, and extract a toll. "In fact," Mac Knight says, "we have one of the lowest *average* life expectancies in all of Canada."

"Nova Scotians had something up their sleeve" that enabled so many of them to reach such an advanced age, says a U.S.-based longevity expert. "Someone had to look into it."

Yet the province's cluster of centenarians has begged for a scientific explanation ever since it came to light several years ago. Dr. Thomas Perls, who conducts research on centenarians at the Boston Medical Center, noticed that people in his study often spoke of very old relatives in Nova Scotia. (To be sure, the two regions have historically close ties; a century ago, young Nova Scotians sought their fortunes in what they called "the Boston States.") At a gerontology meeting, Perls talked to one of MacKnight's Dalhousie colleagues, who reported seeing a centenarian's obituary in a Halifax newspaper nearly every week. "That was amazing," Perls recalls. "Down here, I see obituaries for centenarians maybe once every five or six weeks." Perls says he became convinced that "Nova Scotians had something up their sleeve" that enabled them to reach such advanced ages. "Someone had to look into it."

MacKnight and researcher Margaret Miedzyblocki began by analyzing Canadian census data. They found that the province has about 21 centenarians per 100,000 people (the United States has about 18; the world, 3). More important, MacKnight and Miedzyblocki narrowed the quest to two areas along the southwestern coast where 100-year-olds were extraordinarily common, with up to 50 centenarians per 100,000 people. One concentration is in Yarmouth, a town of 8,000, and the other is in Lunenburg, a town of 2,600.

To the researchers, the notable feature was not that Yarmouth and Lunenburg were started by people from different countries. Rather, the key was what the two towns have in common: each is a world of its own, populated to a significant degree by descendants of original settlers. And as the researchers learned, longevity tends to run in families. Elroy Shand, a 96-year-old in Yarmouth, says he has a 94-year-old aunt and had two uncles who lived into their 90s. Delima Rose d'Entremont's mother died at 95. Betty Cooper's father died at 98. Says MacKnight: "It's very possible that the 100-year-olds in Nova Scotia have some genetic factor that has protected them—even from all the bad effects of the local environment."

ONLY A THREE-HOUR FERRY RIDE from Bar Harbor, Maine, Nova Scotia extends like a long foot into the Atlantic, connected to New Brunswick by a thin ankle. Almost all the stormy weather that roars up the Eastern Seaboard crashes into Nova Scotia. In winter, powerful northeasters batter the province with snow and freezing rain. The windswept shoreline, the vast expanse of ocean beyond, and frequent low hovering clouds make the place *feel* remote.

Unlike most Nova Scotians, whose ancestors were English, Irish and Scottish, Lunenburg residents largely trace their heritage to Germany. In the mid-1700s, the province's British government moved to counteract the threat posed by French settlers, the Acadians, who practiced Catholicism and resisted British rule. The provincial government enticed Protestants in southwestern Germany to immigrate to Nova Scotia by offering them tax-free land grants, surmising they would not sympathize with either the unruly Acadians or the American revolutionaries in the colonies to the south.

Settling predominantly along the south shore of Nova Scotia, the Germans eventually gave up on farming because the soil is so rocky. They turned to fishing and shipbuilding. For generations, they kept mostly to themselves, marrying within the community and hewing to tradition. Lunenburg has so retained its original shipbuilding, seafaring character that the United Nations has named it a World Heritage Site.

Grace Levy, of Lunenburg, is a petite 95-year-old woman with blue eyes, shining white hair and impossibly smooth skin. She has two sisters, both of whom are still living at ages 82 and 89, and five brothers, four of whom drowned in separate fishing accidents. She left school at age 13 to do housework for other families in Lunenburg. The hardships seem not to have dampened her spirit—or health. "My Dad said you've gotta work," she recalls. "He was a kind of a hard taskmaster. He didn't mind using a piece of rope on our back if we did the least little thing. But Mom was so good and kind."

Grace married a man from nearby Tancook. Although the two were not blood relatives, their ancestries so overlapped they had the same last name. "My name has always been Levy," she says with a smile that flashes white teeth. "I had a brother named Harvey Levy and I married a Harvey Levy."

The town of Yarmouth was settled by New Englanders, but areas just to the south and north were settled by the

French, whose plight is dramatized in Henry Wadsworth Longfellow's epic poem *Evangeline*. It tells the story of lovers from Nova Scotia's northern "forest primeval" who were separated during the brutal Acadian expulsion of 1755, when the English governor, fed up with the French peasants' refusal to swear allegiance to Britain, banished them to the American colonies and Louisiana. Later, large numbers of Acadians returned to Nova Scotia and settled the coastline from Yarmouth north to Digby.

After their rough treatment by the English, the Acadians were not inclined to mix with the rest of the province. Today, many people in the Yarmouth area still speak French and display the blue, white and red Acadian flag. Local radio stations play Acadian dance music, a country-French sound not unlike Louisiana zydeco.

"The Yarmouth area would have been settled by only 20 or 30 families," MacKnight says. "Many of the people who live there now are their descendants." The question is, he says, did one of the original ancestors bring a gene or genes that predisposed them to extreme longevity, which have been passed down through the generations?

In Boston, Perls and his colleagues, who have been studying centenarianism for almost a decade, gathered promising evidence to support the notion of a genetic basis for extreme longevity: a woman with a centenarian sibling is at least eight times more likely to live 100 years than a woman without such a sibling; likewise, a man with a centenarian sibling is 17 times more likely to reach 100 than a man without one. "Without the appropriate genetic variations, I think it's extremely difficult to get to 100," Perls says. "Taking better care of yourself might add a decade, but what matters is what you're packin' in your chassis."

Additional evidence comes from recent studies on DNA. Drs. Louis M. Kunkel and Annibale A. Puca of Children's Hospital in Boston—molecular geneticists working with Perls—examined DNA from 137 sets of centenarian siblings. Human beings have 23 pairs of chromosomes (the spindly structures holding DNA strands), and the researchers discovered that many of the centenarians had similarities in their DNA along the same stretch of chromosome No. 4. To Perls and colleagues, that suggested that a gene or group of genes located there contributed to the centenarians' longevity. The researchers are so determined to find one or more such genes that they formed a biotechnology company in 2001 to track them down: Centagenetix, in Cambridge, Massachusetts.

Scientists suspect there may be a handful of age-defying genes, and the competition to pinpoint and understand them is heated. Medical researchers and drug company scientists reason that if they can figure out exactly what those genes do, they may be able to develop drugs or other treatments to enhance or mimic their action. To skeptics, that might sound like the same old futile quest for a fountain of youth. But proponents of the research are buoyed by a little-appreciated fact of life for many of the super old: they're healthier than you might think.

That, too, has been borne out in Nova Scotia. "I'm forgetful, I can't help it," says 96-year-old Doris Smith of Lunenburg. "But I've never had an ache nor a pain."

"I can't remember being sick, not a real sickness," Hildred Shupe says. "But my legs are beginning to get kind of wobbly now. I don't expect to live to be 200."

Alice Strike, who served in the Royal Air Corps in World War I and lives in a veteran's healthcare facility in Halifax, doesn't recall ever being in a hospital before. She is 106.

Scientists suspect there may be a few age-defying genes and hope to develop drugs that mimic their action. To skeptics, that sounds like a futile quest for the fountain of youth.

CENTENARIANS OFTEN ARE HEALTHIER and livelier than many people in their 70s or 80s, according to research by Perls. He says that 40 percent of centenarians avoid chronic illnesses until they're 85 or older, and another 20 percent until they're over 100. "We used to think that the older you were the sicker you were," Perls says. "The fact is, the older you are, the healthier you've *been*."

He speculates that longevity-enabling genes may work via several possible mechanisms, such as protecting against chronic diseases and slowing down the aging process. Then again, those processes may amount to much the same thing. "If you slow down the rate of aging, you naturally decrease susceptibility to illnesses like Alzheimer's, stroke, heart disease and various cancers," he says.

Clues to how such genes might operate come from a centenarian study being conducted by Dr. Nir Barzilai, a gerontologist and endocrinologist at Albert Einstein College of Medicine in the Bronx. Barzilai has found that his research subjects—more than 200 Ashkenazi Jewish centenarians and their children—have abnormally high blood levels of high-density lipoprotein, or HDL, a.k.a. the "good" cholesterol. The average woman has an HDL level of 55, he says, whereas the grown children of his centenarians have levels up to 140.

He believes that a gene or genes are responsible for the extremely high HDL levels, which may have helped the very old people in his studies maintain their sharp minds and clear memories. He says their high HDL levels, which are presumably controlled by genes, might protect them from heart disease; HDL clears fat from coronary arteries, among other things.

Other researchers say that longevity-enabling genes might protect people in much the same manner as caloric restriction, the only treatment or dietary strategy shown experimentally to extend life. Studies with laboratory rats have found that those fed an extremely low-calorie diet live at least 33 percent longer than rats that eat their fill. The restricted animals also seem to avoid ailments connected with aging, such as diabetes, hypertension, cataracts and cancer. Another possibility is that longevity-enabling genes limit the activities of free radicals—unpaired electrons known to corrode human tissue. Medical researchers have suggested that free radicals spur atherosclerosis and Alzheimer's disease, for instance. "Free radicals are a key mechanism in aging," Perls says. "I wouldn't be surprised if something to do with free-radical damage pops up in our genetic studies."

IF MACKNIGHT RECEIVES funding to pursue the research, he and his associates plan to interview Nova Scotian centenarians about their histories as well as examine them and draw blood samples for genetic analysis. He hopes to work with Perls to compare the Nova Scotians' genetic material to that from Perls' New England subjects, with an eye for similarities or differences that might betray the presence of longevity-enabling genes.

Like all students of the extremely old, MacKnight is interested in their habits and practices. "We're trying to look at frailty," MacKnight says, "or, what makes some 100-year-old people seem like they're 60 and some seem like they're 150. What are the differences between those who live in their own homes and cook their own breakfast and those who are blind and deaf and mostly demented and bed-bound? And can we develop some kind of intervention for people in their 50s and 60s to keep them from becoming frail?"

Not all centenarians—not even all of those in Nova Scotia—seem as young as Betty Cooper. And though it could be that the difference between the frail and the strong is determined largely by genes, researchers say it is also true that some people who reach 100 in fine shape have been especially prudent. Among centenarians, smoking and obesity are rare. Other qualities that are common to many centenarians include staying mentally engaged, having a measure of financial security (though not necessarily wealth) and remaining involved with loved ones. And though healthy nonagenarians and centenarians often say they've led physically active lives—"I did a lot of hard labor," says 90-year-old Arthur Hebb, of Lunenburg County, who eagerly reads the newspaper every day—Perls and other researchers haven't definitively answered that question.

Nor do researchers fully understand all the centenarian data, such as why the great majority are women. In the United States, women older than 100 outnumber men by more than four to one. But men at 100 are more likely than women the same age to be in good health and clearheaded.

Perls and his colleague Margery Hutter Silver, a neuropsychologist, have found that about 70 percent of centenarian women show signs of dementia, compared with only 30 percent of the men. A surprisingly high proportion of the women—14 percent—have never married. In contrast, almost all centenarian men are, or have been, married.

Centenarians tend to be healthier than you might think: 40 percent avoid chronic illnesses until they're 85 or older; 20 percent postpone age-related debilities until they're 100.

Whether they've survived so long because they're resilient, or they're resilient because they've survived so long, centenarians are often possessed of exceptional psychological strength. "They're gregarious and full of good humor," Perls says. "Their families and friends genuinely like to be with them, because they're basically very happy, optimistic people." A genial attitude makes it easier for people to handle stress, he adds: "It isn't that centenarians have never suffered any traumatic experiences. They've been through wars, they've seen most of their friends die, even some of their own children. But they get through."

Paradoxically, that centenarians have lived such long and eventful lives makes it all the more difficult to pinpoint any one advantage they may have shared. No matter how much researchers learn about longevity-enabling genes, no matter how well they discern the biological protections that centenarians have in common, the very old will always be an exceptionally diverse group. Each one will have a story to tell—as unique as it is long.

"I started fishing when I was 14," says Shand, of Yarmouth. "Then I built fishing boats for 35 years." He uses a wheelchair because a stroke 18 years ago left him with some disability in his right leg. He is broad-chested, robust—and sharp. "I don't think hard work ever hurt anybody."

"We had a lot of meat and a lot of fish and fowl," says Elizabeth Slauenwhite, 99, of Lunenburg. There were also "vegetables and fruit," she adds. "And sweets galore."

MARY DUENWALD, former executive editor of *Harper's Bazaar,* writes about health.

The Demographic Drivers of Aging

Kevin Kinsella and David R. Phillips

When asked "Why do populations age?," most people intuitively think of changes in longevity. We know that life expectancy has been rising in most countries throughout the world, so it seems reasonable that population aging is an outcome of people living longer. Yet, the most prominent historical factor in population aging has been declining fertility. If we think of population aging as an increase in the percent of people age 65 or older, we realize that, over time, a decline in the number of babies will mean fewer young people and proportionally more people at older ages.

Fertility—The Primary Driver

The decrease in fertility in industrialized nations during the last century has pushed the average number of children per woman in almost all more developed countries below the population replacement level of 2.1 children. Sustained low fertility since the late 1970s has reduced the size of successive birth cohorts and increased the proportion of older people in these countries' populations. Fertility decline in the less developed world has been more recent and more rapid; most regions have seen large reductions in fertility rates during the last 30 years. Although the aggregate total fertility rate (TFR, the average number of children per woman given current birth rates) remains in excess of 4.5 children per woman in Africa and many countries of the Middle East, overall levels in Asia and Latin America decreased by about 50 percent (from 6 to 3 children per woman) between 1965 and 1995. The TFR in many less developed countries is now at or below replacement level—notably in the world's most populous country, China. By 2000, a majority of the world's population lived in countries with near- or below- replacement fertility.[6] The UN projects that, by 2050, three of every four of today's less developed countries will have below-replacement fertility.

At very old ages, the rate of increase in mortality tends to slow.

Populations with high fertility tend to have low proportions of older people and vice versa. The term "demographic transition" is used to describe a gradual process of change from high rates of fertility and mortality to low rates of fertility and mortality. The process is characterized first by declines in infant and childhood mortality, as infectious and parasitic diseases are controlled through expansion of public health services and facilities and disease eradication programs. This improvement in mortality occurs while fertility is still high, resulting in large birth cohorts and an expanding proportion of children relative to adults. Other things being equal, the initial decline in mortality generates a younger population age structure.[7]

Increasing Importance of Mortality

In countries where infant mortality rates are relatively high but declining, most of the improvement in life expectancy at birth results from helping infants survive the high-risk early years of life. Reductions in maternal mortality also contribute to increased life expectancy at birth. As a nation's infant, childhood, and maternal mortality reach low levels, longevity gains at older ages become more prominent contributors to increased life expectancy.[8] Most countries today are experiencing a rise in life expectancy at older ages, which contributes to rising life expectancy at birth. For example, the average Japanese woman reaching age 65 in 2000 could expect to live more than 22 additional years, and the average man more than 17 years. Japanese life expectancy at age 65 for both sexes combined increased 44 percent from 1970 to 2000, while life expectancy at birth increased only 9 percent. Comparative figures for the United States are 19 percent and 9 percent, respectively.

The speed at which death rates at advanced ages decline will play a major role in determining future numbers of older, and especially of very old, populations. The remaining life expectancy of 80-year-old women in England and Wales is about 50 percent higher today than it was in 1950. Hence, the number of female octogenarians is about 50 percent higher than it would have been had oldest-old mortality remained at 1950 levels. In absolute terms, there are more than 500,000 British women age 80 or older alive today who otherwise would have died if death rates for the oldest-old had not improved.[9]

Until the mid-1990s, conventional demographic wisdom held that the human death rate increases with age in an exponential manner. Newer research has documented that, at very old ages, the rate of increase in the mortality rate tends to slow down. A study of 28 countries with reliable data for 1950 to 1990 found not only a decline in mortality rates at ages 80 and older, but also a tendency toward greater decline in more recent years.[10] Other work has confirmed this tendency, and one study in the United States suggests that the age at which mortality deceleration occurs is rising.[11]

There are at least two potential explanations of this deceleration of mortality at the oldest ages. The "heterogeneity" hypothesis, an extension of the notion of "survival of the fittest," posits that the deceleration in old-age mortality is a result of frailer older people dying at younger ages, thus creating a very old population with exceptionally healthy attributes resulting from genetic endowment and/or lifestyle. A second, "individual-risk" hypothesis, suggests that the rate of aging may slow down at very old ages, and/or that certain genes that are detrimental to survival may be suppressed.[12] The observed deceleration in mortality, combined with the fact that human mortality at older ages has declined substantially, has led to the questioning of many of the theoretical tenets of aging. Important insights are being garnered from "biodemographic" research that attempts to crossfertilize the biologic and demographic perspectives of aging and senescence. A clearer picture of the causes of mortality deceleration at very old ages may emerge from the study of evolutionary biology and aging in nonhuman species. But recognition of this slowdown in old-age mortality—at a time when numbers of the very old are growing rapidly—has important policy implications.[13]

Changes in Life Expectancy

The dramatic increases in life expectancy that began in the mid-1800s often are thought to be the result of medical breakthroughs. In fact, the major impact of improvements in medicine and sanitation did not occur until the late 19th century. Prior innovations in industrial and agricultural production and distribution, which improved nutrition for large numbers of people, were more powerful forces in mortality reductions. A growing multidisciplinary research consensus attributes the gain in human longevity since the 1800s to the interplay of advancements in medicine and sanitation against a backdrop of new modes of familial, social, economic, and political organization.[14] Life expectancy at birth in Japan approached 82 years in 2003, the highest level among the world's major countries. Life expectancy is at least 79 years in several other developed nations, including Australia, Canada, Italy, Iceland, Sweden, and Switzerland. Average life expectancy in the United States and most other developed countries ranged between 76 and 78 years.

Throughout the less developed world, there are extreme variations in life expectancy at birth. Some nations have levels equal to or higher than those in many European nations, whereas life expectancy at birth in numerous African countries is less than 45 years. The average person born in a more developed country can now expect to outlive his or her counterpart in the less developed world by 14 years.

In some nations, life expectancy more than doubled during the 20th century (see Table). Increases in life expectancy were more rapid in the first half than in the second half of the century. Between 1900 and 1950, many Western nations added 20 or more years to their average life expectancy. Reliable estimates of life expectancy for less developed countries prior to 1950 are scarce, but changes in life expectancy in these countries have been fairly uniform since then. Practically all nations have shown continued improvement, with some exceptions in Latin America and more recently in Africa, the latter due to the impact of the HIV/AIDS epidemic. The most dramatic gains have occurred in East Asia, where average life expectancy at birth for the region increased from less than 45 years in 1950 to more than 72 years today.

An increasing gender differential in life expectancy was a hallmark of mortality patterns in more developed countries in the 20th century, reflecting the generally lower mortality of females than males in every age group and for most causes of death. In Europe in 1900, women typically outlived men by two or three years. Today, the average gap between the sexes is approximately seven years, and may be as high as 12 years in parts of the former Soviet Union. Gender differentials tend to be smaller (between three and six years) in less developed countries, and are reversed in a few South Asian and Middle Eastern societies in which such cultural factors as low female social status and a preference for male rather than female offspring affect female life expectancy.

Changing Age Structure

Populations begin to age when fertility declines and adult mortality rates improve. Successive birth cohorts eventually become smaller, although the trend may be interrupted by "baby-boom echoes" as women of prior large birth cohorts reach childbearing age. International migration usually does not play a major role in the aging process, but can be important in smaller populations. Some Caribbean nations, for example, have experienced a combination of emigration of working-age adults, immigration of retirees from other countries, and return migration of older former emigrants; all three factors contribute to population aging. Many observers expect international migration to assume a more prominent role in the aging process, particularly in "older" countries where persistently low fertility has led to stable or even declining population size.[15]

Most if not all countries once had a youthful age structure similar to that of less developed countries as a whole in 1950, with a large percentage of the entire population under age 15. Given the comparatively high rates of fertility that prevailed in most less developed countries from 1950 through the early 1970s, the pyramidal shape of the age and sex profile of less developed countries had not changed greatly by 1990. However, the effects of fertility and mortality decline can be seen in the projected

Table

Life Expectancy at Birth in Years, Selected Countries, 1900, 1950, and 2003

Region/country	Circa 1900		Circa 1950		Circa 2003	
	Male	Female	Male	Female	Male	Female
More developed countries						
Western Europe						
Austria	38	40	63	68	75	81
France	45	49	64	70	75	83
Sweden	53	55	70	73	78	83
United Kingdom	46	50	67	72	76	81
Southern and eastern Europe						
Hungary	37	38	62	66	68	76
Italy	43	43	64	68	76	82
Spain	34	36	62	66	76	83
Other						
Australia	53	57	67	72	76	82
Japan	43	44	60	63	78	85
United States	48	51	66	72	74	80
Less developed countries						
Africa						
Egypt	—	—	41	44	67	71
Ghana	—	—	40	44	57	59
Mali	—	—	31	34	48	49
South Africa	—	—	44	46	45	51
Uganda	—	—	39	42	45	47
Asia						
China	—	—	39	42	69	73
India	—	—	39	38	63	65
Kazakhstan	—	—	52	62	61	72
South Korea	—	—	46	49	72	79
Syria	—	—	45	47	71	73
Latin America						
Argentina	—	—	60	65	71	78
Bolivia	—	—	39	43	62	66
Brazil	—	—	49	53	64	73
Costa Rica	—	—	56	59	76	81
Mexico	—	—	49	52	70	76

— Not available.

Note: Average number of years a person born in those years could expect to live.

Source: UN Population Division, *World Population Prospects: The 2002 Revision* (2003); and G. Siampos, *Statistical Journal of the United Nations Economic Commission for Europe 7*, no. 1 (1990): 13–25.

age-sex pyramid for 2030, which loses its strictly triangular shape as the size of younger five-year cohorts stabilizes and the older portion of the total population increases.

The picture in more developed countries has been and will be quite different. In 1950, there was relatively little variation in the size of five-year groups between the ages of 5 and 24. The beginning of the post-World War II baby boom can be seen in the 0-to-4 age group. By 1990, the baby-boom cohorts were ages 25 to 44, and younger cohorts were successively smaller. If projected fertility rates are reasonably accurate through 2030, the aggregate pyramid will start to invert, with more weight on the top than on the bottom, and the size of the oldest-old population (especially women) will increase substantially.

WILL YOU LIVE TO BE 100?

After completing a study of 150 centenarians, Harvard Medical School researchers Thomas Perls, M.D., and Margery Hutter Silver, Ed.D., developed a quiz to help you calculate your estimated life expectancy.

LONGEVITY QUIZ	Score
1 Do you smoke or chew tobacco, or are you around a lot of secondhand smoke? Yes (–20) No (0)	
2 Do you cook your fish, poultry, or meat until it is charred? Yes (–2) No (0)	
3 Do you avoid butter, cream, pastries, and other saturated fats as well as fried foods (eg., French Fries)? Yes (+3) No (–7)	
4 Do you minimize meat in your diet, preferably making a point to eat plenty of fruits, vegetables, and bran instead? Yes (+5) No (–4)	
5 Do you consume more than two drinks of beer, wine, and/or liquor a day? (A standard drink is one 12-ounce bottle of beer, one wine cooler, one five-ounce glass of wine, or one and a half ounces of 80-proof distilled spirits.) Yes (–10) No (0)	
6 Do you drink beer, wine, and/or liquor in moderate amounts (one or two drinks/day)? Yes (+3) No (0)	
7 Do air pollution warnings occur where you live? Yes (–4) No (+1)	
8 **a** Do you drink more than 16 ounces of coffee a day? Yes (–3) No (0) **b** Do you drink tea daily? Yes (+3) No (0)	
9 Do you take an aspirin a day? Yes (+4) No (0)	
10 Do you floss your teeth every day? Yes (+2) No (–4)	
11 Do you have a bowel movement less than once every two days? Yes (–4) No (0)	
12 Have you had a stroke or heart attack? Yes (–10) No (0)	
13 Do you try to get a sun tan? Yes (–4) No (+3)	
14 Are you more than 20 pounds overweight? Yes (–10) No (0)	
15 Do you live near enough to other family members (other than your spouse and dependent children) that you can and want to drop by spontaneously? Yes (+5) No (–4)	
16 Which statement is applicable to you? **a** "Stress eats away at me. I can't seem to shake it off." Yes (–7) **b** "I can shed stress." This might be by praying, exercising, meditating, finding humor in everyday life, or other means. Yes (+7)	
17 Did both of your parents either die before age 75 of nonaccidental causes or require daily assistance by the time they reached age 75? Yes (–10) No (0) Don't know (0)	
18 Did more than one of the following relatives live to at least age 90 in excellent health: parents, aunts/uncles, grandparents? Yes (+24) No (0) Don't know (0)	
19 **a** Are you a couch potato (do no regular aerobic or resistance exercise)? Yes (–7) **b** Do you exercise at least three times a week? Yes (+7)	
20 Do you take vitamin E (400–800 IU) and selenium (100–200 mcg) every day? Yes (+5) No (–3)	

SCORE

STEP 1:   Add the negative and positive scores together. Example: –45 plus +30 = –15. Divide the preceding score by 5 (–15 divided by 5 = –3).

STEP 2:   Add the negative or positive number to age 84 if you are a man or age 88 if you are a woman (example: –3 + 88 = 85) to get your estimated life span.

THE SCIENCE BEHIND THE QUIZ

Question 1   Cigarette smoke contains toxins that directly damage DNA, causing cancer and other diseases and accelerating aging.

Question 2   Charring food changes its proteins and amino acids into heterocyclic amines, which are potent mutagens that can alter your DNA.

Questions 3, 4   A high-fat diet, and especially a high-fat, high-protein diet, may increase your risk of cancer of the breast, uterus, prostate, colon, pancreas, and kidney. A diet rich in fruits and vegetables may lower the risk of heart disease and cancer.

Questions 5, 6   Excessive alcohol consumption can damage the liver and other organs, leading to accelerated aging and increased susceptibility to disease. Moderate consumption may lower the risk of heart disease.

Question 7   Certain air pollutants may cause cancer; many also contain oxidants that accelerate aging.

Question 8   Too much coffee predisposes the stomach to ulcers and chronic inflammation, which in turn raise the risk of heart disease. High coffee consumption may also indicate and exacerbate stress. Tea, on the other hand, is noted for its significant antioxidant content.

Question 9   Taking 81 milligrams of aspirin a day (the amount in one baby aspirin) has been shown to decrease the risk of heart disease, possibly because of its anticlotting effects.

Question 10   Research now shows that chronic gum disease can lead to the release of bacteria into the bloodstream, contributing to heart disease.

Question 11   Scientists believe that having at least one bowel movement every 20 hours decreases the incidence of colon cancer.

Question 12   A previous history of stroke and heart attack makes you more susceptible to future attacks.

Question 13   The ultraviolet rays in sunlight directly damage DNA, causing wrinkles and increasing the risk of skin cancer.

Question 14   Being obese increases the risk of various cancers, heart disease, and diabetes. The more overweight you are, the higher your risk of disease and death.

Questions 15, 16   People who do not belong to cohesive families have fewer coping resources and therefore have increased levels of social and psychological stress. Stress is associated with heart disease and some cancers.

Questions 17, 18   Studies show that genetics plays a significant role in the ability to reach extreme old age.

Question 19   Exercise leads to more efficient energy production in the cells and overall, less oxygen radical formation. Oxygen (or free) radicals are highly reactive molecules or atoms that damage cells and DNA, ultimately leading to aging.

Question 20   Vitamin E is a powerful antioxidant and has been shown to retard the progression of Alzheimer's, heart disease, and stroke. Selenium may prevent some types of cancer.

Adapted from *Living to 100: Lessons in Living to Your Maximum Potential at Any Age* (Basic Books, 1999) by Thomas Perls, M.D., and Margery Hutter Silver, Ed.D., with John F. Lauerman.

THE COMING DEATH SHORTAGE

Why the longevity boom will make us sorry to be alive

CHARLES C. MANN

Anna Nicole Smith's role as a harbinger of the future is not widely acknowledged. Born Vickie Lynn Hogan, Smith first came to the attention of the American public in 1993, when she earned the title Playmate of the Year. In 1994 she married J. Howard Marshall, a Houston oil magnate said to be worth more than half a billion dollars. He was eighty-nine and wheelchair-bound; she was twenty-six and quiveringly mobile. Fourteen months later Marshall died. At his funeral the widow appeared in a white dress with a vertical neckline. She also claimed that Marshall had promised half his fortune to her. The inevitable litigation sprawled from Texas to California and occupied batteries of lawyers, consultants, and public-relations specialists for more than seven years.

Even before Smith appeared, Marshall had disinherited his older son. And he had infuriated his younger son by lavishing millions on a mistress, an exotic dancer, who then died in a bizarre face-lift accident. To block Marshall senior from squandering on Smith money that Marshall junior regarded as rightfully his, the son seized control of his father's assets by means that the trial judge later said were so "egregious," "malicious," and "fraudulent" that he regretted being unable to fine the younger Marshall more than $44 million in punitive damages.

In its epic tawdriness the Marshall affair was natural fodder for the tabloid media. Yet one aspect of it may soon seem less a freak show than a cliché. If an increasingly influential group of researchers is correct, the lurid spectacle of inter generational warfare will become a typical social malady.

The scientists' argument is circuitous but not complex. In the past century U.S. life expectancy has climbed from forty-seven to seventy-seven, increasing by two nearly two thirds. Similar rises happened in almost every country. And this process shows no sign of stopping: according to the United Nations, by 2050 global life expectancy will have increased by another ten years. Note, however, that this tremendous increase has been in *average* life expectancy—that is, the number of years that most people live. There has been next to no increase in the *maximum* lifespan, the number of years that one can possibly walk the earth—now thought to be about 120. In the scientists' projections, the ongoing increase in average lifespan is about to be joined by something never before seen in human history: a rise in the maximum possible age at death.

Stem-cell banks, telomerase amplifiers, somatic gene therapy—the list of potential longevity treatments incubating in laboratories is startling. Three years ago a multi-institutional scientific team led by Aubrey de Grey, a theoretical geneticist at Cambridge University, argued in a widely noted paper that the first steps toward "engineered negligible senescence"—a rough-and-ready version of immortality—would have "a good chance of success in mice within ten years." The same techniques, De Grey says, should be ready for human beings a decade or so later. "In ten years we'll have a pill that will give you twenty years," says Leonard Guarente, a professor of biology at MIT. "And then there'll be another pill after that. The first hundred-and-fifty-year-old may have already been born."

Critics regard such claims as wildly premature. In March ten respected researchers predicted in the *New England Journal of Medicine* that "the steady rise in life expectancy during the past two centuries may soon come to an end," because rising levels of obesity are making people sicker. The research team leader. S. Jay Olshansky, of the University of Illinois School of Public Health, also worries about the "potential impact of infectious disease." Believing that medicine can and will overcome these problems, his "cautious and I think defensibly optimistic estimate" is that the average lifespan will reach eighty-five or ninety—in 2100. Even this relatively slow rate of increase, he says, will radically alter the underpinnings of human existence. "Pushing the outer limits of lifespan" will force the world to confront a situation no society has ever faced before: an acute shortage of dead people.

The twentieth-century jump in life expectancy transformed society. Fifty years ago senior citizens were not a force in electoral politics. Now the AARP is widely said to be the most powerful organization in Washington. Medicare, Social Security, retirement, Alzheimer's, snowbird economies, the population boom, the golfing boom, the cosmetic-surgery boom, the nostalgia boom, the recreational-vehicle boom, Viagra—increasing longevity is entangled in every one. Momentous as these changes have been, though, they will pale before what is coming next.

Instead of helping their juniors begin careers and families, tomorrow's rich oldsters will be expending their disposable income to enhance their memories, senses, and immune systems, refashioning their flesh to ever higher levels of performance.

From religion to real estate, from pensions to parent-child dynamics, almost every aspect of society is based on the orderly succession of generations. Every quarter century or so children take over from their parents—a transition as fundamental to human existence as the rotation of the planet about its axis. In tomorrow's world, if the optimists are correct, grandparents will have living grandparents; children born decades from now will ignore advice from people who watched the Beatles on *The Ed Sullivan Show*. Intergenerational warfare—the Anna Nicole Smith syndrome—will be but one consequence. Trying to envision such a world, sober social scientists find themselves discussing pregnant seventy-year-olds, offshore organ farms, protracted adolescence, and lifestyles policed by insurance companies. Indeed, if the biologists are right, the coming army of centenarians will be marching into a future so unutterably different that they may well feel nostalgia for the long-ago days of three score and ten.

The oldest *in vitro* fertilization clinic in China is located on the sixth floor of a no-star hotel in Changsha, a gritty fly-over city in the south-central portion of the country. It is here that the clinic's founder and director, Lu Guangxiu, pursues her research into embryonic stem cells.

Most cells *don't* divide, whatever elementary school students learn—they just get old and die. The body subcontracts out the job of replacing them to a special class of cells called stem cells. Embryonic stem cells—those in an early-stage embryo—can grow into any kind of cell: spleen, nerve, bone, whatever. Rather than having to wait for a heart transplant, medical researchers believe, a patient could use stem cells to grow a new heart: organ transplant without an organ donor.

The process of extracting stem cells destroys an early-stage embryo, which has led the Bush administration to place so many strictures on stem-cell research that scientists complain it has been effectively banned in this country. A visit to Lu's clinic not long ago suggested that ultimately Bush's rules won't stop anything. Capitalism won't let them.

During a conversation Lu accidentally brushed some papers to the floor. They were faxes from venture capitalists in San Francisco, Hong Kong, and Stuttgart. "I get those all the time," she said. Her operation was short of money—a chronic problem for scientists in poor countries. But it had something of value: thousands of frozen embryos, an inevitable by-product of *in vitro* fertilizations. After obtaining permission from patients, Lu uses the embryos in her work. It is possible that she has access to more embryonic stem cells than all U.S. researchers combined.

Sooner or later, in one nation or another, someone like Lu will cut a deal: frozen embryos for financial backing. Few are the stem-cell researchers who believe that their work will not lead to tissue-and-organ farms, and that these will not have a dramatic impact on the human lifespan. If Organs 'Я' Us is banned in the United States, Americans will fly to longevity centers elsewhere. As Steve Hall wrote in *Merchants of Immortality*, biotechnology increasingly resembles the software industry. Dependence on venture capital, loathing of regulation, pathological secretiveness, penchant for hype, willingness to work overseas—they're all there. Already the U.S. Patent Office has issued 400 patents concerning human stem cells.

Longevity treatments will almost certainly drive up medical costs, says Dana Goldman, the director of health economics at the RAND Corporation, and some might drive them up significantly. Implanted defibrillators, for example, could constantly monitor people's hearts for signs of trouble, electrically regulating the organs when they miss a beat. Researchers believe that the devices would reduce heart-disease deaths significantly. At the same time, Goldman says, they would by themselves drive up the nation's health-care costs by "many billions of dollars" (Goldman and his colleagues are working on nailing down how much), and they would be only one of many new medical interventions. In developed nations anti-retroviral drugs for AIDS typically cost about $15,000 a year. According to James Lubitz, the acting chief of the aging and chronic-disease statistics branch of the CDC National Center for Health Statistics, there is no a priori reason to suppose that lifespan extension will be cheaper, that the treatments will have to be administered less frequently, or that their inventors will agree to be less well compensated. To be sure, as Ramez Naam points out in *More Than Human*, which surveys the prospects for "biological enhancement," drugs inevitably fall in price as their patents expire. But the same does not necessarily hold true for medical procedures: heart bypass operations are still costly, decades after their invention. And in any case there will invariably be newer, more effective, and more costly drugs. Simple arithmetic shows that if 80 million U.S. senior citizens were to receive $15,000 worth of treatment every year, the annual cost to the nation would be $1.2 trillion—"the kind of number," Lubitz says, "that gets people's attention."

The potential costs are enormous, but the United States is a rich nation. As a share of gross domestic product the cost of U.S. health care roughly doubled from 1980 to the present, explains David M. Cutler, a health-care economist at Harvard. Yet unlike many cost increases, this one signifies that people are better off. "Would you rather have a heart attack with 1980 medicine at the 1980 price?" Cutler asks. "We get more and better treatments now, and we pay more for the additional services. I don't look at that and see an obvious disaster."

The critical issue, in Goldman's view, will be not the costs per se but determining who will pay them. "We're going to have a very public debate about whether this will be covered by insurance," he says. "My sense is that it won't. It'll be like cosmetic surgery—you pay out of pocket." Necessarily, a pay-as-you-go policy would limit access to longevity treatments. If high-level anti-aging therapy were expensive enough, it could become a perk for movie stars, politicians, and CEOs. One can envision Michael Moore fifty years from now, still denouncing the rich in political tracts delivered through the next generation's version of the Internet—neural implants, perhaps. Donald Trump, a 108-year-old multibillionaire in 2054, will be firing the children of the apprentices he fired in 2004. Meanwhile, the maids, chauffeurs, and gofers of the rich will stare mortality in the face.

Short of overtly confiscating rich people's assets, it would be hard to avoid this divide. Yet as Goldman says, there will be "furious" political pressure to avert the worst inequities. For instance, government might mandate that insurance cover longevity treatments. In fact, it is hard to imagine any democratic government foolhardy enough not to guarantee access to those treatments, especially when the old are increasing in number and political clout. But forcing insurers to cover longevity treatments would only change the shape of the social problem. "Most everyone will want to take [the treatment]," Goldman says. "So that jacks up the price of insurance, which leads to more people uninsured. Either way, we may be bifurcating society."

Ultimately, Goldman suggests, the government would probably end up paying out right for longevity treatments: an enormous new entitlement program. How could it be otherwise? Older voters would want it because it is in their interest; younger ones would want it because they, too, will age. "At the same time," he says, "nobody likes paying taxes, so there would be constant pressure to contain costs."

To control spending, the program might give priority to people with healthy habits; no point in retooling the genomes of smokers, risk takers, and addicts of all kinds. A kind of reverse eugenics might occur, in which governments would freely allow the birth of people with "bad" genes but would let nature take its course on them as they aged. Having shed the baggage of depression, addiction, mental retardation, and chemical-sensitivity syndrome, tomorrow's legions of perduring old would be healthier than the young. In this scenario moralists and reformers would have a field day.

Meanwhile, the gerontocratic elite will have a supreme weapon against the young: compound interest. According to a 2004 study by three researchers at the London Business School, historically the average rate of real return on stock markets worldwide has been about five percent. Thus a twenty-year-old who puts $10,000 in the market in 2010 should expect by 2030 to have about $27,000 in real terms—a tidy increase. But that happy forty-year-old will be in the same world as septuagenarians and octogenarians who began investing their money during the Carter administration. If someone who turned seventy in 2010 had invested $10,000 when he was twenty, he would have about $115,000. In the same twenty-year period during which the young person's account grew from $10,000 to $27,000, the old person's account would grow from $115,000 to $305,000. Inexorably, the gap between them will widen.

The result would be a tripartite society: the very old and very rich on top, beta-testing each new treatment on themselves; a mass of the ordinary old, forced by insurance into supremely healthy habits, kept alive by medical entitlement; and the diminishingly influential young. In his novel *Holy Fire* (1996) the science-fiction writer and futurist Bruce Sterling conjured up a version of this dictatorship-by-actuary: a society in which the cautious, careful centenarian rulers, supremely fit and disproportionately affluent if a little frail, look down with ennui and mild contempt on their juniors. Marxist class warfare, upgraded to the biotech era!

Increased longevity may add to marital strains. The historian Lawrence Stone noted that divorce was rare in previous centuries partly because people died so young that bad unions were often dissolved by early funerals.

In the past, twenty- and thirty-year-olds had the chance of sudden windfalls in the form of inheritances. Some economists believe that bequests from previous generations have provided as much as a quarter of the start-up capital for each new one— money for college tuitions, new houses, new businesses. But the image of an ingénue's getting a leg up through a sudden bequest from Aunt Tilly will soon be a relic of late-millennium romances.

Instead of helping their juniors begin careers and families, tomorrow's rich oldsters will be expending their disposable income to enhance their memories, senses, and immune systems. Refashioning their flesh to ever higher levels of performance, they will adjust their metabolisms on computers, install artificial organs that synthesize smart drugs, and swallow genetically tailored bacteria and viruses that clean out arteries, fine-tune neurons, and repair broken genes. Should one be reminded of H. G. Wells's *The Time Machine*, in which humankind is divided into two species, the ethereal Eloi and the brutish, underground-dwelling Morlocks? "As I recall," Goldman told me recently, "in that book it didn't work out very well for the Eloi."

When lifespans extend indefinitely, the effects are felt throughout the life cycle, but the biggest social impact may be on the young. According to Joshua Goldstein, a demographer at Princeton, adolescence will in the future evolve into a period of experimentation and education that will last from the teenage years into the mid-thirties. In a kind of *wanderjahr* prolonged for decades, young people will try out jobs on a temporary basis, float in and out of their parents' homes, hit the Europass-and-hostel circuit, pick up extra courses and degrees, and live with different people in different places. In the past the transition from youth to adulthood usually followed an orderly sequence: education, entry into the labor force, marriage, and parenthood. For tomorrow's thirtysomethings, suspended in what Goldstein calls "quasi-adulthood," these steps may occur in any order.

From our short-life-expectancy point of view, quasi-adulthood may seem like a period of socially mandated fecklessness—what Leon Kass, the chair of the President's Council on Bioethics, has decried as the coming culture of "protracted youthfulness, hedonism, and sexual license." In Japan, ever in the demographic forefront, as many as one out of three young adults is either unemployed or working part-time, and many are living rent-free with their parents. Masahiro Yamada, a sociologist at Tokyo Gakugei University, has sarcastically dubbed them *parasaito shinguru*, or "parasite singles." Adult offspring who live with their parents are common in aging Europe, too. In 2003 a report from the British Prudential financial-services group awarded the 6.8 million British in this category the mocking name of "kippers"—"kids in parents' pockets eroding retirement savings."

To Kass, the main cause of this stasis is "the successful pursuit of longer life and better health." Kass's fulminations easily lend themselves to ridicule. Nonetheless, he is in many ways correct. According to Yuji Genda, an economist at Tokyo University, the drifty lives of parasite singles are indeed a by-product, of increased longevity, mainly because longer-lived seniors are holding on to their jobs. Japan, with the world's oldest population, has the highest percentage of working senior citizens of any developed nation: one out of three men over sixty-five is still on the job. Everyone in the nation, Genda says, is "tacitly aware" that the old are "blocking the door."

In a world of 200-year-olds "the rate of rise in income and status perhaps for the first hundred years of life will be almost negligible," the crusty maverick economist Kenneth Boulding argued in a prescient article from 1965. "It is the propensity of the old, rich, and powerful to die that gives the young, poor, and powerless hope." (Boulding died in 1993, opening up a position for another crusty maverick economist.)

Kass believes that "human beings, once they have attained the burdensome knowledge of good and bad, should not have access to the tree of life." Accordingly, he has proposed a straightforward way to prevent the problems of youth in a society dominated by the old: "resist the siren song of the conquest of aging and death." Senior citizens, in other words, should let nature take its course once humankind's biblical seventy-year lifespan is up. Unfortunately, this solution is self-canceling, since everyone who agrees with it is eventually eliminated. Opponents, meanwhile, live on and on. Kass, who is sixty-six, has another four years to make his case.

Increased longevity may add to marital strains. The historian Lawrence Stone was among the first to note that divorce was rare in previous centuries partly because people died so young that bad unions were often dissolved by early funerals. As people lived longer, Stone argued, divorce became "a functional substitute for death." Indeed, marriages dissolved at about the same rate in 1860 as in 1960, except that in the nineteenth century the dissolution was more often due to the death of a partner, and in the twentieth century to divorce. The corollary that children were as likely to live in households without both biological parents in 1860 as in 1960 is also true. Longer lifespans are far from the only reason for today's higher divorce rates, but the evidence seems clear that they play a role. The prospect of spending another twenty years sitting across the breakfast table from a spouse whose charm has faded must have already driven millions to divorce lawyers. Adding an extra decade or two can only exacerbate the strain.

Worse, child-rearing, a primary marital activity, will be even more difficult than it is now. For the past three decades, according to Ben J. Wattenberg, a senior fellow at the American Enterprise Institute, birth rates around the world have fallen sharply as women have taken advantage of increased opportunities for education and work outside the home. "More education, more work, lower fertility," he says. The title of Wattenberg's latest book, published in October, sums up his view of tomorrow's demographic prospects: *Fewer*. In his analysis, women's continuing movement outside the home will lead to a devastating population crash—the mirror image of the population boom that shaped so much of the past century. Increased longevity will only add to the downward pressure on birth rates, by making childbearing even more difficult. During their twenties, as Goldstein's quasi-adults, men and women will be unmarried and relatively poor. In their thirties and forties they will finally grow old enough to begin meaningful careers—the worst time to have children. Waiting still longer will mean entering the maelstrom of reproductive technology, which seems likely to remain expensive, alienating, and prone to complications. Thus the parental paradox: increased longevity means *less* time for pregnancy and child-rearing, not more.

Even when women manage to fit pregnancy into their careers, they will spend a smaller fraction of their lives raising children than ever before. In the mid nineteenth century white women in the United States had a life expectancy of about forty years and typically bore five or six children. (I specify Caucasians because records were not kept for African-Americans.) These women literally spent more than half their lives caring for offspring. Today U.S. white women have a life expectancy of nearly eighty and bear an average of 1.9 children—below replacement level. If a woman spaces two births close together, she may spend only a quarter of her days in the company of offspring under the age of eighteen. Children will become ever briefer parentheses in long, crowded adult existences. It seems inevitable that the bonds between generations will fray.

Purely from a financial standpoint, parenthood has always been a terrible deal. Mom and Dad fed, clothed, housed, and educated the kids, but received little in the way of tangible return. Ever since humankind began acquiring property, wealth has flowed from older generations to younger ones. Even in those societies where children herded cattle and tilled the land for their aged progenitors, the older generation consumed so little and died off so quickly that the net movement of assets and services was always downward. "Of all the misconceptions that should be banished from discussions of aging," F. Landis MacKellar, an economist at the International Institute for Applied Systems Analysis, in Austria, wrote in the journal *Population and Development Review* in 2001, "the most persistent and egregious is that in some simpler and more virtuous age children supported their parents."

This ancient pattern changed at the beginning of the twentieth century, when government pension and social-security schemes spread across Europe and into the Americas. Within the family parents still gave much more than they received, according to MacKellar, but under the new state plans the children in effect banded together outside the family and collectively reimbursed the parents. In the United States workers pay less to Social Security than they eventually receive; retirees are subsidized by the contributions of younger workers. But on the broadest level financial support from the young is still offset by the movement of assets within families—a point rarely noted by critics of "greedy geezers."

Increased longevity will break up this relatively equitable arrangement. Here concerns focus less on the super-rich than on middle-class senior citizens, those who aren't surfing the crest of compound interest. These people will face a Hobson's choice. On the one hand, they will be unable to retire at sixty-five, because the young would end up bankrupting themselves to support them—a reason why many would-be reformers propose raising the retirement age. On the other hand, it will not be feasible for most of tomorrow's nonagenarians and centenarians to stay at their desks, no matter how fit and healthy they are.

The case against early retirement is well known. In economic jargon the ratio of retirees to workers is known as the "dependency ratio," because through pension and Social Security payments people who are now in the work force funnel money to people who have left it. A widely cited analysis by three economists at the Organization for Economic Cooperation and Development estimated that in 2000 the overall dependency ratio in the United States was 21.7 retirees for every 100 workers, meaning (roughly speaking) that everyone older than sixty-five had five younger workers contributing to his pension. By 2050 the dependency ratio will have almost doubled, to 38 per 100; that is, each retiree will be supported by slightly more than two current workers. If old-age benefits stay the same, in other words, the burden on younger workers, usually in the form of taxes, will more than double.

This may be an underestimate. The OECD analysis did not assume any dramatic increase in longevity, or the creation of any entitlement program to pay for longevity care. If both occur, as gerontological optimists predict, the number of old will skyrocket, as will the cost of maintaining them. To adjust to these "very bad fiscal effects," says the OECD economist Pablo Antolin, one of the report's co-authors, societies have only two choices: "raising the retirement age or cutting the benefits." He continues, "This is arithmetic—it can't be avoided." The recent passage of a huge new prescription-drug program by an administration and Congress dominated by the "party of small government" suggests that benefits will not be cut. Raising the age of retirement might be more feasible politically, but it would lead to a host of new problems—see today's Japan.

Novelist Brace Sterling conjured up a vision of dictatorship-by-actuary: a society in which the cautious, careful centenarian rulers, supremely fit and disproportionately affluent if a little frail, look down with mild contempt on their juniors.

In the classic job pattern, salaries rise steadily with seniority. Companies underpay younger workers and over-pay older workers as a means of rewarding employees who stay at their jobs. But as people have become more likely to shift firms and careers, the pay increases have become powerful disincentives for companies to retain employees in their fifties and sixties. Employers already worried about the affordability of older workers are not likely to welcome calls to raise the retirement age; the last thing they need is to keep middle managers around for another twenty or thirty years. "There will presumably be an elite group of super-rich who would be immune to all these pressures," Ronald Lee, an economic demographer at the University of California at Berkeley, says. "Nobody will kick Bill Gates out of Microsoft as long as he owns it. But there will be a lot of pressure on the average old person to get out."

In Lee's view, the financial downsizing need not be inhumane. One model is the university, which shifted older professors to emeritus status, reducing their workload in exchange for reduced pay. Or, rather, the university *could* be a model: age-discrimination litigation and professors' unwillingness to give up their perks, Lee says, have largely torpedoed the system. "It's hard to reduce someone's salary when they are older," he says. "For the person, it's viewed as a kind of disgrace. As a culture we need to get rid of that idea."

The Pentagon has released few statistics about the hundreds or thousands of insurgents captured in Afghanistan and Iraq, but one can he almost certain that they are disproportionately young. Young people have ever been in the forefront of political movements of all stripes. University students protested Vietnam, took over the U.S. embassy in Tehran, filled Tiananmen Square, served as the political vanguard for the Taliban. "When we are forty," the young writer Filippo Marinetti promised in the 1909 *Futurist Manifesto*, "other younger and stronger men will probably throw us in the wastebasket like useless manuscripts—we want it to happen!"

The same holds true in business and science. Steve Jobs and Stephen Wozniak founded Apple in their twenties; Albert Einstein dreamed up special relativity at about the same age. For better and worse, young people in developed nations will have less chance to shake things up in tomorrow's world. Poorer countries, where the old have less access to longevity treatments, will provide more opportunity, political and financial. As a result, according to Fred C. Iklé, an analyst with the Center for Strategic and International Studies, "it is not fanciful to imagine a new cleavage opening up in the world order." On one side would be the "'bioengineered' nations," societies dominated by the "becalmed temperament" of old people. On the other side would be the legions of youth—"the protagonists," as the political theorist Samuel Huntington has described them, "of protest, instability, reform, and revolution."

Because poorer countries would be less likely to be dominated by a gerontocracy, tomorrow's divide between old and young would mirror the contemporary division between rich northern nations and their poorer southern neighbors. But the consequences might be different—unpredictably so. One assumes, for instance, that the dictators who hold sway in Africa and the Middle East would not hesitate to avail themselves of longevity treatments, even if few others in their societies could afford them. Autocratic figures like Arafat, Franco, Perón, and Stalin often leave the scene only when they die. If the human lifespan lengthens greatly, the dictator in Gabriel García Márquez's *The Autumn of the Patriarch*, who is "an indefinite age somewhere between 107 and 232 years," may no longer be regarded as a product of magical realism.

Bioengineered nations, top-heavy with the old, will need to replenish their labor forces. Here immigration is the economist's traditional solution. In abstract terms, the idea of importing young workers from poor regions of the world seems like a win-win solution: the young get jobs, the old get cheap service. In practice, though, host nations have found that the foreigners in their midst are stubbornly … foreign. European nations are wondering whether they really should have let in so many Muslims. In the United States, traditionally hospitable to migrants, bilingual education is under attack and the southern border is increasingly locked down. Japan, preoccupied by *Nihonjinron* (theories of "Japaneseness"), has always viewed immigrants with suspicion if not hostility. Facing potential demographic calamity, the Japanese government has spent millions trying to develop a novel substitute for immigrants: robots smart and deft enough to take care of the aged.

According to Ronald Lee, the Berkeley demographer, rises in life expectancy have in the past stimulated economic growth. Because they arose mainly from reductions in infant and child mortality, these rises produced more healthy young workers, which in turn led to more-productive societies. Believing they would live a long time, those young workers saved more for retirement than their forebears, increasing society's stock of capital—another engine of growth. But these positive effects are offset when increases in longevity come from old people's neglecting to die. Older workers are usually less productive than younger ones, earning less and consuming more. Worse, the soaring expenses of entitlement programs for the old are likely, Lee believes, "to squeeze out government expenditures on the next generation," such as education and childhood public-health programs. "I think there's evidence that something like this is already happening among the industrial countries," he says. The combination will force a slowdown in economic growth: the economic pie won't grow as fast. But there's a bright side, at least potentially. If the fall in birth rates is sufficiently vertiginous, the number of people sharing that relatively smaller pie may shrink fast enough to let everyone have a bigger piece. One effect of the longevity-induced "birth dearth" that Wattenburg fears, in other words, may be higher per capita incomes.

For the past thirty years the United States has financed its budget deficits by persuading foreigners to buy U.S. Treasury bonds. In the nature of things, most of these foreigners have lived in other wealthy nations, especially Japan and China. Unfortunately for the United States, those other countries are marching toward longevity crises of their own. They, too, will have fewer young, productive workers. They, too, will be paying for longevity treatments for the old. They, too, will be facing a grinding economic slowdown. For all these reasons they may be less willing to finance our government. If so, Uncle Sam will have to raise interest rates to attract investors, which will further depress growth—a vicious circle.

Longevity-induced slowdowns could make young nations more attractive as investment targets, especially for the cash-strapped pension-and-insurance plans in aging countries. The youthful and ambitious may well follow the money to where the action is. If Mexicans and Guatemalans have fewer rich old people blocking their paths, the river of migration may begin to flow in the other direction. In a reverse brain drain, the Chinese coast guard might discover half-starved American postgraduates stuffed into the holds of smugglers' ships. Highways out of Tijuana or Nogales might bear road signs telling drivers to watch out for *norteamericano* families running across the blacktop, the children's Hello Kitty backpacks silhouetted against a yellow warning background.

Given that today nobody knows precisely how to engineer major increases in the human lifespan, contemplating these issues may seem premature. Yet so many scientists believe that some of the new research will pay off, and that lifespans will stretch like taffy, that it would be short-sighted not to consider the consequences. And the potential changes are so enormous and hard to grasp that they can't be understood and planned for at the last minute. "By definition." says Aubrey de Grey, the Cambridge geneticist, "you live with longevity for a very long time."

Charles C. Mann is an Atlantic *correspondent. His book* 1491, *which grew out of his April 2002* Atlantic *cover story, will be published in August.*

UNIT 2
The Quality of Later Life

Unit Selections

Key Points to Consider

- What are the stable unchanging factors in women's sexuality as they age?

- What factors do Kevin Kinsella and David Phillips believe are critical to successful aging?

- What advantages do those who exercise regularly gain over time?

- How do men and women differ in their reactions to life's ups and downs?

- What are the critical factors that Lou Ann Walker identifies as contributing to a long healthy life?

Student Website
www.mhcls.com/online

Internet References
Further information regarding these websites may be found in this book's preface or online.

Aging with Dignity
http://www.agingwithdignity.org/
The Gerontological Society of America
http://www.geron.org
The National Council on the Aging
http://www.ncoa.org

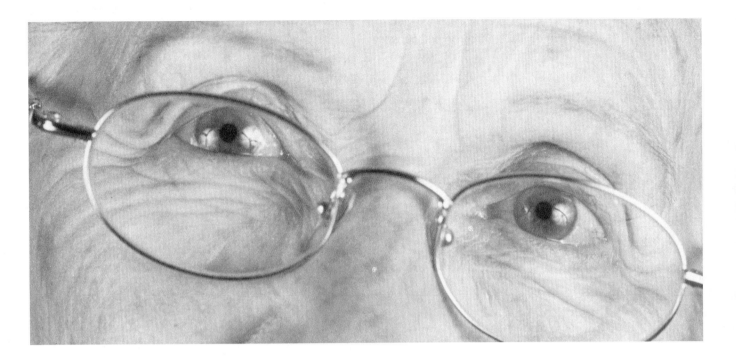

Although it is true that one ages from the moment of conception to the moment of death, children are usually considered to be "growing and developing" while adults are often thought of as "aging." Having accepted this assumption, most biologists concerned with the problems of aging focus their attention on what happens to individuals after they reach maturity. Moreover, most of the biological and medical research dealing with the aging process focuses on the later part of the mature adult's life cycle. A commonly used definition of senescence is "the changes that occur generally in the post-reproductive period and that result in decreased survival capacity on the part of the individual organism" (B. L. Shrehler, Time, Cells and Aging, New York: Academic Press, 1977).

As a person ages, physiological changes take place. The skin loses its elasticity, becomes more pigmented, and bruises more easily. Joints stiffen, and the bone structure becomes less firm. Muscles lose their strength. The respiratory system becomes less efficient. The individual's metabolism changes, resulting in different dietary demands. Bowel and bladder movements are more difficult to regulate. Visual acuity diminishes, hearing declines, and the entire system is less able to resist environmental stresses and strains.

Increases in life expectancy have resulted largely from decreased mortality rates among younger people, rather than from increased longevity after age 65. In 1900, the average life expectancy at birth was 47.3 years; in 2000, it was 76.9 years. Thus, in the last century the average life expectancy rose by 29.6 years. However, those who now live to the age of 65 do not have an appreciably different life expectancy than did their 1900 cohorts. In 1900, 65-year-olds could expect to live approximately 11.9 years longer, while in 2000 they could expect to live approximately 17.9 years longer, an increase of 6 years. Although more people survive to age 65 today, the chances of being afflicted by one of the major killers of older persons is still about as great for this generation as it was for their grandparents.

While medical science has had considerable success in controlling the acute diseases of the young—such as measles, chicken pox, and scarlet fever—it has not been as successful in controlling the chronic conditions of old age, such as heart disease, cancer, and emphysema. Organ transplants, greater knowledge of the immune system, and undiscovered medical technologies will probably increase the life expectancy for the 65-and-over population, resulting in longer life for the next generation. Although people 65 years of age today are living only slightly longer than 65-year-olds did in 1900, the quality of their later years has greatly improved. Economically, Social Security and a multitude of private retirement programs have given most older persons a more secure retirement. Physically, many people remain active, mobile, and independent throughout their retirement years. Socially, most older persons are married, involved in community activities, and leading productive lives. While they may experience some chronic ailments, most are able to live in their own homes, direct their own lives, and involve themselves in activities they enjoy.

The articles in this section examine health, psychological, social, and spiritual factors that affect the quality of aging. All of us are faced with the process of aging, and by putting a strong emphasis on health, both mental and physical, a long, satisfying life is much more attainable.

In "Women's Sexuality As They Age: The More Things Change, The More They Stay the Same," the authors attempt to determine the effect of the women's menstrual status and aging on their sexuality.

Kevin Kinsella and David Phillips in "Successful Aging" review past theories of aging and give their beliefs about what critical factors contribute to successful aging.

In "The Do or Die Decade," Susan Brink examines the basic differences in the attitudes and values of men in comparison to women as they approach diverse life events. She believes these differences help to explain why women have a longer life expectancy than men do.

Lou Ann Walker, in "We Can Control How We Age," gives specific recommendations for what the individual can do to improve his or her chances of aging well.

WOMEN'S SEXUALITY AS THEY AGE: THE MORE THINGS CHANGE, THE MORE THEY STAY THE SAME

Patricia Barthalow Koch, Ph.D.
Associate Professor, Biobehavioral Health & Women's Studies

Phyllis Kernoff Mansfield, Ph.D.
Professor, Women's Studies & Health Education

Pennsylvania State University State College, PA

With the aging of the baby boomers and the development and hugely successful marketing of Viagra® to treat erectile dysfunction, attention from sexologists, pharmaceutical companies, and the public has become focused on the sexuality of aging women.[1]

Some of the burning questions that are currently being pursued are: Does women's sexual functioning (sexual desire, arousal, orgasm, activity, and/or satisfaction) decrease with age and/or menopausal status? And what can be done to enhance aging women's sexual functioning?

As researchers try to provide answers for women, pharmaceutical companies, and other interested parties, what is becoming crystal clear is that we (the scientific community, health care professionals, and society at large) don't understand women's sexuality as they age because we don't understand women's sexuality. Therefore, we may not even be pursuing the right questions. For example, are specific elements of sexual "functioning" the most important aspects of women's sexuality or do we need to shift our focus?

MODELS OF FEMALE SEXUALITY: THE IMPORTANCE OF CONTEXT

Much of the information accumulated about women's sexuality has been generated from theories, research methodologies, and interpretation of data based on male models of sexuality, sexual functioning, and scientific inquiry.

As explained by Ray Rosen, Ph.D., at a recent conference on "Emerging Concepts in Women's Health," sexology has pursued a path of treating male and female functioning as similar, as evidenced by Masters and Johnson's development of the human sexual response cycle.[2]

What has resulted is a lack of appreciation for and documentation of the unique aspects of women's sexual functioning and expression. There is a growing chorus of sexologists acknowledging that women's sexuality, including their sexual response, merits different models than those developed for men.[3]

As Leonore Tiefer, Ph.D., has advocated, what is needed is a model of women's sexuality that is more "psychologically-minded, individually variable, interpersonally oriented, and socioculturally sophisticated."[4] Such models are beginning to emerge.[5]

The new models of female sexual response have been developed from quantitative and qualitative research findings and clinical practice assessments that more accurately reflect women's actual experiences than previous male-centered models.

A key component of these models is the importance of context to women's sexual expression. Context has been defined as "the whole situation, background, or environment relevant to some happening."[6] For example, unlike men whose sexual desire often is independent of context, women's sexual desire is often a responsive reaction to the context (her partner's sexual arousal, expressions of love and intimacy) rather than a spontaneous event.[7] Jordan identified the central dynamic of female adolescent sexuality as the relational context.[8] She described young women's sexual desire as actually being "desire for the experience of joining toward and joining in something that thereby becomes greater than the separate selves."[9]

So throughout women's development and the transitions in their lives (adolescence, pregnancy, parenthood, menopause) context is a key factor in their sexual expression. Thus, the more things change (their bodies, their relationships, their circumstances), the more they stay the same (the importance of context to their sexual expression).

INSIGHTS FROM THE MIDLIFE WOMEN'S HEALTH SURVEY

Applying the new models of women's sexuality that emphasize the importance of context helps us to better understand women's sexuality as they age. Findings from the Midlife Women's Health Survey (MWHS), a longitudinal study of the menopausal transition that is part of the broader Tremin Trust Research Program on Women's Health, support these new models.[10]

The Tremin Trust is a longitudinal, intergenerational study focusing on menstrual health that first enrolled 2,350 university women in 1934 and a second cohort of 1,600 young women between 1961 and 1963. (See the Tremin Trust Web site at www.pop.psu.edu/tremin/). In 1990, an additional 347 mid-life women were enrolled in order to better study various aspects of the menopausal transition, including sexual changes.

All the participants complete a daily menstrual calendar, recording detailed information about their menstrual health. They also complete a yearly comprehensive survey, assessing biopsychosocial information about their health and aging, life experiences, and sexuality, among other factors. These surveys collect both quantitative and qualitative data. Throughout the years, some of the women have been called upon to participate in special qualitative studies in which they have been interviewed. One hundred of the perimenopausal women who are not taking hormone replacement therapy have also supplied daily morning urine specimens so that hormonal analysis could be conducted.

The Tremin Trust participants are incredibly dedicated to the project. For example, they keep daily records throughout their lives (for some almost 70 years) and enlist participation from their daughters, granddaughters, and great-granddaughters. The study's potential for providing a greater understanding of women's sexuality throughout their lives, and the factors that affect sexual changes, is unparalleled. The greatest limitation is the lack of diversity among the participants, since over 90 percent are well-educated white women. However, data collection has been conducted with additional samples of African-American and Alaskan women as well as lesbians. More diverse cohorts may be enlisted in the future.

Analysis of the sexuality data is ongoing, with more data being collected each year. Interesting findings have emerged regarding midlife women's sexuality (ages 35 through 55 years of age) as they progress through menopausal transition. The average age of menopause is 51, with perimenopause beginning as early as the late thirties. In an open-ended question asking what they enjoyed most about their sexuality, more than two-thirds of the women referred to aspects of their relationships with their partners.[11] Most of these responses described some

aspect of intimacy, including love, closeness, sharing, companionship, affection, and caring, as described below. About 15 percent of the women noted feeling comfortable and secure in their relationship, emphasizing feelings of mutual trust and honesty.

> It is the most healthy relationship I've ever been in. Sex in the context of a respectful, caring, non-exploitative relationship is very wonderful.

> Wow! The sexual experience is another heightened way we share the humor that comes from shared experiences such as canoeing, fine music, backyard work, scuba trips. It makes the "union" a joyous and complete one!

Many of the lesbian participants felt that the intimacy they shared in their relationships was even greater than what they had experienced or observed in male-female relationships.

> Many straight women in 20-to-25-year marriages are distant and emotionally separate from their husbands. I think this is a time when lesbian women and their partners really come into their own—their best time together. There's much greater emotional intimacy with less emphasis on sex. It's very nurturing and increases the bond between us.

Another very important contextual feature that at least one in ten women enjoyed about their sexuality was a newly-found sexual freedom they experienced as they aged, either from their children leaving home or from being with a new partner.

> Freedom and ability to be spontaneous with our sexual desires due to the "empty nest."

> The freedom to have sex at his apartment. The growing intimacy and closeness that goes along with sex itself. The sexual playfulness and frivolity that threads itself through regular daily activities (teasing, sexual nuances, private jokes, and touches).

Approximately 20 percent of the women discussed some particular aspect to their sexual interactions, with mutual sexual satisfaction, continuing sexual interest, desire, and attraction, and lessened inhibitions and increased experimentation mentioned most often.

> We seem to enjoy sex more and more as the years go by. The orgasms seem even better. We both respond well to each other sexually since we feel safe in our loving monogamous relationship.

One-third of these discussions emphasized that touching, kissing, hugging, and cuddling were the most important aspects of the sexual interactions.

> You may not consider it sexual, but sleeping together in a queen-sized bed in the last year and a half. While the kids were growing up, we had twin beds. We enjoy the cuddling this provides daily.

Qualities exhibited by their sexual partners, who are most often the women's husbands, have been found to significantly impact the women's sexual responding.[12] Specifically, the more love, affection, passion, assertiveness, interest, and equality expressed by the sexual partners, the higher the women's sexual desire, arousal, frequency, and enjoyment. Women also expressed appreciation for a non-demanding partner who was responsive to their needs.

> My partner is very accepting about how I feel and what I like and what I don't like even though it changes often. I also appreciate that he doesn't expect me to have an orgasm every time we make love.

SEXUAL CHANGES AS WOMEN AGE

Each year the women report many changes in their sexual responding. Some women have reported enjoying sex more (8.7 percent), easier arousal (8.7 percent), desiring sexual relations more (7 percent), easier orgasm (6.7 percent), and engaging in sexual relations more often (4.7 percent).[13] The women attribute their improved sexuality most often to changes in life circumstances (new partner, more freedom with children leaving home), improved emotional well-being, more positive feelings toward partner, and improved appearance.[14]

However, two to three times more women have reported declines in their sexual responding, including: desiring sexual relations less (23.1 percent), engaging in sexual relations less often (20.7 percent), desiring more non-genital touching (19.7 percent), more difficult arousal (19.1 percent), enjoying sexual relations less (15.4 percent), more difficult orgasm (14 percent), and more pain (10 percent).

Women are much more likely to attribute declining sexual response to physical changes of menopause than to other factors.[15] Analysis of the health data has found a statistically significant relationship between having vaginal dryness and decreased sexual desire and enjoyment.[16] However, no statistically significant relationship between menopausal status and decreased sexual desire, enjoyment, or more difficulty with orgasm was found. On the other hand, sexual desire and enjoyment were significantly related to marital status, with decreases associated with being married. The woman's age was also significantly related to her sexual enjoyment, with enjoyment decreasing as the woman became older. Further, a significant relationship has been found between poor body image and decreased sexual satisfaction.[17]

Other studies among general populations of aging women have failed to find clear associations between menopausal status and declines in sexual functioning.[18] Similar to the MWHS findings, they found psychosocial factors to be more important determinants of sexual responding among midlife (perimenopausal and menopausal) women than menopausal status.[19] The factors include sexual attitudes and knowledge; previous sexual behavior and enjoyment; length and quality of relationship; physical and mental health; body image and self-esteem; stress; and partner availability, health, and sexual functioning.

SEXUAL SATISFACTION AND THE IMPORTANCE OF SEX FOR WOMEN

Even with many aging women in the MWHS identifying declines in their sexual desire, frequency, or functioning, about three-quarters of them reported overall sexual satisfaction (71 percent), including being physically and emotionally satisfied (72 percent).

> Even though sex is less frequent and it takes much longer to feel turned on, it is still very satisfying.

> I have been a very fortunate person. The man I married I still love dearly. We both respect each other and try to keep each other happy. We don't have sex as much as we used to but we kiss and hug and hold each other a lot.

The importance of sexual expression varied in the midlife women's lives and was affected by the circumstances in which they found themselves (married, divorced, widowed, in a same-sex relationship). Once again, women evaluated the importance of sexuality in the overall context of their lives. Some women who had lost their sexual partners to death or divorce reported missing a sexual relationship, mostly because of the lack of intimacy.

> I find being a widow at a young age to be very lonely. I find that I miss the desire to have a sexual closeness with a man. I also feel very sad and confused as my husband was the only man I have ever been with. Having lost him, I fear beginning a new relationship.

> I have been alone for 18 years after a 14 year marriage and three children. I miss regular sex, but *most* of all I miss touching, cuddling, body-to-body contact, not the sex act.

Yet many women without partners had decided that having sexual relations was not worth the price if the overall relationship was not fulfilling.

> I am single by choice (heterosexual) and have never wanted children. I am finding it difficult to meet men as I get older and my relationships are further apart. My sexual response is still very strong, but I am not willing to compromise what I want in a relationship just for sex. My attitude is that if that doesn't happen, I am doing fine, and am happy with my life.

> I find myself wishing for a "partner" but only if he's a real friend. My celibacy is comfortable at the moment. It has become apparent to me that our culture has taught most females to sacrifice themselves to their partner's desires and not to defend themselves. I hope I don't fall in that trap again. I find that I satisfy my physical sexual desires better than my husband ever did.

On the other hand, sexual interaction is very important to many of the aging women.

> I am 58 and as horny as ever…. The sex urge is still with me, not much different from my earlier years. Maybe I am too physically active and healthy! I can't seem to get it into my head that I am approaching a different time of life…. There is little or no speaking about a situation like mine in books or media. Yet women my age say the same thing: "Where are the men? Men want only younger women. The 'good men' are married or in relationships."…. My request to you is—listen to the voice of the horny women. When we hear each other and gain our dignity, solutions will come!

CONCLUSION

Results from the MWHS, some of which have been shared in this article, illustrate that women experience their sexuality as complex and holistic. Thus, it is doubtful that a particular drug or other substance or device that could improve physical functioning (increase libido or vasocongestion) would be the "magic bullet" to transform women's sexuality as they age. In order to understand and enhance women's sexuality throughout their lives, we must listen to their voices, learn from their experiences, and appreciate the importance of context to their sexual expression.

REFERENCES

1. R. Basson, J. Berman, et al., "Report on the International Consensus Development Conference on Female Sexual Dysfunction: Definitions and Classifications," *Journal of Urology*, vol. 163, pp. 888–93; J. Hitt, "The Second Sexual Revolution," *The New York Times Magazine*, February 20, 2000, pp. 34–41, 50, 62, 64, 68–69; J. Leland, "The Science of Women and Sex," *Newsweek*, May 29, 2000, pp. 48–54; P. K. Mansfield, P. B. Koch, and A. M. Voda, "Qualities Midlife Women Desire in Their Sexual Relationships and Their Changing Sexual Response," *Psychology of Women Quarterly*, vol. 22, pp. 285–303.
2. R. Rosen, *Major Issues in Contemporary Research in Women's Sexuality.* (Roundtable discussion at the Women's Health Research Symposium, Baltimore, MD.)
3. R. Basson, "The Female Sexual Response: A Different Model," *Journal of Sex and Marital Therapy*, vol. 26, pp. 51–65. S. R. Leiblum, "Definition and Classification of Female Sexual Disorders," *International Journal of Impotence Research*, vol. 10, pp. S102–S106; R. Rosen, *Major Issues in Contemporary Research in Women's Sexuality.*
4. L. Tiefer, "Historical, Scientific, Clinical and Feminist Criticisms of the Human Sexual Response Cycle," *Annual Review of Sex Research*, vol. 2, p. 2.
5. R. Basson, "The Female Sexual Response: A Different Model," pp. 51–65; L. Tiefer, "A New View of Women's Sexual Problems: Why New? Why Now?," *The Journal of Sex Research*, vol. 38, no. 2, pp. 89–96.
6. *Webster's New World Dictionary of the American Language: College Edition* (New York: The World Publishing Company, 2000).
7. R. Basson, "The Female Sexual Response: A Different Model," pp. 51–65.
8. J. Jordan, *Clarity in Connection: Empathic Knowing, Desire and Sexuality*, work in progress (Wellesley, MA: Stone Center Working Papers Series, 1987).
9. J. Jordan, *Clarity in Connection: Empathic Knowing, Desire and Sexuality.*
10. A. M. Voda and P. K. Mansfield, *The Tremin Trust and the Midlife Women's Health Survey: Two Longitudinal Studies of Women's Health and Menopause.* (Paper presented at the Society for Menstrual Cycle Research Conference, Montreal, June 1995.); A. M. Voda, J. M. Morgan, et al., "The Tremin Trust Research Program" in N. F. Taylor and D. Taylor, editors, *Menstrual Health and Illness* (New York: Hemisphere Press, 1991), pp. 5–19.
11. *Midlife Women's Health Survey*, 1992, unpublished data.
12. P. K. Mansfield, P. B. Koch, et al., "Qualities Midlife Women Desire in Their Sexual Relationships and Their Changing Sexual Response," *Psychology of Women Quarterly*, vol. 22, pp. 285–303.
13. Ibid.
14. P. K. Mansfield, P. B. Koch, et al., "Midlife Women's Attributions for Their Sexual Response Changes," *Health Care for Women International*, vol. 21, pp. 543–59.
15. Ibid.
16. P. K. Mansfield, A. Voda, et al., "Predictors of Sexual Response Changes in Heterosexual Midlife Women," *Health Values*, vol. 19, no. 1, pp. 10–20.
17. D. A. Thurau, *The Relationship between Body Image and Sexuality among Menopausal Women.* (Unpublished master's thesis, Pennsylvania State University, 1996).
18. N. E. Avis, M. A. Stellato, et al., "Is There an Association between Menopause Status and Sexual Functioning?," *Menopause*, vol. 7, no. 5, pp. 297–309; K. Hawton, D. Gaith, et al., "Sexual Function in a Community Sample of Middle-aged Women with Partners: Effects of Age, Marital, Socioeconomic, Psychiatric, Gynecological, and Menopausal Factors, *Archives of Sexual Behavior*, vol. 23, no. 4, pp. 375–95.
19. N. E. Avis, M. A. Stellato, et al., "Is There an Association between Menopause Status and Sexual Functioning?," pp. 297–309; I. Fooken, "Sexuality in the Later Years—The Im-

pact of Health and Body-Image in a Sample of Older Women," *Patient Education and Counseling*, vol. 23, pp. 227–33; K. Hawton, D. Gaith, et al., "Sexual Function in a Community Sample of Middle-aged Women with Partners: Effects of Age, Marital, Socioeconomic, Psychiatric, Gynecological, and Menopausal Factors," *Archives of Sexual Behavior*, vol. 23, no. 4, pp. 375–95; B. K. Johnson, "A Correlational Framework for Understanding Sexuality in

Women Age 50 and Older," *Health Care for Women International*, vol. 19, pp. 553–64.

(Dr. Mansfield is director of the Tremin Trust Research Program on Women's Health. Dr. Koch is assistant director. Dr. Koch is also adjunct professor of human sexuality at Widener University in West Chester, PA.)

—**Editor**

HALF OF AMERICANS OVER 60 HAVE SEXUAL RELATIONS AT LEAST ONCE A MONTH

Nearly half of all Americans over the age of 60 have sexual relations at least once a month, and 40 percent would like to have it more often. In addition, many seniors say their sex lives are more emotionally satisfying now than when they were in their forties.

These findings were part of the latest Roper-Starch Inc. survey of 1,300 men and women over the age of 60 conducted by the National Council on the Aging.

"This study underscores the enduring importance of sex among older men and women—even among those who report infrequent sexual activity," said Neal Cutler, director of survey research for the Council. "When older people are not sexually active, it is usually because they lack a partner or because they have a medical condition."

As most people might expect, the survey found that sexual relations taper off with age, with 71 percent of men and 51 percent of women in their sixties having sex once a month or more and 27 percent of men and 18 percent of women in their eighties saying they do. Cutler said women had sex less often in part because women are more likely to be widowed.

Thirty-nine percent of people said they were happy with the amount of sexual relations they currently have—even if it is none—while another 39 percent said they would like to make love more often. Only four percent of the people surveyed said they would like to have sexual relations less frequently. The people who had sex at least once a month said it was important to their relationship.

The survey also found that 74 percent of men and 70 percent of women find their sex lives more emotionally satisfying now that they are older than when they were in their forties. As to whether it is physically better, 43 percent say it is just as good as or better than in their youth, while 43 percent say sex is less satisfying.

"When it comes to knowledge about sex, older people are not necessarily wiser than their children. A third of the respondents believed it was natural to lose interest in sex as they got older," said Cutler.

Successful Aging

Kevin Kinsella and David R. Phillips

Aging is not merely a matter of accumulating years but also, as a popular catch-phrase states, a process of "adding life to years, not years to life." People grow old in a social and economic context that affects their psychosocial development: their feelings of self-esteem, value, and place in family and society. These factors have a combined effect on the morale of older people, and a number of models have been developed to explain why some people remain more active and healthier at older ages than other people. These are generalized models and cannot account for differences in the genetic makeup of individuals, although the models can identify factors that favor healthy lifestyles and ways in which a society can assist its members to grow old with dignity and comfort. Underpinning these concepts or models are several decades of study by gerontologists who have offered a number of social theories of aging.

The concept of *successful aging* has recently attracted a great deal of policy and research attention and is related to the broad issues of coping and adaptation in later life. Growing numbers of older people do not exhibit the chronic health problems and declining cognitive skills that were assumed to accompany aging. Successful aging is viewed as maximizing desired outcomes and minimizing undesired ones. As demonstrated in the Berlin Aging Study, adaptation is a key component to successful aging: Older adults can compensate for losses and declines and retain the potential for further growth. Aging experts John Rowe and Robert Kahn view successful aging as the confluence of three functions: decreasing the risk of diseases and disease-related disability; maintaining physical and mental functioning; and being actively engaged with life. There is debate, however, about how those who age successfully differ from others and about the role of external factors in the process.

In addition to *successful aging*, concepts such as *productive aging* (the ability to contribute directly and indirectly in older age) and *healthy aging* (the ability to remain physically and mentally fit) have been identified. These concepts come together in the WHO's policy framework of *active aging* developed between the late 1990s and 2002. The word "active" refers to continuing participation in social, economic, cultural, spiritual, and civic affairs, not just being physically or economically active. Active aging encompasses those who have retired as well as people who are frail, disabled, or in need of care; and it takes place within a broad social context of friends, family, neighbors, associates, and the workplace. Active aging recognizes the UN's principles of independence, participation, dignity, care and self-fulfillment. It shifts strategic planning away from a needs-based approach (which implies older people are passive recipients) to a rights-based approach of equality and opportunity. The WHO advocates a life-course approach to active aging that recognizes older people not as a homogeneous group but as individuals who, collectively, are as diverse as younger members of a society. The strategy promotes supportive environments and fosters healthy life choices at all stages of life. Finally, it recognizes that a collective approach to aging and older people will ultimately determine how we and our children and grandchildren experience life in later years.

Box 6

Social Theories of Aging

Theory building—the cumulative development of explanation and understanding of observations and findings—lies at the core of scientific inquiry and knowledge. In areas such as social gerontology, social theories are essential for providing coherent and valid bases for policies, programs, and activities. Social theories are not proved or disproved; rather, they represent a cumulative and evolutionary understanding as parts of the explanations are better understood, improved, or rejected.

Role theory is one of the oldest social gerontological theories, dating back to the 1940s.[1] Individuals play a variety of roles during their lives—child, adult, spouse, parent, employer, employee, grandparent, retiree. Roles are often sequential, some are concurrent, and individuals lose and gain roles throughout life. Chronological age often determines some changes (such as attaining voting age or retirement age), but age norms—assumptions that people should do or cease certain activities at certain ages—underpin much of role theory. Some role images and changes can be challenged legally (such as formal retirement ages) or by public perceptions (older people as athletes, astronauts, entertainers, and other positive images).

Activity theory (from the 1960s) suggests that older people who take on a large number and variety of activities and roles will have a more positive older age, adjust to aging better, and be more satisfied with their lives.[2] Activity theory tends to promote old age as a social problem or issue that individuals can tackle. A differing perspective to this was **disengagement theory**, which found a mutual withdrawal between the older person and society.[3] Disengagement theory sees society withdrawing from the aging person as much as the older person withdrawing from society, and disengagement is viewed as adaptive behavior. Assumptions about disengagement of older people—which was seen by some as unavoidable and universal—have prompted much debate, research, and modification.

Continuity theory holds that middle-aged and older adults often attempt to preserve ties with their own past experiences by substituting new roles that are similar to lost ones.[4] The theory suggests that people are most satisfied in their older years when their new roles and activities are consistent with previous experiences. This approach tends to emphasize individual behavior and neglects the societal constraints that deter older people from continuing some activities, but it nevertheless looks positively at continuation of activities such as sports, religion, reading, or teaching.

While these theories have been sometimes portrayed as challenging one another, they also represent an evolution of understanding of aging and the place of older people in society. A number of alternative and additional theories have focused on the interaction between an individual and the environment.[5] The **subculture of aging theory** views older people as maintaining their self-concepts and identities through membership in social groups. Subcultures might form within political, religious, and professional groups, or from "membership" that accrues from living in, say, a retirement home or retirement community. Within such potentially closed communities, residents may act and behave in collective ways that perhaps they would not do if living in the wider community.

Other more general theories such as **modernization theory** discuss negative effects on the roles and status of older people if their knowledge, traits, and skills are deemed less relevant or valuable as modernization proceeds. **Exchange theory** helps explain why most older people, in spite of reduced resources, seek to maintain some degree of reciprocity while remaining independent and active. **Feminist gerontology** criticizes the male-centered views inherent in much theory on aging, even though older people are predominantly women.[6]

References

1. Leonard S. Cottrell, "The Adjustment of the Individual to His Age and Sex Roles," *American Sociological Review* 7 (1942): 617–20.

2. Cary S. Kart and Jennifer M. Kinney, *The Realities of Aging: An Introduction to Gerontology* (Boston: Allyn and Bacon, 2001).

3. Elaine Cumming and William E. Henry, *Growing Old* (New York: Basic Books, 1961).

4. Robert C. Atchley, *The Social Forces in Later Life* (Belmont, CA: Wadsworth, 1972); and Robert C. Atchely, "A Continuity Theory of Normal Aging," *The Gerontologist* 29, no. 2 (1989): 183–90.

5. Nancy R. Hooyman and H. Asuman Kiyak, *Social Gerontology: A Multidisciplinary Perspective*, 6th ed. (Boston: Allyn and Bacon, 2002).

6. Robert J. Lynott and Patricia Passuth Lynott, "Tracing the Course of Theoretical Development in the Sociology of Aging," *The Gerontologist* 36, no. 6 (1996): 749–60.

THE DO OR DIE DECADE

Men plummet into poor health when they hit their 50s. They don't have to.

By Susan Brink

It's largely a guy thing, the willingness to run like an un-stoppable locomotive into a moving wall of beefy giants. So, too, is the sportsmanlike hostility, the blasé attitude about bodily harm—in short, the traits on display in February's Super Bowl XXXVI. For better or worse, those professional football players can thank the uniquely male mix of chemicals circulating in their bodies for their un-shakable sense of invulnerability. At least they're getting some decent exercise out of the bargain.

Not so for the 50 or so men watching the game on a pair of big-screen TVs at St. Luke's Hospital and Health Network in Bethlehem, Pa. These men are sitting on their duffs, eating chips and dip and buffalo wings, though they also had been offered carrots and broccoli and strips of lean chicken breast. Many are drinking beer, lots of it, though they also could have chosen sodas or bottled water. Six of them are having their blood pressure and heart rate monitored during the ups and downs of the closely fought contest. Those lucky half dozen are seated in re-cliners, and even though they're sprawled out, smiling, and look to be relaxed, their bodies' reactions sometimes place them in a danger zone. Indeed, five of the six had el-evated blood pressure before the game started. Five saw their blood pressure spike to its highest level of the evening—one as high as 165/106—when New England Patriot Adam Vinatieri kicked the winning field goal. All six reached their highest heart rate of the evening as the clock ran out.

Longevity gap. This scene of male camaraderie was also a loosely run experiment being conducted by physicians establishing a men's health center, to open this summer. It will be one of only a handful around the country. Increasing evidence indicates that simply being male carries significant health costs, and the doctors doing the Super Bowl Sunday monitoring are developing hypothe-ses for future studies of men's health risks. The hard truth is that women, for all the unsolved mysteries about their health, will live an average of six years longer than men.

A woman's lifetime risk of getting cancer is 1 in 3, a man's 1 in 2. Men have twice the rate of liver disease as women. Most heart attacks happen in women after 75. Most men are dead by then. Even at the age of 85, the men who are still alive can expect to live 5.2 more years, while surviv-ing women can look forward to 6.4 years.

Given these fundamental differences in health, it's per-haps not surprising that the women's health movement stands in stark contrast to the men's—such that it exists at all. The women's health movement grew from a ground-swell of concern from women themselves about breast cancer, ovarian cancer, childbirth, and menopause. The men's health effort by comparison is struggling to pro-ceed, basically because actual men don't much care. The Department of Health and Human Services has had an Office on Women's Health for 10 years. A proposal for a counterpart office for men still sits in committees in the House and Senate. "You've got a segment of the popula-tion identifiable by a certain trait—maleness—dying pre-maturely, and no one is paying attention," says David Gremillion, associate professor of medicine at the Univer-sity of North Carolina—Chapel Hill, who specializes in men's health.

It's a lifelong heartbreak, this dying off of men, and the human race loses a lot of its young males to accident, war, disease, and violence. But even those who survive the perils of youth still push the extremities of human nature: They drink too much, drive too fast, inhale too deeply, shun vitamin pills and sunscreen, eat too much fat and not enough fiber.

It's the sixth decade when men's health really tanks, though the decline starts even earlier. "At 40, you know you're not as young as you used to be. At 50, you realize it almost every day," says Ardmore, Pa., resident Brian King, 52. Forgetting that reality can be painful. Recently, while coaching the high school rugby team, King joined in the scrum. A young man tossed him to the ground, leaving him breathless and in need of emergency treat-ment at the hospital. It took weeks to recover. "I had to have my wife dress me, had to pee in a bottle. That kid left me for dead," says King. "I expected solace, but instead, my family said, 'What? Are you crazy?' "

The rugby field may be the least of middle-aged men's concerns. By the age of 50, once robust men have a 50/50 chance of erectile dysfunction. That's also about when they start succumbing to diseases of the vascular system, diseases that affect not only the heart but the brain as well. The dying off from all kinds of disease begins in earnest at about the start of men's sixth decade. Indeed, the longevity gap has been around so long that many men have become fatalistic about it. "When it's time to go, it's time to go, so you might as well enjoy yourself," reasons David Keech, 48, of York, Pa. As a kid, he enjoyed himself by jumping out of trees, riding motorcycles, and driving fast cars. Both of his grandfathers died of strokes, something he sees as part of his pedigree, along with thrill seeking. "I figure I'll go from a car crash or a stroke," he says.

But is it really inevitable? In 1900, the life expectancy for both men and women was equally poor, about 48 years. Back then, diseases like diphtheria, tuberculosis, dysentery, pneumonia, and flu wiped out many more children than adults, lowering the overall life-span statistics. But men and women who managed to survive to the age of 50 could look forward to about another 20 years. It was only at the mid-20th century that the gap between the life spans of men and women became obvious. And it has gradually widened ever since.

No fate. A handful of researchers, unwilling to take the early demise of men as a biological given, are starting to look at males as a total package of biology, psychology, and culture. They are concluding that male gender alone is not, as the American Heart Association calls it, an "uncontrollable risk factor" for half the population. Anatomy, they say, is not destiny.

But preventive healthcare is a hard sell to men. When family practitioner Samuel Harrell set up a men's health center in Bellevue, Wash., he tried marketing to stereotypical manliness. Called The Garage, the center advertised checkups, impotence treatment, smoking cessation, and prostate care as "tuneups, spark plug, emission control, and fuel-injector services." When only seven men showed up in six months, it closed up shop.

But Bob Martin, senior vice president of network development at St. Luke's, and a man "rapidly approaching 50," likes that kind of structure. "Men are very basic in some respects. If I take my car in, there's a 30,000-mile checkup. I need that in my healthcare. I need to get a letter saying, 'Hey, Bob, it's time for an oil change,' " he says. One goal of the men's center is to reach the 1 in 4 men ages 45 to 64 who do not even have a regular physician, nearly twice the number of women who do not. "Aside from prison, there's probably no more threatening place for a man to be than naked in an exam room," says urologist Ken Goldberg of Dallas, founder of the first male health center in the country. "They think someone is going to find a chink in their armor."

Men are so consistently no-shows at doctors' offices that insurers have come to count on it. "An HMO representative told me recently that if men actually sought healthcare as frequently as women, they'd have to change the premium structure. It's like the airlines overbooking. Insurers have way overbooked, assuming that men won't show up," says Gremillion. That translates into millions of men who are not being screened for prostate, skin, and colon cancer. They may be overlooking early signs of diabetes. No health professional is advising them about diet, exercise, weight, smoking, or drinking. And they don't have a clue what their blood pressure or cholesterol levels are, much less a plan or prescription to lower it.

Men have traditionally gotten health services for two reasons: One, an accident, act of violence, or health crisis brought them to the emergency room. Or, two, a loved one made them go. The latter saved Charles Hargrove's life in 1984, when he was 44. He had been having chest pains on and off for a few days but ignored them. Then he and his wife, Judy, went water skiing, and within minutes he dropped the rope and fell like a rock into the water. Judy jumped in and swam to her husband, but what he did next is classically male. "He said, go away. Leave me alone. I just need a little time alone," Judy recalls.

She didn't go away. She insisted he see a doctor. He dug in, wanting to go with his son on a planned hiking trip to the Sierra Nevada first. "I thought I didn't need to see a doctor, that I could wait till I got back," he says. This despite knowing his father had died of a massive heart attack at the age of 58, and despite a feeling in his own chest of being completely out of breath, as if he had run too hard. He finally conceded, but grudgingly. The doctor immediately admitted him to the hospital for a coronary angioplasty to open an artery that was 98 percent blocked. "The doctor said, had I gone up into the mountains, I probably never would have walked back down," says Hargrove.

But now there's a third reason men are making appointments to see a doctor: Viagra. "It's extraordinary. Men will come in for a prescription for Viagra, having ignored their impotence for many years. They'll nervously come in, wishing only to have a script," says Gremillion. An astute doctor will use the visit to probe for some of the underlying causes of impotence: untreated diabetes, hypertension, alcohol abuse, or chronic depression. "When men are at that visit, they've admitted their vulnerability, which takes a lot of courage on their part. A doctor can accomplish a lot with that visit."

Viagra has given men an entree into the healthcare world to talk about a nearly universal underlying fear. What will their sex lives be as they grow old? "Being able to do it. I worry about that. I think every man does. No one ever tells you as a man, 'You know, son, you'll still be able to do it when you're 100.' When you're a teenager, sex is all the guys talk about. Then all of a sudden, you don't talk about it," said Wayne Neveling, 48, of Bethlehem, Pa.

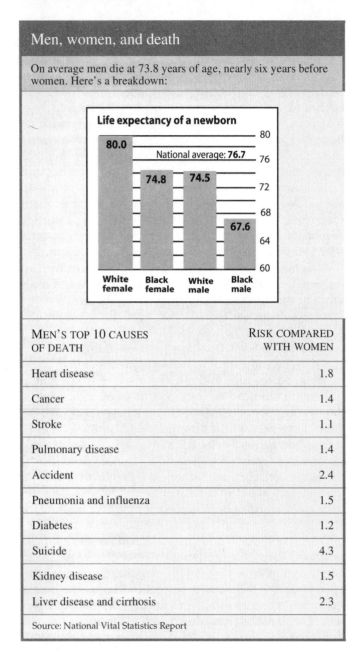

Men, women, and death

On average men die at 73.8 years of age, nearly six years before women. Here's a breakdown:

Life expectancy of a newborn

White female	Black female	White male	Black male
80.0	74.8	74.5	67.6

National average: 76.7

MEN'S TOP 10 CAUSES OF DEATH	RISK COMPARED WITH WOMEN
Heart disease	1.8
Cancer	1.4
Stroke	1.1
Pulmonary disease	1.4
Accident	2.4
Pneumonia and influenza	1.5
Diabetes	1.2
Suicide	4.3
Kidney disease	1.5
Liver disease and cirrhosis	2.3
Source: National Vital Statistics Report	

rector of Men's Health Consulting and lecturer at McLean Hospital and Harvard Medical School.

The reasons behind men's greater, and earlier, rate of heart disease are still not fully understood. But it is clear that men, compared with women, have lower levels of HDL, the good cholesterol that protects against heart disease. That may be due in part to men's lack of estrogen, although experts doubt that accounts for all the difference. Exercise, which is known to raise levels of protective HDL, may be a factor. The perception is that men are more physically active than women, but in reality women 35 and older get more consistent, healthful exercise than do men of that age, who are more likely to work out sporadically. Even before that age, men are already getting less exercise through activities like daily household chores. "Men come home and sit and relax, whereas women keep going," says Gerdi Weidner, director of research for the Preventive Medicine Research Institute in Sausalito, Calif.

What frustrates physicians is that exercise (or lack of it) is a choice, so men are in effect choosing poor health. The same is true of diet. Middle-aged men have higher levels of the protein homocysteine in their blood—a recently proven risk factor for heart disease. They could lower their homocysteine quite easily, either through a diet rich in fruits, vegetables, and unprocessed grains, or with supplementary vitamins B6, B12, and folate. But men are also less likely than women to eat a healthful diet and less likely again to take a supplementary vitamin pill.

The litany goes on. Men also have a greater physiological response to stress. A 2001 study in *Health Psychology* found that, when faced with a stressful situation like public speaking or timed math problems, the blood pressures of men rose more and stayed elevated longer than did the blood pressure of women. No one is sure quite why, but it may be because women are subjected to more everyday stress—lower income, child-rearing issues—so their bodies adapt and can handle episodes of acute stress better.

Almost all men do experience a gradual drop-off in testosterone as they age. For some men, it happens faster and sooner than for others. And lower levels of testosterone are associated with a number of losses: libido, muscle mass, memory, bone mass. The good news is that healthy behaviors—exercise, good diet, not smoking, moderate drinking—can slow the decline.

Same vein. Impotence can actually be an early signal of other diseases, including heart disease. The penis is fueled by the same system of blood vessels as the heart, only the vessels are much smaller and might become blocked sooner. Coronary artery disease could show up first as impotence. "The penis is just like the heart. The things that we do that are good for the heart are also good for the penis. There's no reason why it can't function well for men into their 70s and on," says Will Courtenay, di-

Stress and snacks. Once again, the male heart suffers. A study in the January journal *Psychophysiology* found that increased stress causes triglycerides, a type of fat linked to heart disease, to linger in the bloodstream longer. "If a person has a high-fat snack during a time of stress, that fat is going to be circulating in the blood for a longer time," says Ohio State University researcher Catherine Stoney. "That means it may be more likely to be deposited in the arteries, where it can contribute to heart disease."

That's not good news for those guys kicking back in their recliners, munching chips and wings, on Super Bowl Sunday. And now it's becoming clear that those who neglect their hearts are also neglecting their brains. Even if they don't suffer a full-blown stroke, they could suffer a kind of ministroke, recently understood to cause a form of depression in older people. And—guess what?—it's more common in men than in women. "Having high blood pressure, diabetes, and smoking puts a person at higher risk for developing silent strokes, strokes that the person is not aware they've had," says Ranga Krishnan, a psychiatrist at Duke University Medical Center. Such ministrokes can affect the brain's frontal lobe and cause a mental disorder called vascular depression, though it causes none of the usual stroke symptoms like loss of motor skills. Most victims have never been depressed before in their lives.

PREVENTION

Surviving middle age

Doctors urge men to have these screenings performed:

RECOMMENDED PROCEDURES	40-49	50+
Physical exam	Every 2 years	Annually
Blood pressure	Annually	Annually
Blook tests & urinalysis	Every 2 years	Annually
EKG	Every 4 years	Every 3 years
Rectal exam	Annually	Annually
PSA blood test Prostate screening		Annually
Hemoccult Screens the stool for blood	Annually	Annually
Sigmoidoscopy Proctoscopy		Every 3-4 years
Chest X-ray For smokers	Annually	Annually

Depression may in fact be what's behind the phenomenon known as midlife crisis. "Men having pain, men running away, men having affairs—it's all really a depressive experience," says William Pollack, editor of the book *New Psychotherapy for Men*. Pollack believes that men not only can but need to change some of their attitudes at midlife. "All their lives, men are put in a gender straight jacket," he explains. "Now zoom ahead 50 years. They have a family they don't know how to interact with. In their careers, one of two things can happen. Their dream of becoming the best and the strongest has come true, but they think, 'So what?' Or they've played the game but it hasn't really helped them, and they feel like losers. Middle-aged men are four to five times more likely to kill themselves than women. If that's happening, they've got to be depressed. There's no way they can enjoy their next 20 or 30 years unless they rethink who they are."

A handful of mental health experts are so concerned about the male frame of mind that they are rethinking the very definition of depression. They believe the disorder should include an expanded set of symptoms for what Pollack, director of the Centers for Men and Young Men at McLean Hospital in Boston, calls "depressive disorder-male type." Men, in general, have far fewer close friends and tight family ties than women. When depressed, they become even more socially isolated. "Men don't get weepy; they don't ask for help," Pollack says. Instead, they are more inclined to pull away from loved ones, throw themselves into work or alcohol or affairs as a coverup to pain, and run from help to the point of becoming rigidly autonomous. They deny they're sad and don't even have the vocabulary to put words to feelings.

Two lives.   It's not too late, even at 50, to start making more wholesome choices, but there's a lot to change. The fall 2000 issue of the *Journal of Men's Studies* lists 30 behaviors that increase the risk of disease, injury, and death. On every single measure, women are bad, but men are worse. Men are less likely than women to stay in bed when they're sick. They're less likely to restrict their use of salt when they know they have high blood pressure, but they often don't know they have it because they're less likely to go to the doctor. They're less likely to get suspicious moles examined or to buckle their seat belts. They're less likely to do a testicular self-exam for cancer than women are to do a breast self-exam. When men and women smoke, men smoke more cigarettes and inhale more deeply. Men sleep less, floss less, stay in the sun longer, use less sunscreen, and eat more fast foods and fewer breakfasts than do women.

"Men come home and sit and relax, whereas women keep going."

PREVENTION SPECIALIST GERDI WEIDNER

Getting men to improve their health, says Martin, requires knowing what makes them tick. The schemes that work for women may not work for men. Women trying to lose weight, for example, respond well to an organization like Weight Watchers with its group support and gold stars for pounds shed. Men thrive on competition. "If we have a group of men and we're trying to reduce their stress, one of the best ways to do it is to create a competition. Who can reduce stress the most? Or who can reduce their weight the most? Who can prove they're eating better? Take something that's programmed into us and work with it," Martin says. "If we create a competition, men respond."

That truth was brought home on Super Bowl Sunday in Bethlehem. Two of the men leaving St. Luke's after the game walked up to a police officer—there to ensure ev-

An unhealthy combo

When Louis Brothers was diagnosed with prostate cancer, his reaction was, cancer of my what? "I think it's a sin that I didn't even know I had a prostate until I had prostate cancer." Ten years later, he's now an advocate for men's health in his Dorchester neighborhood in Boston.

Accidents, disease, and early death can happen to anyone. But they happen sooner and more often to black men. African-American men like Brothers are at such increased risk of prostate cancer that the American Cancer Society recommends they begin screening for the disease at age 40, rather than the generally recommended age 50. By middle age, black men are more likely than white men to die of complications of diabetes, cancer, and heart disease. They are at increased risk of high blood pressure and glaucoma.

That adds up to a life expectancy of 67.6 years—nearly seven years less than for white men and black women, and 12 years less than for white women. Part of the problem is that a lot of African-Americans don't trust the healthcare system. "The doctors and nurses, they don't like black men," says a 47-year-old Baltimore man who was forced to seek public care for his kidney problems when he lost his insurance. "When you walk in there, you're treated like a bum who never worked a day in his life. They just think you want a handout. It's very insulting."

Poor, urban black men are the most difficult for the healthcare system to reach. In 1992, Martha Hill, director of the Center for Nursing Research at Johns Hopkins University, set out to see if she could prove conventional wisdom wrong by lowering and controlling the blood pressure of a vulnerable group of East Baltimore men. Middle-aged men in that impoverished area have a mortality rate among the highest in the state of Maryland. Many of them were unemployed, homeless, drug addicted, or alcoholic.

Nurses visted the men at home, helped them get medications, and enlisted the help of community workers to help the men look for jobs, get off drugs or alcohol, or find a place to live. They didn't perform miracles, but they proved that these men would show up for appointments, take their medications, and change some diet habits. Overall, the men lowered their blood pressure a few points. As a bonus, some of the 40 percent who were unemployed found jobs.

Poverty can't take all the blame. Recent research points a finger at genetics. For example, black people are more likely to have genes that cause the body to process salt differently, making them more sensitive to the salty American diet. That, in turn, puts them at greater risk for high blood pressure. Black people also appear to process nicotine and cigarette carcinogens in more harmful ways. That could help explain why black smokers have higher rates of lung cancer, even though they smoke fewer cigarettes than do white. –S.B.

eryone got home safely—and blew into a breathalyzer. One had had 11 beers, the other only six. The latter failed the breath test but said he was sure he would have no problem driving. The former passed but said he felt too inebriated to drive. The two men compared blood-alcohol numbers, high-fiving each other and shouting "way to go." The aura of friendly competition continued all the way out the door, as they climbed into the passenger seats of waiting vehicles and were driven off into the night by their designated drivers.

A PRACTICAL GUIDE TO BETTER HEALTH

What does it take to age successfully—to maintain both a sound body and mind?
A landmark Harvard study has followed individuals from their teens into their 80s.
It arrives at some optimistic conclusions:

We Can Control How We Age

BY LOU ANN WALKER

HOW DO SOME PEOPLE AGE SO successfully? Many of us assume it takes genes or dumb luck. So here's the surprise. Arguably the longest and most comprehensive study of human development ever undertaken is just revealing its final results: *We are very much in control of our own aging.* The secret to a long and happy life, it seems, does not lie as much in our stars as in ourselves.

The Study of Adult Development at Harvard Medical School comprises three projects begun in the 1920s, '30s, and '40s. These careful scientific studies analyze three very different demographic groups: one of Harvard men (the Grant Study), another of inner-city Boston men and the third of gifted California women. In all, 824 men and women have been followed from their teens into their 80s. Over the decades, these people were given psychological tests and asked to evaluate their lives and feelings. They responded to numerous questionnaires, interviews by psychiatrists and physical examinations by doctors.

The study is a medical rarity because it examines the lives of the well, not the sick. "Old age is like a minefield," the study's director, Dr. George E. Vaillant, told PARADE. "If you see footprints leading to the other side, step in them." These results show a clear path that Baby Boomers and Gen X-ers can follow to lead a long, happy life.

The study divides individuals between 60 and 80 years old into two main groups: (1) the "Happy-Well," those who are physically healthy and find life satisfying; and (2) the "Sad-Sick," those with various ailments who do not seem to enjoy life. And it analyzes those who died during the course of the study (the "Prematurely Dead").

Living With A Full Heart

The Harvard study found these four attributes vital to successful aging:

- ORIENTATION TOWARD THE FUTURE. The ability to anticipate, to plan and to hope.
- GRATITUDE, FORGIVENESS AND OPTIMISM. We need to see the glass as half-full, not half-empty.
- EMPATHY. The ability to imagine the world as it seems to the other person.
- THE ABILITY TO REACH OUT. "We should want to do things *with* people, not do things *to* people or ruminate that they do things to us," says Dr. George E. Vaillant. In other words, we need to "leave the screen door unlatched."

It's *not* in our genes...

A major finding was that good genes did not account for better aging. Nor did income. Good care obviously is important, said Dr. Vaillant, "but the trick is not going to the hospital in the first place."

The study disputes the assumption that with aging comes decay. When 30- and 55-year-old brains are compared, the older one is better developed. Advancing age

Seven Keys To Aging Well

What are the secrets to a long, happy life? Dr. George E. Vaillant points out seven major factors that, at 50, predict what life's outcome will be at 80:

1 NOT SMOKING OR QUITTING EARLY: Those who quit the habit before 50 were, at 70, as healthy as those who had never smoked. And heavy smoking was 10 times more prevalent among the Prematurely Dead than among the Happy-Well. "Smoking," said Vaillant, "is probably the most significant factor in terms of health."

Coping With Life's Stresses
Those who learn early how to roll with the punches are much happier in their later years, despite real problems.

2 THE ABILITY TO TAKE LIFE'S UPS AND DOWNS IN STRIDE: If you can make lemonade out of lemons, then you have an adaptive coping style, also known as "mature defenses." Mature defenses don't actually ensure good health at an older age. But a person will suffer less from life's real problems if he or she has the ability to roll with the punches. "Life ain't easy," Vaillant said. "Terrible things happen to everyone. You have to keep your sense of humor, give something of yourself to others, make friends who are younger than you, learn new things and have fun."

An Active Lifestyle
The long-term results of regular exercise are both physical and psychological well-being.

3 ABSENCE OF ALCOHOL ABUSE: "Abusing alcohol destroys both your physical and mental health," Vaillant noted. (He added that a partner's alcoholism can destroy a marriage, which also may have an impact on how one ages.)

4 HEALTHY WEIGHT: Obesity is a risk factor for poor health in later life.

A Strong Marriage
A good marriage contributes to a long and happy life. The study also found that, overall, marriages improved with time—if people were willing to work out the bumps.

5 A SOLID MARRIAGE: This is important for both physical and psychological health. Happy-Well people were six times more likely to be in good marriages than were the Sad-Sick.

6 PHYSICAL ACTIVITY: The study specified that the Happy-Well usually did "some exercise." The benefits of fitness also extended to mental health.

Continuing Education
The more years of school people have, the more they tend to age successfully.

7 YEARS OF EDUCATION: Vaillant speculated that people to whom "self-care and perseverance" are important are also more likely to continue their educations. These individuals, he surmised, are able to take the long view. "People seek education because they believe it is possible to control the course of their lives," he said. In the study, people with less education also were more likely to be obese. Their physical health at age 65 was close to that of the more-educated group at 75.

People who had four or more of these seven factors at age 50 were one-third less likely to be dead by 80. People who had three or fewer of these factors at 50—even though they were in good physical shape—were three times as likely to die during the following 30 years.

impairs some motor skills, but maturation can make people sharper at emotional tasks.

...but in ourselves.

Many of the study's findings focus on psychological health. As we age, we should try to develop more mature coping styles, Vaillant concluded from the results. "Our defenses are always more mature when we are not hungry, angry, lonely, tired or drunk," he noted.

"Taking people inside oneself" emotionally is important, he said, adding, "Popular people can be extraordinarily lonely and depressed. The paradox is that they starve, yet there's plenty of food." He pointed to the example of Marilyn Monroe, who made Arthur Miller and others feel cared for yet was unable to feel that love within herself.

Although developmental psychologists often say that personality is formed by age 5, the study found otherwise. By 70, it's how we nurture ourselves throughout our lifetimes that takes precedence over nature. Interestingly, Vaillant discovered that many people who aged well unconsciously reinterpreted early events in their lives in a more positive light as they grew older. Those who clung to negative events were less happy adults. Forever blaming parents for a rotten childhood seems to impede maturity.

"What goes *right* in childhood predicts the future far better than what goes wrong," he noted. Especially important was a feeling of acceptance.

As one ages, remaining connected to life is crucial—as is learning the rules of a changing world. On the other hand, Vaillant said, "One task of living out the last half of life is excavating and recovering those whom we loved in the first half. The recovery of lost loves becomes an important way in which the past affects the present."

The study's results will be published by Little, Brown in January in a book titled *Aging Well: Surprising Guideposts to a Happier Life from the Landmark Harvard Study of Adult Development.* In addition to facts and figures, the book is filled with life stories of the men and women studied.

Vaillant, who has been called "a big, handsome, humorous psychiatrist," looks a decade younger than his 67 years. He and his wife of 30 years, Caroline, live in Vermont. In addition to his research, he maintains a small clinical practice at Boston's Brigham and Women's Hospital. He calls himself an "oppositional character" who loves "proving other people wrong."

I asked Vaillant what he hopes the results of this study will accomplish. "A heightened appreciation of the positive," he shot back. Then he added: "Worry less about cholesterol and more about gratitude and forgiveness."

UNIT 3

Societal Attitudes Toward Old Age

Unit Selections

12. **Society Fears the Aging Process**, Mary Pipher
13. **Ageism in America**, David Crary
14. **The Activation of Aging Stereotypes in Younger and Older Adults**, Alison L. Chasteen, Norbert Schwarz, and Denise C. Park
15. **The Under-Reported Impact of Age Discrimination and Its Threat to Business Vitality**, Robert J. Grossman

Key Points to Consider

- What are the prevalent images Americans have of older people?

- Why do most Americans fear getting old?

- What are the basic arguments made by Erdman Palmore against the widespread negative views of older Americans?

- As the work force ages, what changes in employer attitudes toward older workers will have to take place in order for business to keep and maintain the critical skills of these workers?

Student Website

www.mhcls.com/online

Internet References

Further information regarding these websites may be found in this book's preface or online.

Adult Development and Aging: Division 20 of the American Psychological Association
    http://www.iog.wayne.edu/APADIV20/APADIV20.HTM
American Society on Aging
    http://www.asaging.org/index.cfm
Canadian Psychological Association
    http://www.cpa.ca/contents.html

There is a wide range of beliefs regarding the social position and status of the aged in American society today. Some people believe that the best way to understand the problems of the elderly is to regard them as a minority group, faced with difficulties similar to those of other minority groups. Discrimination against older people, like racial discrimination, is believed to be based on a bias against visible physical traits. Since the aging process is viewed negatively, it is natural that the elderly try to appear and act younger. Some spend a tremendous amount of money trying to make themselves look and feel younger.

The theory that old people are a minority group is weak because too many circumstances prove otherwise. The U.S. Congress, for example, favors its senior members and delegates considerable prestige and power to them. The leadership roles in most religious organizations are held by older persons. Many older Americans are in good health, have comfortable incomes, and are treated with respect by friends and associates.

Perhaps the most realistic way to view the aged is as a status group, like other status groups in society. Every society has some method of "age grading," by which it groups together individuals of roughly similar age. ("Preteens" and "senior citizens" are some of the age-grade labels in American society.)

Because it is a labeling process, age grading causes members of the age group, as well as others, to perceive themselves in terms of the connotations of the label. Unfortunately, the tag "old age" often has negative connotations in American society.

The readings included in this section illustrate the wide range of stereotypical attitudes toward older Americans. Many of society's typical assumptions about the limitations of old age have been refuted. A major force behind this reassessment of the elderly is that there are so many people living longer and healthier lives and in consequence playing more of a role in all aspects of our society. Older people can remain productive members of society for many more years than has been traditionally assumed.

Such standard stereotypes of the elderly as frail, senile, childish, and sexually inactive are topics discussed in this section. Mary Pipher, in "Society Fears the Aging Process," contends that young people often avoid interacting with older persons because it reminds them that someday they will get old and die. She further argues that the media most often portrays a negative and stereotypical view of the elderly.

David Crary, in "Ageism in America," outlines the basic arguments made by Dr. Palmore, a retired professor from Duke, against the widespread negative stereotypes of older Americans. Then, in "The Activation of Aging Stereotypes in Younger and Older Adults," the authors compare and contrast how a

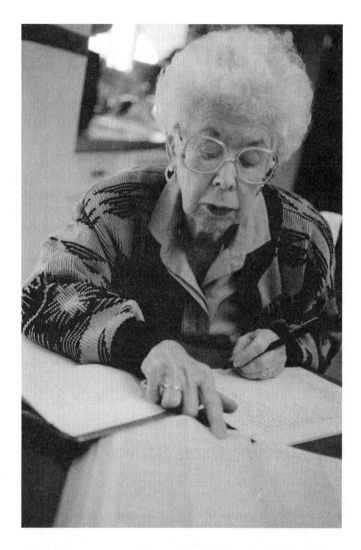

sample of young and old people view older persons. Robert Grossman in "The Under-Reported Impact of Age Discrimination and Its Threat to Business Vitality" believes that the legal system is slanted toward the employers who perpetuate many of the negative stereotypes and views of the older workers. He sees age discrimination in the workplace as a more serious problem in the future when labor shortages will make older workers and their skills more critical and more in demand.

Society Fears the Aging Process

Americans fear the processes of aging and dying, Mary Pipher contends in the following viewpoint. She claims that younger and healthier adults often avoid spending time around the aging because they want to avoid the issues of mortality and loss of independence. In addition, she contends that negative views of the aging process are portrayed in the media and expressed through the use of pejorative words to describe the elderly. Pipher is a psychologist and author of several books, including *Another Country: Navigating the Emotional Terrain of Our Elders*, the book from which this viewpoint was excerpted.

Mary Pipher

We segregate the old for many reasons—prejudice, ignorance, a lack of good alternatives, and a youth-worshiping culture without guidelines on how to care for the old. The old are different from us, and that makes us nervous. Xenophobia means fear of people from another country. In America we are xenophobic toward our old people.

How Greeting Cards Reflect Culture

An anthropologist could learn about us by examining our greeting cards. As with all aspects of popular culture, greeting cards both mirror and shape our realities. Cards reflect what we feel about people in different roles, and they also teach us what to feel. I visited my favorite local drugstore and took a look.

There are really two sets of cards that relate to aging. One is the grandparent/grandchild set that is all about connection. Even a very dim-witted anthropologist would sense the love and respect that exist between these two generations in our culture. Young children's cards to their grandparents say, "I wish I could hop on your lap," or, "You're so much fun." Grandparents' cards to children are filled with pride and love.

There is another section of cards on birthdays. These compare human aging to wine aging, or point out compensations. "With age comes wisdom, of course that doesn't make up for what you lose." We joke the most about that which makes us anxious. "Have you picked out your bench at the mall yet?" There are jokes about hearing loss, incontinence, and losing sexual abilities and interest. There are cards on saggy behinds, gray hair, and wrinkles, and cards about preferring chocolate or sleep to sex. "You know you're getting old when someone asks if you're getting enough and you think about sleep."

Fears of Aging and Dying

Poking fun at aging isn't all bad. It's better to laugh than to cry, especially at what cannot be prevented. However, these jokes reflect our fears about aging in a youth-oriented culture. We younger, healthier people sometimes avoid the old to avoid our own fears of aging. If we aren't around dying people, we don't have to think about dying.

We baby boomers have been a futureless generation, raised in the eternal present of TV and advertising. We have allowed ourselves to be persuaded by ads that teach that if we take good care of ourselves, we will stay healthy. Sick people, hospitals, and funerals destroy our illusions of invulnerability. They force us to think of the future.

Carolyn Heilbrun said, "It is only past the meridian of fifty that one can believe that the universal sentence of death applies to oneself." Before that time, if we are healthy, we are likely to be in deep denial about death, to feel as if we have plenty of time, that we have an endless vista ahead. But in hospitals and at funerals, we remember that we all will die in the last act. And we don't necessarily appreciate being reminded.

When I first visited rest homes, I had to force myself to stay. What made me most upset was the thought of myself in a place like that. I didn't want to go there, literally or figuratively. Recently I sat in an eye doctor's office surrounded by old people with white canes. Being in this room gave me intimations of mortality. I thought of Bob Dylan's line: "It's not dark yet, but it's getting there."

We know the old-old will die soon. The more we care and the more involved we are with the old, the more pain we feel at their suffering. Death is easier to bear in the abstract, far away and clinical. It's much harder to watch someone we love fade before our eyes. It's hard to visit an uncle in a rest home and realize he no longer knows who we are or even who he is. It's hard to see a grandmother in pain or drugged up on morphine. Sometimes it's so hard that we stay away from the people who need us the most.

Our culture reinforces our individual fears. To call something old is to insult, as in *old hat* or *old ideas*. To call something young is to compliment, as in *young thinking* or *young acting*. It's considered rude even to ask an old person's age. When we meet an adult we haven't seen in a long time, we compliment her by saying, "You haven't aged at all." The taboos against acknowledging age tell us that aging is shameful.

Many of the people I interviewed were uncomfortable talking about age and were unhappy to be labeled old. They said, "I don't feel old." What they meant was, "I don't act and feel like the person who the stereotypes suggest I am." Also, they were trying to avoid being put in a socially undesirable class. In this country, it is unpleasant to be called old, just as it is unpleasant to be called fat or poor. The old naturally try to avoid being identified with an unappreciated group....

The Elderly Are Treated Poorly

Nothing in our culture guides us in a positive way toward the old. Our media, music, and advertising industries all glorify the young. Stereotypes suggest that older people keep younger people from fun, work, and excitement. They take time (valuable time) and patience (in very short supply in the 1990s). We are very body-oriented, and old bodies fail. We are appearance-oriented, and youthful attractiveness fades. We are not taught that old spirits often shimmer with beauty.

Language is a problem. Old people are referred to in pejorative terms, such as *biddy, codger,* or *geezer,* or with cutesy words, such as *oldster, chronologically challenged,* or *senior citizen.* People describe themselves as "eighty years young." Even *retirement* is an ugly word that implies passivity, uselessness, and withdrawal from the social and working world. Many of the old are offended by ageist stereotypes and jokes. Some internalize these beliefs and feel badly about themselves. They stay with their own kind in order to avoid the harsh appraisals of the young.

Some people do not have good manners with the old. I've seen the elderly bossed around, treated like children or simpletons, and simply ignored. Once in a cafe, I heard a woman order her mother to take a pill and saw the mother wince in embarrassment. My mother-in-law says she sees young people but they don't see her. Her age makes her invisible.

In our culture the old are held to an odd standard. They are admired for not being a bother, for being chronically cheerful. They are expected to be interested in others, bland in their opinions, optimistic, and emotionally generous. But the young certainly don't hold themselves to these standards.

Accidents that old drivers have are blamed on age. After a ninety-year-old friend had his first car accident, he was terrified that he would lose his license. "If I were young, this accident would be perceived as just one of those things," he pointed out. "But because I am old, it will be attributed to my age." Now, of course, some old people are bad drivers. But so are some young people. To say "He did that because he's old" is often as narrow as to say, "He did that because he's black" or "Japanese." Young people burn countertops with hot pans, forget appointments, and write overdrafts on their checking accounts. But when the old do these same things, they experience double jeopardy. Their mistakes are not viewed as accidents but rather as loss of functioning. Such mistakes have implications for their freedom.

Media Stereotypes

As in so many other areas, the media hurts rather than helps with our social misunderstandings. George Gerbner reported on the curious absence of media images of people older than sixty-five. Every once in a while a romantic movie plot might involve an older man, but almost never an older woman. In general, the old have been cast as silly, stubborn, and eccentric. He also found that on children's programs, older women bear a disproportionate burden of negative characteristics. In our culture, the old get lumped together into a few stereotyped images: the sweet old lady, the lecherous old man, or the irascible but soft-hearted grandfather. Almost no ads and billboards feature the old. Every now and then an ad will show a grandparent figure, but then the grandparent is invariably youthful and healthy.

In *Fountain of Age,* Betty Friedan noted that the old are portrayed as sexless, demented, incontinent, toothless, and childish. Old women are portrayed as sentimental, naive, and silly gossips, and as troublemakers. A common movie plot is the portrayal of the old trying to be young—showing them on motorbikes, talking hip or dirty, or liking rock and roll. Of course there are exceptions, such as *Nobody's Fool, On Golden Pond, Mr. and Mrs. Bridge, Driving Miss Daisy, Mrs. Brown,* and *Twilight.* But we need more movies in which old people are portrayed in all their diversity and complexity.

The media is only part of much larger cultural problems. We aren't organized to accommodate this developmental stage. For example, being old-old costs a lot of money. Assisted-living housing, medical care, and all the other services the old need are expensive. And yet, most old people can't earn money. It's true that some of our elders are wealthy, but many live on small incomes. Visiting the old, I heard tragic stories involving money. I met Arlene, who, while dying of cancer, had to fear losing her house because of high property taxes. I met Shirley, who lived on noodles and white rice so that she could buy food for her cat and small gifts for her grandchildren. I met people who had to choose between pills and food or heat.

The American Obsession with Independence

Another thing that makes old age a difficult stage to navigate is our American belief that adults need no one. We think of independence as the ideal state for adults. We associate independence with heroes and cultural icons such as the Marlboro man and the Virginia Slims woman, and we associate dependence with toxic families, enmeshment, and weakness. To our postmodern, educated ears, a psychologically healthy but dependent adult sounds oxymoronic.

We all learn when we are very young to make our own personal declarations of independence. In our culture, *adult* means "self-sufficient." Autonomy is our highest virtue. We want relationships that have no strings attached instead of understanding, as one lady told me, "Honey, life ain't nothing but strings."

These American ideas about independence hurt families with teens. Just when children most need guidance from parents, they turn away from them and toward peers and media. They are socialized to believe that to be an adult, they must break away from parents. Our ideas about independence also hurt families with aging relatives. As people move from the young-old stage into the old-old stage, they need more help. Yet in our culture we provide almost no graceful ways for adults to ask for help. We make it almost impossible to be dependent yet dignified, respected, and in control.

As people age, they may need help with everything from their finances to their driving. They may need help getting out of bed, feeding themselves, and bathing. Many would rather pay strangers, do without help, or even die than be dependent on those they love. They don't want to be a burden, the greatest of American crimes. The old-old often feel ashamed of what is a natural stage of the life cycle. In fact, the greatest challenge for many elders is learning to accept vulnerability and to ask for help.

If we view life as a time line, we realize that all of us are sometimes more and sometimes less dependent on others. At certain stages we are caretakers, and at other stages we are cared for. Neither stage is superior to the other. Neither implies pathology or weakness. Both are just the results of life having seasons and circumstances. In fact, good mental health is not a matter of being dependent or independent, but of being able to accept the stage one is in with grace and dignity. It's an awareness of being, over the course of one's lifetime, continually interdependent.

Rethinking Dependency

In our culture the old fear their deaths will go badly, slowly, and painfully, and will cost lots of money. Nobody wants to die alone, yet nobody wants to put their families through too much stress. Families are uneasy as they negotiate this rocky terrain. The trick for the younger members is to help without feeling trapped and overwhelmed. The trick for older members is to accept help while preserving dignity and control. Caregivers can say, "You have nurtured us, why wouldn't we want to nurture you?" The old must learn to say, "I am grateful for your help and I am still a person worthy of respect."

As our times and circumstances change, we need new language. We need the elderly to become elders. We need a word for the neediness of the old-old, a word with less negative connotations than *dependency,* a word that connotes wisdom, connection, and dignity. *Dependency* could become mutuality or *interdependency.* We can say to the old: "You need us now, but we needed you and we will need our children. We need each other."

However, the issues are much larger than simply which words to use or social skills to employ. We need to completely rethink our ideas about caring for the elderly. Like the Lakota, we need to see it as an honor and an opportunity to learn. It is our chance to repay our parents for the love they gave us, and it is our last chance to become grown-ups. We help them to help ourselves.

We need to make the old understand that they can be helped without being infantilized, that the help comes from respect and gratitude rather than from pity or a sense of obligation. In our society of disposables and planned obsolescence, the old are phased out. Usually they fade away graciously. They want to be kind and strong, and, in America, they learn that to do so means they should ask little of others and not bother young people.

Perhaps we need to help them redefine kindness and courage. For the old, to be kind ought to mean welcoming younger relatives' help, and to be brave ought to mean accepting the dependency that old-old age will bring. We can reassure the old that by showing their children how to cope, they will teach them and their children how well this last stage can be managed. This information is not peripheral but rather something everyone will need to know.

Further Readings

Henry J. Aaron and Robert D. Reischauer. *Countdown to Reform: The Great Social Security Debate.* New York: Century Foundation Press, 2001.

Claude Amarnick. *Don't Put Me in a Nursing Home.* Deerfield Beach, FL: Garrett, 1996.

Dean Baker and Mark Weisbrot. *Social Security: The Phony Crisis.* Chicago: University of Chicago Press, 1999.

Margret M. Baltes. *The Many Faces of Dependency in Old Age.* Cambridge, England: Cambridge University Press, 1996.

Sam Beard. *Restoring Hope in America: The Social Security Solution.* San Francisco: Institute for Contemporary Studies, 1996.

Robert H. Binstock, Leighton E. Cluff, and Otto von Mering, eds. *The Future of Long-Term Care: Social and Policy Issues.* Baltimore: Johns Hopkins University Press, 1996.

Robert H. Binstock and Linda K. George, eds. *Handbook of Aging and the Social Sciences.* San Diego: Academic Press, 1996.

Jimmy Carter. *The Virtues of Aging.* New York: Ballantine, 1998.

Marshall N. Carter and William G. Shipman. *Promises to Keep: Saving Social Security's Dream.* Washington, DC: Regnery, 1996.

Martin Cetron and Owen Davies. *Cheating Death: The Promise and the Future Impact of Trying to Live Forever.* New York: St. Martin's Press, 1998.

William C. Cockerham. *This Aging Society.* Upper Saddle River, NJ: Prentice-Hall, 1997.

Peter A. Diamond, David C. Lindeman, and Howard Young, eds. *Social Security: What Role for the Future?* Washington, DC National Academy of Social Insurance, 1996.

Ursula Adler Falk and Gerhard Falk. *Ageism, the Aged and Aging in America: On Being Old in an Alienated Society.* Springfield, IL: Charles C. Thomas, 1997.

Peter J. Ferrara and Michael Tanner. *A New Deal for Social Security.* Washington, DC Cato Institute, 1998.

Arthur D. Fisk and Wendy A. Rogers, eds. *Handbook of Human Factors and the Older Adult.* San Diego: Academic Press, 1997.

Muriel R. Gillick. *Lifelines: Living Longer: Growing Frail, Taking Heart.* New York: W. W. Norton, 2000.

Margaret Morganroth Gullette. *Declining to Decline: Cultural Combat and the Politics of the Midlife.* Charlottesville: University Press of Virginia, 1997.

Charles B. Inlander and Michael A. Donio. *Medicare Made Easy.* Allentown, PA: People's Medical Society, 1999.

Donald H. Kausler and Barry C. Kausler. *The Graying of America: An Encyclopedia of Aging, Health, Mind, and Behavior.* Urbana: University of Illinois Press, 2001.

Eric R. Kingson and James H. Schulz, eds. *Social Security in the Twenty-First Century* New York: Oxford University Press, 1997.

Thelma J. Lofquist. *Frail Elders and the Wounded Caregiver.* Portland, OR: Binford and Mort, 2001.

Joseph L. Matthews. *Social Security, Medicare, and Pensions.* Berkeley, CA: Nolo, 1999.

E. J. Myers. *Let's Get Rid of Social Security: How Americans Can Take Charge of Their Own Future.* Amherst, NY: Prometheus Books, 1996.

Evelyn M. O'Reilly. *Decoding the Cultural Stereotypes About Aging: New Perspectives on Aging Talk and Aging Issues.* New York: Garland, 1997.

S. Jay Olshansky and Bruce A. Carnes. *The Quest for Immortality: Science at the Frontiers of Aging.* New York: W. W. Norton, 2001.

Fred C. Pampel. *Aging, Social Inequality, and Public Policy.* Thousand Oaks, CA: Pine Forge Press, 1998.

Peter G. Peterson. *Gray Dawn: How the Coming Age Wave Will Transform America—And the World.* New York: Times Books, 1999.

Peter G. Peterson. *Will America Grow Up Before It Grows Old?: How the Coming Social Security Crisis Threatens You, Your Family, and Your Country.* New York: Random House, 1996.

John W. Rowe and Robert L. Kahn. *Successful Aging.* New York: Pantheon Books, 1998.

Sylvester J. Schieber and John B. Shoven. *The Real Deal: The History and Future of Social Security.* New Haven, CT: Yale University Press, 1999.

Ken Skala. *American Guidance for Seniors—And Their Caregivers.* Falls Church, VA: K. Skala, 1996.

Max J. Skidmore. *Social Security and Its Enemies: The Case for America's Most Efficient Insurance Program.* Boulder, CO: Westview Press, 1999.

Richard D. Thau and Jay S. Heflin, eds. *Generations Apart: Xers vs. Boomers vs. the Elderly.* Amherst, NY: Prometheus Books, 1997.

Dale Van Atta. *Trust Betrayed: Inside the AARP.* Washington, DC: Regnery, 1998.

James W. Walters, ed. *Choosing Who's to Live: Ethics and Aging.* Urbana: University of Illinois Press, 1996.

David A. Wise, ed. *Facing the Age Wave.* Stanford, CA: Hoover Institutional Press, Stanford University, 1997.

Periodicals

W. Andrew Achenbaum. "Perceptions of Aging in America," *National Forum,* Spring 1998. Available from the Honor Society of Phi Kappa Phi, Box 16000, Louisiana State University, Baton Rouge, LA 70893.

America. "Keep an Eye on the Third Age," May 16, 1998.

Robert Butler. "The Longevity Revolution," *UNESCO Courier,* January 1999.

Issues and Controversies on File. "Age Discrimination," May 21, 1999. Available from Facts on File News Services, 11 Penn Plaza, New York, NY 10001-2006.

Margot Jefferys. "A New Way of Seeing Old Age Is Needed," *World Health,* September/October 1996.

Ann Monroe. "Getting Rid of the Gray: Will Age Discrimination Be the Downfall of Downsizing?" *Mother Jones,* July/August 1996.

Bernadette Puijalon and Jacqueline Trincaz. "Sage or Spoilsport?" *UNESCO Courier,* January 1999.

Jody Robinson. "The Baby Boomers' Final Revolt," *Wall Street Journal,* July 31, 1998.

Dan Seligman. "The Case for Age Discrimination," *Forbes,* December 13, 1999.

Ruth Simon. "Too Damn Old," *Money,* July 1996.

John C. Weicher. "Life in a Gray America," *American Outlook,* Fall 1998. Available from 5395 Emerson Way, Indianapolis, IN 46226.

Ron Winslow. "The Age of Man," *Wall Street Journal,* October 18, 1999.

Ageism in America

As boomers become seniors, bias against the elderly becomes hot topic

By David Crary

Greeting-card and novelty companies call them "Over the Hill" products: the 50th Birthday Coffin Gift Boxes featuring prune juice and anti-aging soap; the "Old Coot" and "Old Biddy" bobblehead dolls; the birthday cards mocking the mobility, intellect and sex drive of the no-longer-young.

Many Americans chuckle at such humor. Others see it as offensive, as one more sign of pervasive ageism in America.

It's a bias some also see in substandard conditions at nursing homes, in pension-plan cutbacks by employers, in the relative invisibility of the elderly on television shows and in advertisements.

"Daily we are witness to, or even unwitting participants in, cruel imagery, jokes, language, and attitudes directed at older people," contends Dr. Robert Butler, president of the International Longevity Center-USA and the person who coined the term "ageism" 35 years ago.

That ageism exists in a society captivated by youth culture and taut-skinned good looks is scarcely debatable.

But as the oldest of the 77 million baby boomers approach their 60s, the elderly and their concerns will inevitably move higher on the national agenda.

Already, there is lively debate as to whether ageism will ease or grow

worse in the coming decades of boomer senior citizenship. Erdman Palmore, a professor emeritus at Duke University who has written or edited more than a dozen books on aging, counts himself—cautiously—among the optimists.

"One can say unequivocally that older people are getting smarter, richer and healthier as time goes on," Palmore said. "I've dedicated most of my life to combating ageism, and it's tempting for me to see it everywhere. ... But I have faith that as science progresses, and reasonable people get educated about it, we will come to recognize ageism as the evil it is."

Palmore, 74, lives what he preaches—challenging the stereotypes of aging by skydiving, whitewater rafting, bicycling his age in miles each birthday. He recently got a tattoo on his shoulder, though the image he chose was the relatively discreet symbol of the American Humanist Association.

"What makes me mad is how aging, in our language and culture, is equated with deterioration and impairment," Palmore said. "I don't know how we're going to root that out, except by making people more aware of it."

To the extent that ageism persists, there will soon be many more potential targets. The number of Americans 65 and older is projected

to double over the next three decades from 35.9 million to nearly 70 million, comprising 20 percent of the population in 2030 compared to less than 13 percent now.

The 85-and-over population is the fastest growing segment—projected to grow from 4 million in 2000 to 19 million in 2050 as part of an unprecedented surge in longevity. Americans now turning 65 will live, on average, an additional 18 years.

Some researchers believe that ageism, in the form of negative stereotypes, directly affects longevity. In a study published by the American Psychological Association, Yale School of Public Health professor Becca Levy and her colleagues concluded that old people with positive perceptions of aging lived an average of 7.5 years longer than those with negative images of growing older.

Levy said many Americans start developing stereotypes about the elderly during childhood, reinforce them throughout adulthood, and enter old age with attitudes toward their own age group as unfavorable as younger people's attitudes.

"It's possible to overcome the stereotypes, but they often operate without people's awareness," Levy said. "Look at all the talk about plastic surgery, Botox—the message is, 'Don't get old.'"

For thousands of American workers, it's the same message they claim to hear on the job. The U.S. Equal Employment Opportunity Commission has received more than 19,000 age discrimination complaints in each of the past two years, and has helped win tens of millions of dollars in settlements. However, attorneys say age discrimination often is hard to prove. Only about one-seventh of the EEOC age cases were settled to the complainant's benefit.

New Yorker Bill DeLong, 84, was fired three years ago from his long-time job as a waiter at a Shea Stadium restaurant, but he continues to seek out charitable volunteer assignments and still works as a waiter occasionally at special events.

"I didn't give up," he said. "A lot of my contemporaries give up too soon."

Seventy-eight-year-old Catherine Roberts stays active with New York City's Joint Public Affairs Committee for Older Adults, a coalition that encourages seniors to advocate on their own behalf on legislative and community issues.

"I don't have time to get old," said Roberts, who came to New York from Maine in 1955. "I'm too busy."

Yet despite her upbeat outlook, she resents how some of her peers are treated. "We're a culture that worships youth," she said. "Seniors are getting pushed aside. I see people in my building whose families ignore them—they fall through the cracks."

For many older people, ageism surfaces most painfully in the context of health care. A report by the Alliance for Aging Research, pre-sented to a Senate committee last year, said the elderly are less likely to receive preventive care and often lack access to doctors trained in their needs.

Only about 10 percent of U.S. medical schools require work in geriatric medicine. The American Geriatrics Society says there are only about 7,600 physicians nationwide certified as geriatric specialists—not enough to meet demand and far below the 36,000 the society says will be needed by 2030.

While the society says the best way to attract more doctors to the field is to make Medicare practice more lucrative, some experts believe that many medical students also have negative attitudes toward the elderly that should be challenged.

In one such effort, the National Institute on Aging, working with Johns Hopkins Medical School and a Baltimore museum, teamed elderly people and first-year medical students in an art program in which they drew, made collages, sang songs and shared stories. A survey showed the students gained a more positive view of seniors and of geriatrics as a possible specialty.

Ageism also manifests itself in advertising. Though adults of all ages drink beer and buy cars, for example, TV and print ads for those products almost invariably feature youthful actors and models.

According to AARP, the lobbying group for people 50 and over, Americans in that age bracket account for half of all consumer spending but are targeted by just 10 percent of marketing. The dynamic is particularly potent in television, where network executives gear programming toward 18-to-34-year-olds because advertisers will pay more to reach those viewers. Jim Fishman, group publisher for AARP Publications oversees the organization's three magazines. He predicts advertisers will increasingly tilt their messages toward older consumers as the baby boomers enter their 60s.

"By and large, the wealth that resides in the older segment of the population is disposable wealth—the kids are done with college, the mortgage is paid off," Fishman said. "This older market is huge and feeling largely ignored."

Looking ahead, Fishman foresees people of all ages, elderly included, gaining the ability to look more attractive than in the past thanks to developments ranging from Botox to fitness programs. He also expects a more deep-rooted change in society's view of aging as the 65-and-older ranks are filled with increasing numbers of computer-savvy boomers, eager for civic engagement and lifelong education programs.

Still, David Wolfe, whose book "Ageless Marketing" advises advertisers how to reach over-50 consumers, says ageism is likely to persist. "There will always be people in society who can't come to terms with other people's aging because they can't come to terms with their own aging," he said.

The Activation of Aging Stereotypes in Younger and Older Adults

The activation of ageism and aging stereotypes in younger and older adults was investigated by manipulating both the valence and the stereotypicality of trait stimuli. Participants completed a lexical decision task in which the stimulus onset asynchronies (SOAs) between the prime and target stimuli were varied to examine the effects of automatic and controlled processing (300 and 2,000 ms, respectively). Both younger and older adults demonstrated strong stereotype activation for elderly stereotypes but relatively weak activation for young stereotypes. Both younger and older adults also demonstrated a positive bias toward older people, which was not moderated by SOA. These findings suggest that younger and older adults do not differ in their accessibility to aging stereotypes or to their age-based biases, which appear to be positive toward elderly people.

Alison L. Chasteen,[1] Norbert Schwarz,[2] and Denise C. Park[2]

> I will not make age an issue of this campaign. I am not going to exploit for political purposes my opponent's youth and inexperience.
> —Ronald Reagan, 1984 presidential debate against Walter Mondale

WHEN we think about age, we often do so in terms of how we feel toward older adults. As Ronald Reagan demonstrated so adroitly, however, age is a two-way street. When we investigate people's age-related attitudes, it is important to examine attitudes toward both young and old. Although younger adults' attitudes toward older people have received considerable attention, less is known about older adults' attitudes toward young people. The present study addresses this gap by examining both younger and older adults' accessibility of attitudes toward and stereotypes of both age groups.

Most studies of age-related attitudes and stereotyping have relied on self-report questionnaires, often referred to as *explicit measures* (for recent reviews, see Crockett & Hummert, 1987; Hummert, 1999; Hummert, Shaner, & Garstka, 1995; Kite & Johnson, 1988). In general, this research has suggested that people's perceptions of elderly adults are mixed. People associate both positive and negative traits with older people as a group, although there tend to be more negative trait associations than positive ones (Hummert et al., 1995). Research on the cognitive organization of traits has shown there are multiple stereotypes or subcategories of elderly people, some positive and some negative (Brewer, Dull, & Lui, 1981; Hummert, Garstka, Shaner, & Strahm, 1994; Schmidt & Boland, 1986). Finally, Hummert and colleagues (1994) found a fair degree of overlap in the organization of the subcategories across young, middle-aged, and older adults, although elderly people had the most complex representations of older people, followed by middle-aged and young adults. Thus, research using explicit measures has shown that aging stereotypes are complex, with both positive and negative traits and subtypes being associated with elderly people.

As for attitudes toward older people, the literature has suggested that perceptions of elderly individuals *as a group* are more negative compared with perceptions of young or middle-aged adults, although ratings of older people rarely fall at the negative end of most scales (Crockett & Hummert, 1987; Lutsky, 1980). Perceptions of elderly individuals, however, tend to be as positive as perceptions of younger adults, and when age differences are observed those differences have been inconsistent in favoring either age group (Hummert et al., 1985). Hummert and her colleagues (Crockett & Hummert, 1987; Hummert et al., 1995) contended that this inconsistency between attitudes toward elderly individuals versus older people as a group might be due to the multiple stereotypes of older adults that people hold. Compatible with this assumption, research on ambivalent stereotypes suggests that attitudes toward elderly people may be marked by both positive and negative perceptions (Fiske, Cuddy, Glick, & Xu, 2002). Fiske and colleagues proposed that people's attitudes toward different groups are driven by their perceptions of a group's competence and warmth. These perceptions lead people to place most groups into one of two categories: (a) groups they respect for their competence but dislike for their lack of warmth or (b) groups they disrespect for their incompetence but like and patronize for their warmth. It is this second category of groups under which elderly people fall. Fiske and associates found that groups that were similar in terms of perceived frailty (e.g., disabled people, elderly people) were clustered together with regard to perceived incompetence and warmth. In combination, these lines of research suggest that when people think of the concept *old*, positive associations might be just as likely to come to mind as negative associations.

As with other domains of stereotyping (e.g., race, gender), using explicit measures of age-based attitudes and stereotyping can pose problems because participants may be unaware of their beliefs and sentiments or reluctant to reveal any negativity they might feel (Fazio, Jackson, Dunton, & Williams, 1995; Greenwald, McGhee, & Schwartz, 1998). To avoid these difficulties, researchers in social cognition have begun using implicit measures of attitudes and stereotypes in order to assess people's mental representations of various groups, as well as people's feelings toward those groups (e.g., Kawakami, Dion, & Dovidio, 1998; Wittenbrink, Judd, & Park, 1997). Implicit measures usually involve priming paradigms in which participants are first exposed to stimuli that activate the target group and then respond either to adjectives or to traits. Either the primes are presented at a subthreshold rate, such that participants are unaware of the presence of the primes, or a short stimulus onset asynchrony (SOA) is chosen to prevent participants from controlling their initial responses when they are aware of the primes.

Perdue and Gurtman (1990) reported one of the few studies that investigated the activation of age-related attitudes using implicit measures. In their experiment, young adult participants were presented with the subthreshold primes young and old, which were then followed by either a positive or a negative trait. Participants indicated whether each trait was good or bad for someone to possess. Perdue and Gurtman found that young adults made faster responses when positive traits were preceded by the young prime compared with the old prime. Conversely, participants made faster responses when negative traits were preceded by the old prime compared with the young prime. Perdue and Gurtman concluded from these results that there is an automatic ageism that influences the way people process trait information. Hence, subliminal presentation of the word *old* facilitated the processing of negative trait information, and subliminal presentation of the word *young* facilitated the processing of positive information. Perdue and Gurtman suggested that labeling a person as old could automatically activate primarily negative constructs that might then be applied in evaluating that individual.

Unfortunately, the interpretation of this study is hampered by Perdue and Gurtman's (1990) selection of personality traits. Intending to examine age-based prejudice, the authors selected extremely positive or negative traits from Anderson's (1968) list of trait valence ratings, but did not consider the issue of trait stereotypicality (i.e., trait descriptiveness). As a result, their stimulus set overrepresented positive traits that have been shown to be more descriptive of younger adults than older adults (e.g., studious, tolerant). Conversely, their set of negative traits overrepresented traits that have been shown to be more descriptive of older adults (e.g., stubborn, forgetful). Because of this confound of valence and stereotypicality, it is unclear whether Perdue and Gurtman's (1990) findings are due solely to age-based prejudice, to the differential stereotypicality of the selected positive (young) and negative (old) traits, or a mix of both influences. The present study addresses this ambiguity.

Since Perdue and Gurtman's (1990) study, it has become common practice to measure the separate effects of trait valence and stereotypicality in research on stereotype activation (typically addressing the domains of gender and race; e.g., Blair & Banaji, 1996; Kawakami et al., 1998; Wittenbrink et al., 1997). This research refers to *implicit stereotyping* to describe the automatic accessibility to mental representations of groups. Effects of implicit stereotyping are usually seen in the form of faster responses to traits that are descriptive of a group when those traits are preceded by the group label (e.g., old followed by wise or frail). These stereotype facilitation effects are independent of trait valence. *Implicit prejudice*, however, describes facilitation effects that depend on valence and not on trait descriptiveness.

Because of the above confound of valence and stereotypicality, Perdue and Gurtman's findings may reflect either, or both, of these phenomena. The present study addresses this issue with a stimulus set that permits examination of *both* implicit prejudice and implicit stereotyping for the domain of age and extends previous research by examining the activation of aging stereotypes and attitudes in both younger and older people.

The purpose of the present study was to address four basic questions. First, do younger and older adults hold the same stereotypes about the young and old? Although Perdue and Gurtman (1990) examined young adults' age-based prejudices, no study has addressed whether the accessibility of aging stereotypes differs in younger and older adults. Evidence suggesting that both age groups hold the same stereotypes would be in the form of finding no age differences in responses when a group label matches the descriptiveness of the trait.

Second, are people more positive about their own age group than another age group? Research on intergroup relations suggests that people will favor their own group over another (Tajfel, 1981), and some research using explicit measures of age-related attitudes has found age differences in how younger and older people feel about one another (e.g., Celejewski & Dion, 1998). However, to date, the accessibility of age-related attitudes has not been assessed in both younger and older adults. In the present study, intergroup biases would be evident if each age group responded faster when their own group label was paired with positive traits and the other group label was paired with negative traits.

Third, who is prejudiced against whom? It may be that only one age group holds negative attitudes toward the other age group. Some research has suggested that only young adults hold negative attitudes toward older adults and that older adults have positive attitudes toward the young (Speas & Obenshain, 1995). It is also possible that older adults not only feel favorably toward younger adults but also share young people's negative views of older people. That is, older adults might also feel positively toward the young and negatively toward their own age group. We sought to determine which of these patterns of age-based prejudice most accurately describes younger and older adults' views of one another.

Fourth, do people "correct" their automatic response when they have a chance to do so? To address this issue, we examined whether younger and older adults would attempt to inhibit their age-related associations if given the chance. By manipulating SOA, we sought to determine whether younger and older adults form different age-related associations if they are permitted more control over their responses.

METHODS

Overview

The present study examined the activation of age-based stereotypes and prejudice in younger and older adults. Participants completed a lexical decision task in which the primes young, old, or XXXX were presented, followed by a target word or nonword. To examine stereotyping and prejudice, both the valence and the stereotypicality of the target words were varied. To see whether participants would show different response patterns under conditions of automatic and controlled processing, the SOA was varied (300 ms or 2,000 ms).

Table 1. Experimental Trait Stimuli

	Stereotypically Old		Stereotypically Young	
	Positive	Negative	Positive	Negative
	Experienced	Senile	Energetic	Inexperienced
	Wise	Forgetful	Healthy	Reckless
	Sage	Fragile	Adventurous	Rebellious
	Sentimental	Feeble	Excited	Lazy
	Generous	Tired	Carefree	Wasteful
	Patient	Neglected	Curious	Greedy
	Cautious	Inflexible	Eager	Disrespectful
	Learned	Afraid	Vigorous	Vain
	Knowledgeable	Bitter	Ambitious	Loud
	Practical	Lonely	Optimistic	Irresponsible
	Mature	Helpless	Flexible	Impatient
Mean				
Typicality	3.88	4.12	2.06	2.10
Valence	4.10	2.08	4.07	1.74

Notes: Stereotypicality ratings ranged from 1 (characteristic of young adults) to 5 (characteristics of older adults). Valence ratings ranged from 1 (negative) to 5 (positive).

Participants and Design

Participants were 72 younger adults (M_{age} = 18.86 years; M_{edu} = 13.43 years) and 59 older adults (M_{age} = 70.58 years; M_{edu} = 15.00 years). In the young adult sample, 68% of the participants were female, 79% were Caucasian, and the mean health rating was 4.37 (scale ranged from 1, very poor to 5, excellent). In the older adult sample, 67% were female, 97% were Caucasian, and the mean health rating was 3.98. The younger adults were recruited from the introductory psychology course at the University of Michigan and received course credit for their participation. The older adults were recruited from the greater Ann Arbor, Michigan area and were paid $10 for their participation. Data from 2 participants who did not follow instructions (1 young, 1 old) were excluded from the analyses.

A 2 (age: young or old) × 2 (SOA: 2,000 or 300 ms) × 3 (prime: young, old, or XXXX) × 2 (stereotypicality: young or old traits) × 2 (valence: positive or negative traits) factorial design was used. Age and SOA were between-subjects factors, and the rest were within-subject factors.

Stimuli

An initial pool of 60 traits was developed by selecting items from studies in which words describing young and/or elderly people had been pretested (Bargh, Chen, & Burrows, 1996; Hummert et al., 1994; Levy, 1996; Rothbaum, 1983; Schmidt & Boland, 1986). The 60 selected traits were pilot tested for valence and stereotypicality by having 10 older and 8 younger adults rate the traits on each dimension (e.g., 1 = characteristic of young adults to 5 = characteristic of older adults). Forty-four traits (11 per category; see Table 1) were selected on the basis of the mean ratings of stereotypicality and valence. The selected traits were approximately equal in word frequently (Ku-cera & Francis, 1967) and word length across the four conditions (*ps* > .12 and .68, respectively). Moreover, the young traits differed significantly from the old traits in stereotypicality, $t(17)$ = 11.95,

$p < .001$, and the positive traits differed significantly from the negative traits when rated for valence, $t(17) = 10.19, p < .001$.

A second pilot study ensured that the differences in stereotypicality ratings were not due to the use of a bipolar scale in which participants were forced to rate the words as either characteristically young or characteristically old. Ten young and 10 older adults rated the traits using a unipolar scale ranging from 1 (not at all characteristic) to 5 (very characteristic). Half of the participants rated the traits for their descriptiveness of young adults, and the other half rated them for their descriptiveness of older adults. Note that in the first pilot test we obtained the expected effect for stereotypicality, with young traits rated closer to the young end of the scale and old traits rated closer to the old end of the scale. In the second study, because two versions of the scale were used (Young or Old scale), we expected to find a Scale Version × Stereotypicality interaction. Analyses revealed a main effect for scale version, $F(1,16) = 8.08, p < .05$. Participants who used the Young scale rated the traits as more stereotypical ($M = 3.17$) than those who used the Old scale ($M = 2.71$). However, this main effect was moderated by the predicted Scale Version × Stereotypicality interaction, $F(1,16) = 124.42, p < .001$. Participants receiving the Young scale rated the young traits as more typical of young adults than the old traits ($Ms = 3.72$ and 2.61, respectively, $p < .001$). Participants receiving the Old scale rated the old traits as more typical of older adults than the young traits ($Ms = 3.16$ and 2.26, respectively, p .001). Also, old traits were rated as more typical in the old version than in the young version ($Ms = 3.16$ vs 2.61, $p < .001$), and young traits were rated as more typical in the young version than in the old version ($Ms = 3.72$ vs. 2.26, $p < .001$). Participant age did not moderate the two-way interaction, $F(1,16) = 2.85, p > .11$ (Appendix, Note 1).

Procedure

After completing some cognitive tasks unrelated to the present study, participants completed a lexical decision task.

The word stimuli included the four types of traits shown in Table 1, which were paired with three primes (young, old, or XXXX). The nonword stimuli were pronounceable nonwords (e.g., *garlant, fronge*) that were paired with the three primes.

The trial sequence was based on a procedure used by Kawakami and colleagues (1998). On each trial, a fixation point (+) appeared in the center of the screen for 300 ms and was followed by a blank screen for 500 ms. For participants in the short SOA condition (300 ms), the prime then appeared for 250 ms followed by a blank screen for 50 ms before the onset of the target word or nonword. For participants in the long SOA condition (2,000 ms), the prime appeared for 1,950 ms followed by a blank screen for 50 ms before the onset of the target. The target remained on the screen until participants made a key-press to indicate their lexical decision. Key-press responses were counterbalanced across participants. Half of the participants were instructed to press the *z* key if the target was a word and to press the / key if the target was a nonword, and the other half were instructed to do the opposite.

Participants completed a total of 176 trials, which were divided into four blocks of 44 trials each. There were 44 traits (11 per trait type; see Table 1) that were paired with each of the three primes, yielding a total of 132 word trials. The word and nonword trials were presented randomly across the four blocks.

Before beginning the task, participants were told that they would see a series of three things on the computer screen: a plus sign; the word *young, old,* or *XXXX*; and then a second word. They were instructed that their job was to decide whether the second word was a real word or a nonsense word and to press the yes key if it was a real word and the no key if it was not. Thus, although participants were not told specifically to ignore the prime, they were instructed to make a decision about the second word (Kawakami et al., 1998). Next, participants were given two examples and then completed 10 practice trials. At the end of the practice trials, the experimenter checked to see if there were any additional questions, and then participants began the main set of trials.

Following the lexical decision task, participants completed a demographic questionnaire and then two explicit measures of their attitudes toward older people. One was the five-item Fear of Old People subscale from the Anxiety About Aging scale (e.g., *I enjoy being around old people;* Lasher & Faulkender, 1993), which ranged from –2 (*strongly disagree*) to 2 (*strongly agree*). The other measure was a 5-item affective scale that assessed people's liking for older people (e.g., *I admire older people a great deal*) and ranged from – 3 to 3. These two scales were highly correlated, $r(129) = .69, p < .001$. Scores on the two scales were transformed to z scores and then combined to form a composite aging attitude score for each participant (α for combined scale = .93), with higher scores indicating positive views of elderly people. Finally, participants were debriefed and compensated.

RESULTS

Explicit Aging Attitude Measure

A 2 (age group: young or old) × 2 (SOA: short or long) analysis of variance (ANOVA) was conducted on participants' scores on the aging attitude scale. Only a marginal age group difference was found, $F(1,125) = 2.96, p = .09$. Young adults were slightly more negative than older adults (mean z scores = – .11 and .13, respectively). No other effects were significant.

Implicit Measure

Each participant's response times from the lexical decision task were checked for errors and outliers. We defined an outlier as a latency that was 2.5 standard deviations above the mean for that condition. All errors and outliers were excluded from the analyses and treated as missing values. The mean error and outlier rates were 2.11% and 2.45%, respectively. All analyses were conducted on the log-transformed latencies, although the untransformed means are presented in the text and in the figures so that the presented metric is familiar to the reader. In line with other studies (Blair & Banaji, 1996; Kawakami et al., 1998), we used mean response latencies rather than facilitation scores in which the means from the young and old prime conditions were first subtracted from the baseline prime condition (for a methodological discussion, see Fazio, Sanbonmatsu, Powell, & Kardes, 1986; Jonides & Mack, 1984).

A 2 (age: young or old) × 2 (SOA: short or long) × 2 (prime: young or old) × 2 (stereotypicality: young or old) × 2 (valence: positive or negative) repeated-measures ANOVA was conducted on the log-transformed latencies. Age and SOA were between-subjects factors and prime, stereotypicality, and valence were within-subject factors. The ANOVA revealed a significant main effect for age, $F(1,125) = 26.30, p < .001$, with the younger adults responding faster ($M = 714$ ms) than the older adults ($M = 867$ ms). In addition, participants in the short SOA condition made faster responses ($M = 727$ ms) than participants in the long SOA condition ($M = 855$ ms; $F(1,125) = 15.77, p < .001$). In the next two sections, we report the findings regarding age-based stereotyping and age-based prejudice that resulted from the repeated-measures ANOVA.

Age-Based Stereotyping

One objective of this study was to assess the influence of old and young primes on the identification of stereotypically old or young traits, independent of the valence of these traits. Theoretically, the observation that participants respond faster to Trait X when it is preceded by the old prime rather than the young prime would indicate that Trait X is part of a well-defined aging stereotype. Figure 1 shows the respective latencies.

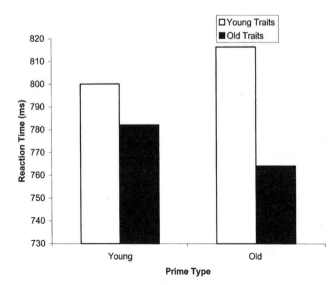

Figure 1. Mean response latency as a function of prime type and trait stereotypicality.

Overall, participants responded faster to traits descriptive of older people (*M* = 773 ms) than to traits descriptive of younger people (*M* = 808 ms), independent of the preceding prime, $F(1,125)$ = 29.02, $p < .001$, for the main effect of trait stereotypicality. More important, the ANOVA revealed a significant Prime × Stereotypicality interaction, $F(1,125)$ = 8.07, $p < .01$. Comparisons within each trait type indicate that participants responded faster to stereotypically old traits when they were preceded by the old prime (*M* = 764 ms) rather than the young prime (*M* = 782 ms; $p < .05$). Conversely, they responded faster to the young traits when these were preceded by the young prime (*M* = 800 ms) rather than the old prime (*M* = 816 ms; $p < .06$). Comparisons within each prime type further indicated that participants responded faster to stereotypically old traits than to stereotypically young traits after the old prime (*M*s = 764 and 816 ms, respectively, $p < .001$). Surprisingly, however, this facilitation effect did not hold for the young prime. Following the young prime, participants were faster to respond to the stereotypically old traits than to the stereotypically young traits (*M*s = 782 and 800 ms, respectively, $p < .05$).

If older and younger respondents differ in the stereotypes they hold about these age groups, the above patterns should be qualified by participants' age. Empirically, this was not the case, and the above Prime × Stereotypicality interaction was not moderated by participants' age ($F < 1$ for the three-way interaction). As shown in Table 2, younger and older adults had similar patterns of reaction times, which suggests that older and younger respondents share the same stereotypes, particularly with regard to elderly people.

Finally, the Prime × Stereotypicality interaction was not moderated by SOA ($F < 1$ for the three-way interaction). Theoretically, participants' responses under short SOA conditions are based on automatic processes, whereas long SOAs allow for deliberate corrections before to the overt response, which may be motivated by social desirability concerns. The absence of an interaction with SOA therefore suggests that participants did not edit their responses even under conditions where this would have been possible.

Table 2. Mean Reaction Times (in Milliseconds) as a Function of Age Group and Prime Type for Trait Stereotypicality and Trait Valence

Prime	Trait Stereotypicality		Trait Valence	
	Young	Old	Positive	Negative
Young Adults				
Young	716	712	710	718
Old	742	693	703	731
Older Adults				
Young	887	855	868	874
Old	894	839	850	884

Age-Based Prejudice

A second objective of our study was to examine the influence of old and young primes on the identification of positive and negative traits, independent of the stereotypicality of these traits. Theoretically, the observation that participants respond

faster to a negative trait when it is preceded by the old prime rather than the young prime, for example, would indicate implicit prejudice.

Overall, participants produced faster responses to positive traits (*M* = 781 ms) than to negative traits (*M* = 800 ms), $F(1,125)$ = 13.52, $p < .001$, for the main effect of trait valence. The Prime × Valence interaction was not significant, $F(1,125)$ = 2.66, $p > .10$. To examine whether Perdue and Gurtman's (1990) results replicate with a stimulus set that eliminates the previous confound of stereotypicality and valence, we conducted planned comparisons (see Figure 2; all tests were one tailed). These analyses revealed a pattern of responses that was *opposite* to the one found by Perdue and Gurtman, with both younger and older participants showing more positive attitudes toward elderly people than toward young people. For example, Perdue and Gurtman observed faster responses to positive traits after the young prime rather than the old prime; however, a marginally significant pattern ($p < .08$) that was opposite in direction was found in the present data (*M*s = 787 ms and 775 ms for the young and old primes, respectively). Perdue and Gurtman also found faster responses to negative traits when they were preceded by the old prime rather than young prime, but there was no difference between those means in the present study (*M*s = 806 ms and 794 ms for old and young primes, respectively, $p > .17$). In short, Perdue and Gurtman's pattern did not hold up when the effects of trait valence were separated from the effects of trait typicality.

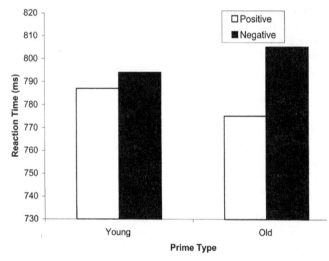

Figure 2. Mean response latency as a function of prime type and trait valence.

Comparisons within each prime type further indicated that participants made faster responses to positive traits (*M* = 775 ms) than to negative traits (*M* = 806 ms) when they were preceded by the old prime ($p < .001$). Note that this finding indicates that positive traits are more closely associated with elderly people than are negative traits, in contrast to what the implicit prejudice hypothesis would predict. These results again differ from those of Perdue and Gurtman (1990), who found no difference for this comparison with a stimulus set that confounded valence and stereotypicality, Finally, the present data did replicate Perdue and Gurtman's finding of faster responses to positive than to negative traits that followed the young prime, although the difference was less pronounced (*M*s = 787 and 794 ms for positive and negative traits, respectively, $p < .05$) compared with that for the old prime.

As in the preceding stereotyping analysis, participants' age did not moderate the prejudice effects ($F < 1$ for the Age × Prime × Trait Valence interaction). This suggests that the younger and older adults shared similar attitudes toward elderly adults (see Table 2). Moreover, those attitudes are positive rather than negative, in contrast to what an implicit prejudice hypothesis would suggest. In addition, SOA did not qualify these effects ($F < 1$ for the three-way interaction), again suggesting that participants felt no need to modify their responses. Finally, none of the other three-way interactions, nor any higher order interactions, were significant, with participant age and SOA only producing main effects and qualifying no interactions.

DISCUSSION

The present study examined the activation of age prejudice and aging stereotypes in younger and older adults. The small amount of research that has been conducted in this area has suggested that younger adults associate negative traits with the concept *old* and positive traits with the concept *young* (Chasteen & Pratt, 1999; Perdue & Gurtman, 1990). Unfortunately, however, previous studies did not separate the contributions of trait valence and trait stereotypicality. It is therefore unclear whether their results reflected the activation of stereotypes or of attitudes (Blair & Banaji, 1996; Wittenbrink et al., 1997). The current research addressed this ambiguity by manipulating trait valence and trait stereotypicality independently, thus permitting an examination of the activation of aging stereotypes and age-based prejudice in younger and older people. The results provided compelling evidence for automatic stereotyping, but not for automatic prejudice.

Automatic Stereotyping

With regard to automatic stereotyping, we found that younger and older adults shared the same stereotypes of younger and older people. Age did not moderate the significant Prime × Stereotypicality interaction. Moreover, the data indicated that all participants had stronger stereotypes of older people than of younger people. This was evident in the strong patterns of facilitation regarding the old traits: (a) Participants responded faster to old traits when they followed the old versus the young prime and (b) participants responded faster to old traits than to young traits when they followed the old prime. In contrast, there was only weak evidence supporting the notion of activation of a young stereotype: (a) Participants did respond faster to young traits when those traits followed the young versus the old prime, but (b) participants responded faster to the old traits rather than to the young traits that followed the young prime.

Besides the evidence demonstrating a weaker association between the concept of young and young traits, the present data also raise the possibility of differential patterns of dissociation. Responses to young traits following the old prime were the slowest of all pairings, reflecting the greatest degree of dissociation. Perhaps it is the case that young traits are viewed as more atypical of the concept *old* than old traits are of the concept *young*. This notion is consistent with the data from the second pilot study, in which there was a greater difference in typicality ratings for young traits across the two scale versions ($M = 1.46$)

compared with old traits ($M = 0.55$). Thus, the slower response times in response to the old prime-young trait pairing might reflect some sort of inhibitory response resulting from greater dissociation.

Although the lack of a strong association between the young prime and young traits was unexpected, it is unlikely that it reflects problems with the trait selection. One potential problem might have been that the traits were unequal in their frequency or length. Yet, we found no differences in word frequency and length across the four types of words. Another potential problem might have been that we selected young words that were not as strongly associated with the young stereotype as the old words were associated with the old stereotype. The results from the second trait rating study, however, show that the young traits were rated as characteristic of young people ($M = 3.72$) as the old traits were of old people ($M = 3.16$). Thus, we believe the weak activation pattern we observed for the young stereotype was not due to our selection of traits. Rather, we believe it is more likely that people hold better defined stereotypes of older adults and that these stereotypes are more frequently activated than the stereotypes people have of young adults. When the two types of stereotypes are pitted against one another, as they were in the present study, the elderly stereotypes are more accessible and thus show a stronger pattern of activation than the young stereotypes.

Our finding of the same response patterns in young and old participants suggests that aging stereotypes do not change as people grow older and that both age groups have similar mental representations of each other and of their own age group. As seen in Table 2, younger and older adults showed similar patterns of stereotype activation. Further, SOA did not moderate the Prime × Stereotypicality interaction, suggesting that this pattern of age-based stereotyping exists under conditions of either automatic or controlled processing.

Automatic Prejudice

Whereas our findings make a compelling case for age-based stereotyping of elderly people, they provide only weak support for the presence of age-based prejudice. First, the Prime × Valence interaction was not significant. Second, planned comparisons revealed that the only pattern of means that was consistent with the results of Perdue and Gurtman (1990) was the finding that participants responded faster to positive traits than to negative traits that followed the young prime. However, this same pattern was observed for the old prime, and the effect was even stronger. Taken together, the results from the planned comparisons suggest that perceptions of elderly individuals are relatively favorable. Moreover, the lack of a significant Age × Prime × Valence interaction supports the notion that younger and older adults view each other similarly (see Table 2). As with the Prime × Stereotypicality interaction, SOA did not moderate this pattern of results, indicating that people showed the same pattern of responses whether they were under automatic or controlled processing conditions.

The results regarding age-based prejudice suggest that both younger and older adults have positive associations for the concept *old* and do not show signs of automatic ageism. This finding is consistent with many others that have shown people can access multiple stereotypes of elderly individuals, including positive stereotypes (Brewer et al., 1981; Brewer & Lui, 1984; Hummert, 1990; Hummert et al., 1994; Schmidt & Boland, 1986). Moreover, these findings are also in line with work on ambivalent stereotypes, which suggests that groups like elderly individuals might be disrespected but are also regarded with relative warmth (Fiske et al., 2002). Our findings are incompatible, however, with Perdue and Gurtman's (1990) conclusion of automatic ageism. We propose that their findings can be traced to the confounding of trait valence and trait stereotypicality in their stimulus set. From this perspective, their findings indicate automatic stereotyping, as observed in the present study, rather than automatic prejudice.

In light of participants' positive perceptions of elderly people, the absence of effects for SOA is not surprising. The fact that participants in the long SOA condition did not respond differently suggests that they might not have been motivated to show a different attitude even though they had more control over their responses (see Appendix, Note 2). Indeed, our own explicit measure of aging attitudes revealed only a marginal age difference, suggesting that younger and older people do not differ strongly in their views of elderly individuals and actually hold moderately favorable attitudes toward older people (Crockett & Hummert, 1987; Hummert et al., 1995).

In conclusion, the present study contributed to research on aging stereotypes by examining younger and older adults' accessibility to stereotypic and nonstereotypic traits under automatic and controlled processing situations. Our findings indicate that younger and older adults share similar mental representations or stereotypes of younger and older people. In addition, the present data show that ageism is not automatic in younger or older people, and in fact both age groups access their positive aging attitudes faster than their negative ones. Future research will need to address the conditions under which the accessibility of the concept *old* affects people's subsequent behavior toward older adults in daily life.

Acknowledgments

This research was supported in part by National Institute of Aging (NIA) National Research Service Aware Postdoctoral Fellowship 1F32AG05808 and Social Sciences and Humanities Research Council of Canada Research Grant 410-2000-0017 awarded to Alison L. Chasteen; by NIA Grant AG11715 awarded to Denise C. Park and Norbert Schwarz; and by a fellowship from the Center for Advanced Study in the Behavioral Sciences awarded to Norbert Schwarz. We thank Suzette Baez, Hajera Rostam, and Sudipa Bhattacharyya for their assistance with data collection and coding. We also thank the anonymous reviewers for their helpful comments. Denise Park is now at the Department of Psychology and Beckman Institute, University of Illinois at Urbana-Champaign.

References

Anderson, N. H. (1968). Likeableness ratings of 555 personality-trait words. *Journal of Personality and Social Psychology, 9,* 272–279.

Bargh, J. A., Chen, M., & Burrows, L. (1996). Automaticity of social behavior: Direct effects of trait construct and stereotype activation on action. *Journal of Personality and Social Psychology, 71,* 230–244.

Blair, I., & Banaji, M. (1996). Automatic and controlled processes in stereotype priming. *Journal of Personality and Social Psychology, 70,* 1142–1163.

Brewer, M. B., Dull, V., & Lui, L. (1981). Perceptions of the elderly: Stereotypes as prototypes. *Journal of Personality and Social Psychology, 41,* 656–670.

Brewer, M. B., & Lui, L. (1984). Categorization of the elderly by the elderly: Effects of perceiver's category membership. *Personality and Social Psychology Bulletin, 10,* 585–595.

Celejewski, I., & Dion, K. K. (1998). Self-perception and perception of age groups as a function of the perceiver's category membership. *International Journal of Aging and Human Development, 47,* 205–216.

Chasteen, A. L., & Pratt, J. (1999). The effect of age-related stereotypes on response initiation and execution. *Journal of General Psychology, 126,* 17–36.

Crockett, W. H., & Hummert, M. L. (1987). Perceptions of aging and the elderly. In K. W. Schaie & C. Eisdorfer (Eds.), *Annual review of gerontology and geriatrics* (Vol. 7, pp. 217–241). New York: Springer.

Fazio, R. H., Jackson, J. R., Dunton, B. C., & Williams, C. J. (1995). Variability in automatic activation as an unobtrusive measure of racial attitudes: A bona fide pipeline? *Journal of Personality and Social Psychology, 69,* 1013–1027.

Fazio, R. H., Sanbonmatsu, D., Powell, M., & Kardes, F. (1986). On the automatic activation of attitudes. *Journal of Personality and Social Psychology, 50,* 229–238.

Fiske, S. T., Cuddy, A. C., Glick, P., & Xu, J. (2002). A model of (often mixed) stereotype content: Competence and warmth respectively follow from perceived status and competition. *Journal of Personality and Social Psychology, 82,* 878–902.

Greenwald, A. G., McGhee, D. E., & Schwartz, J. L. K. 91998). Measuring individual differences in implicit cognition: The implicit association test. *Journal of Personality and Social Psychology, 74,* 1464–1480.

Hummert, M. L. (1990). Multiple stereotypes of elderly and young adults: A comparison of structure and evaluations. *Psychology and Aging, 5,* 182–193.

Hummert, M. L. 1999). A social cognitive perspective on age stereotypes. In T. M. Hess & F. Blanchard-Fields (Eds.), *Social cognition and aging* (pp. 175–196). San Diego, CA: Academic Press.

Hummert, M. L., Garstka, T. A., Shaner, J. L., & Strahm, S. (1994). Stereotypes of the elderly held by young, middle-aged, and elderly adults. *Journal of Gerontology: Psychological Sciences, 49,* P240–P249.

Hummert, M. L., Shaner, J. L., & Garstka, T. A. 91995). Cognitive processes affecting communication with older adults: The case for stereotypes, attitudes, and beliefs about communication. In J. F. Nussbaum & J. Coupland (Eds.), *The handbook of communication and aging research* (pp. 105–132). Mahwah, NJ: Erlbaum.

Jonides, J., & Mack, R. (1984). On the cost and benefit of cost and benefit. *Psychological Bulletin, 96,* 29–44.

Kawakami, K., Dion, K. L., & Dovidio, J. F. (1998). Racial prejudice and stereotype activation. *Personality and Social Psychology Bulletin, 24,* 407–416.

Kite, M. E., & Johnson, B. T. (1988). Attitudes toward older and younger adults: A meta-analysis. *Psychology and Aging, 3,* 233–244.

Kucera, H., & Francis, W. N. 91967). *Computational analysis of present day American English.* Providence, RI: Brown University Press.

Lasher, K. P., & Faulkender, P. J. (1993). Measurement of aging anxiety: Development of the anxiety about aging scale. *International Journal of Aging and Human Development, 37,* 247–259.

Levy, B. (1996). Improving memory in old age through implicit self-stereotyping. *Journal of Personality and Social Psychology, 71,* 1092–1107.

Lutsky, N. (1980). Attitudes toward old age elderly persons. In C. Eisdorfer (Ed.), *Annual review of gerontology and geriatrics* (Vol. 1, pp. 287–336). New York: Springer.

Perdue, C. W., & Gurtman, M. B. (1990). Evidence for the automaticity of ageism. *Journal of Experimental Social Psychology, 26*, 199–216.

Rothbaum, F. (1983). Aging and age stereotypes. *Social Cognition, 2*, 171–184.

Schmidt, D. F., & Boland, S. M. (1986). Structure of perceptions of older adults: Evidence for multiple stereotypes. *Psychology and Aging, 1*, 255–260.

Speas, K., & Obenshain, B. (1995). *Images of aging in America.* Washington, DC: American Association of Retired Persons.

Tajfel, H. (1981). *Human groups and social categories: Studies in social psychology.* Cambridge, England: University Press.

Wittenbrink, B., Judd, C. M., & Park, B. (1997). Evidence for racial prejudice at the implicit level and its relationship with questionnaire measures. *Journal of Personality and Social Psychology, 72*, 262–274.

Appendix

Notes

1. Additional results pertaining to the valence of the traits, which was not of concern in this analysis, can be obtained from Alison L. Chasteen.

2. It should be noted that if we had found that both younger and older adults had demonstrated age prejudice, SOA, also might not have had an effect. At present it is unclear whether individuals feel the same societal pressure to mask prejudiced feelings toward elderly people as they do for other groups (e.g., visible minorities, women). If that were the case, then no differences between SOA conditions might have been observed for that pattern of results.

3. An examination of the raw means for each subscale revealed the ratings were well over the neutral point of the two scales (Anxiety About Aging subscale, $M = .89$; Liking scale, $M = 1.91$).

[1]Department of Psychology, University of Toronto, Ontario, Canada.

[2]Department of Psychology and Institute for Social Research, University of Michigan, Ann Arbor.

Address correspondence to Alison L. Chasteen, Department of Psychology, 100 St. George Street, University of Toronto, Toronto, Ontario M5S 3G3, Canada. E-mail; chasteen@psych.utoronto.ca

The under-reported impact of age discrimination and its threat to business vitality

Abstract The Age Discrimination in Employment Act (ADEA, 29 USCA, 621) is credited with helping eliminate many blatant forms of age discrimination in employment. For example, before the ADEA was enacted 37 years ago, it was common for employment ads to list age limitations, indicating people over 40 need not apply. Across the board, mandatory retirement policies went unchallenged. Despite advancements in these areas since the founding of the Age Discrimination in Employment Act, it remains to be seen whether the ADEA has completed the job it set out to do. Has it proven to be an effective tool for eliminating the unreasonable prejudices that make it difficult for older workers to achieve their full potential? Has it provided adequate compensation for victims of discrimination? The following article takes a snapshot of the current work environment to gain a perspective. Based on extensive interviews with academics, employment lawyers, advocates for older workers, and older workers themselves, it reveals the need for reforms. It finds that, in a legal environment slanted toward employers, older workers continue to face bias and stereotyping, that most victims of discrimination are not made whole, and that society's lack of concern for this type of discrimination may prove more costly in the future as employers look more to older workers to fill projected workforce gaps.

Robert J. Grossman

School of Management, Marist College, Poughkeepsie, NY 12601, United States

1. The ADEA: an introduction

Thirty-seven years ago, Congress passed the Age Discrimination in Employment Act (ADEA) which makes it illegal for an employer or union to discharge, refuse to hire, or otherwise discriminate on the basis of age. Looking back, it is easy to forget the overt discrimination faced by older workers at the time. It was common for employment ads prior to 1967 to list age limitations, indicating people over 40 need not apply. Mandatory retirement policies, applicable to almost everyone but Supreme Court Justices, went unchallenged. Although some states had antidiscrimination laws on the books, they were not enforced, giving employers a free hand to discriminate. But now, almost four decades later, it bears asking whether the ADEA has done more than address age dis-

crimination in its most blatant manifestations. Is it really effective in preventing age bias? Has it been successful in "alleviating serious economic and psychological suffering of persons between the ages of 40 and 65 caused by unreasonable prejudice?" (Polstorff v. Fletcher (1978, ND Ala) 452 F Supp 17). What role has it played in transforming the U.S. culture to be more accepting and appreciative of older workers?

2. Stereotypes survive

Despite protestations to the contrary, there seems to be little indication that attitudes have changed significantly since the enactment of the ADEA. The notion that older people have had their day and should make room for the next generation continues to be deeply ingrained. "We think maybe it's okay because it's an economic issue, not a civil rights issue," says Laurie McCann, Senior Attorney for AARP in Washington, D.C. "Until we view it as just as wrong and serious, we may not be making the inroads we need to address the intractable, subtle discrimination that is so pervasive. I don't think employers want to discriminate; they don't hate older workers. It's the stereotypes. They may not even know they harbor these biases, but they do" (McCann, 2003).

Such attitudes are evident in the case of Ann Klingert, a 64-year-old resident of the Bronx, who recalled with astonishment the public response to an article in a local New York City newspaper regarding an EEOC lawsuit she had filed. Klingert filed with the EEOC after she was fired by Woolworths and then prohibited from applying for newly created part-time jobs which were filled mostly by student applicants. "When the lawsuit was reported in a local New York City newspaper, *Our Town,* people were outraged," she said. "They wrote letters to the editor saying things like 'why don't you just retire and just take your social security and go away'" (Klingert, 2003).

Although most employers are sensitive to the issues of sexism and racism, "the idea that you cannot teach an old dog new tricks does not seem to carry the same taboo status in society and the workplace," says Todd Maurer, Associate Professor of Industrial-Organization Psychology at the Georgia Institute of Technology. Maurer says that generalizing is dangerous in the range of older workers; perhaps even more so than in other categories. "One size does not fit all," he says. "There can be older individuals who are both interested and able when it comes to learning. Research has found large differences within older groups in things like training performance and in abilities like memory and reaction time" (Maurer, 2003). However, too often, as in the case of Maryland resident Mort Beres, employers are influenced more by stereotypes than skills or experience. When Beres, then in his late 50s, lost his job, the prior owner of small businesses and successful salesman in the auto parts manufacturing industry knew he had skills that should have been in demand, yet he was turned away repeatedly. Any offers he did receive were salaried at much less than he had earned previously, and the positions were often demeaning in nature. Beres held on as long as he could, but admitted that, out of desperation, he took some sketchy jobs. "You take every jerky job you can get just to have some income; some of them make you nauseous" (Beres, 2003).

Eventually, Beres found his niche, working as a trainer and sales rep for Irvine, California-based BDS Marketing. Assigned to the Canon account at a Best Buy in Maryland, his job was to help store personnel sell Canon printers, for which he was paid a salary plus commission. After 5 years on the job, working with a series of regional supervisors, at age 67, Beres achieved a noteworthy record by helping his store become one of the top five in the terri-

tory. However, when a new supervisor took over, Beres's star began to fall. "He'd call me and make stupid comments about my age, like 'you're too old, I think it's time for a change." Finally, Beres got the axe. When he asked why he had been fired, the manager told him, "I'm not telling you and I don't have to." Beres recalls hanging up and thinking about what had happened. "I got angry; really angry. It was a little, unimportant job, but they had no right to treat me that way." *(BDS Marketing's Vice President for Human Resources, Jeffrey Sopko, refused to comment specifically but denied Beres's version of what happened and claimed that there were other reasons for Beres's dismissal).*

Beres's plight is not uncommon, yet society appears to be less outraged at age bias than other types of discrimination. "It seems more politically correct to discriminate against older people," says Mindy Farber, Managing Partner at Farber Taylor, LL.C. in Rockville, Maryland. Farber recalls hiring a new associate for the firm who was in her mid-fifties. "It was shocking. I was surprised how open people were about talking about the wisdom of my decision in light of her age. If I had hired an African American, they would have been silent. Here they told me straight out that I had made a mistake" (Farber, 2003).

3. Perspective: how older workers see it

From their perspectives, older workers see little evidence that they are competing on a level playing field. Sixty-seven percent of employed workers aged 45 to 74 surveyed by AARP in 2003's *Staying Ahead of the Curve* said that age discrimination is a fact of life in the workplace (AARP, 2003) (Table 1). This percentage is even higher among African Americans and Hispanics, both at 72%. Age is viewed as so critical to employees that respondents listed it, along with education, as more important in how workers are treated than are gender, race, sexual orientation or religion. Sixty percent said they believe that older workers are the first to go when employers make cuts.

A 2002 Conference Board survey of 1,600 workers aged 50 and older found that 31 percent of workers intending to retire within five years said they would stay on if given more responsibilities. Twenty-five percent said they were leaving because they were being held back or marginalized because of their age (The Conference Board, 2002). Linda Barrington, Labor Economist at The Conference Board, says the high percentage of dissatisfied workers is cause for concern. "It's twice as big as I might have expected," she says. Perceptions, of course, are not necessarily reality, but Barrington says that does not matter. "Perceptions affect the way you work; if you're feeling undervalued, that discouragement will affect your work. Is it perception or reality? Either way, it has to be dealt with" (Barrington, 2003).

It also bears noting that far fewer of the respondents said they have suffered personally from ageism. About 9% say

Table 1. Workers over age 45 reporting presence of age discrimination (*n*=1500)

Do not Know	2%
No	31%
Yes	67%

Source: AARP Work and Careers Study Summary (2002).

they believe they have been passed up for a promotion because of their age, 6% said they were fired or laid off because of age, 5% said they were passed up for a raise because of age, and 15% attributed their not being hired for a job to their age. However, the survey only queried current workers and did not include individuals in the same age category who were no longer in the workforce.

4. Advantage: employers

Compared to its sister statutes aimed at race, religion, gender, and disability, the ADEA offers less protection. Court interpretations have proven to be less rigorous and more employer-friendly, ceding to employers the right to make bonafide business decisions even when age is linked. In practice, instead of preventing discrimination, the law serves as a roadmap for employers, enabling all but the obtuse to avoid liability and shield all but the most egregious ageist actions from public scrutiny.

Under the ADEA, if there is a valid reason for an action, it is considered acceptable if age happens to be an accompanying factor. "If you can show you would have done it anyway, you're off the hook," says Harlan Miller, an employment attorney with Miller, Billips, and Ates (Miller et al., 2003) in Atlanta, Georgia. As a result, it is almost impossible to catch a crafty employer discriminating. "I can always get around it if I'm smart. Only idiots get nailed," agrees David Neumark, a nationally recognized expert on the ADEA and Senior Fellow at the Public Policy Institute of California in San Francisco (Neumark, 2003).

Employers are not infallible, however, and they still mess up on occasion. Often when they do, it is because of retaliation: reacting badly to an employee whose initial complaint does not rise above the threshold set by the ADEA. "We tell them to go back and complain about their treatment," says James Rubin, an employment attorney with Farber Taylor. "Then the employer does something really bad. It's not the original claim; it's the reprisal. You can bring an action based on the reprisal even if the original claim is weak" (Rubin, 2003).

Employers also get caught when the rationale for their business decision falls apart. "Typically, the employer comes in with some kind of bogus selection process that says they're trying to keep the most competent," Miller says. "Gulfstream Aerospace's decision to cut from 200 to 230 of its nearly 2000 management-level employees during the period from August through December, 2000, is a

case in point. Gulfstream had a rating device based on flexibility and adaptability; code words for old or young…and not subject to any kind of objective analysis. Our analysis showed a complete correlation between age and those factors" (Miller et al., 2003).

On the other hand, if it is legitimate, an employer's business argument can carry the day. "Is it discrimination to fire someone if it is based on economic foundations?" asks Bob Smith, Professor of Labor Economics, ILR at Cornell University in Ithaca, New York. "It's not a slam dunk that they've been mistreated just because they say they are. There may be good reasons why they're singled out. They often are paid too much and have shorter time to work, making them a poorer investment. Why should I expect my employer to invest more in me than someone who will be there longer? Just because they complain, doesn't mean there's discrimination" (Smith, 2003).

5. Avoiding scrutiny

Employers' incentives to avoid litigation are compelling from financial and public relations perspectives. Generally, when employers get wind that employees are disgruntled and plan to complain or sue, they move to settle by enticing them into retirement with incentives and buyouts, awarded contingent upon their agreeing to confidentiality clauses that prevent discussion of the situation.

The Older Worker Protection Act clarified for employers what they need to say and do when they reach termination agreements with workers. The act requires an employer to give workers 21 days to consider a buyout proposal, to advise them of their right to seek legal counsel, and even to rescind the agreement 10 days after the fact if they have a change of heart. Until recently, a properly negotiated settlement would foreclose a former employee from further litigation. Now, there has been at least one case where the EEOC has been able to sue on behalf of workers who previously signed releases.

In a typical settlement, the employer denies discrimination, attributing the settlement to "business decisions." In a recent survey by Jury Verdict Research, plaintiffs' lawyers estimated that 84% of their clients' claims were settled, while defense lawyers reported 79% (Jury Verdict Research, 2002).

Often, employees are relieved to accept the face-saving exit. In reality, their options are meager. They are scared if they are still working or owed pensions, and lack money if they have been terminated. According to Howard Eglit, Professor of Law at Chicago-Kent College, it costs, on average, about $50,000 for a lawyer if cases go beyond early negotiations with an employer. Most attorneys will not handle such cases on a contingent basis because they know the chances of winning are slim. Employers, on average, can count on spending $100,000 in legal fees from the time a complaint is filed with the EEOC until trial (Eglit, 2003).

Although the amounts paid to ease workers into retirement or silence complaints are private, high-profile EEOC settlements reveal just how well workers actually do when they press the ADEA to the limit. In March, 2003, the EEOC announced a class action settlement with Gulfstream Aerospace, owned by General Dynamics, on behalf of 66 workers for $2.1 million dollars, an average of approximately $33,000 for each manager the EEOC claimed had been wrongfully terminated. Ninety-three percent, many of whom may never work again full-time, accepted the deal and faded away, careers in shambles.

As meager as the settlement proved to be, there would not have been a case without former Gulfstream Aerospace manager Eddie Cosper of Rincon, Georgia. His role suggests that, behind every major class action, there is an activist who serves as a catalyst in pushing for remediation.

When Gulfstream Aerospace cut more than 200 of its nearly 2000 management employees, most of whom worked in Savannah, it had not bargained on Cosper's pride and persistence. Aged 54 and with the company for 28 years, Eddie Cosper was proud, professional, and still moving up. "I was still ambitious. Every time I put out a fire, I kept getting a promotion," he recalls. However, Cosper reached a dead-end when General Dynamics took over the company in 1999. His seasoning suddenly turned sour. "The VP would tell me, 'You're like father time; you've been here forever. Wouldn't you like to retire and do something different?'" Soon Cosper found himself reassigned to nights, with responsibility for 40 people instead of the 300 he usually had. Then, 30 days later, he was terminated. "My performance reviews were all above average," he says. "I had the highest ranking of all the four managers in my category." How did he feel when his career went up in smoke? "It's like a burning sensation in your gut. You say, why me? I put my whole life into something and it's been taken away for no reason. In the beginning, I felt sorry for myself, then I got angry. I did the numbers and realized I wasn't the only older person being targeted. So I started talking to others and built a network and database." Communication was key. "People who don't have that network have no clue," he says. "Every Joe Blow could get hit cold and not know what's happening. Probably half the people in our suit were along for the ride. If I hadn't reached them, they wouldn't have realized they were discriminated against and would have gotten nothing."

The EEOC's settlement with Footlocker is another example of a remedy that fell short of the mark. When the company settled with 764 former Woolworth employees, the complainants, mostly low-paid hourly workers, walked off with an average of $4,000 per person. Overall, the $3.4 million was a small price to pay for a 40,000-worker retailing giant like Footlocker (EEOC, 2002). A tougher question is why they let the matter fester as long as they did. Many companies buy themselves out of trouble, right or wrong (Eglit,

2003). According to Jury Verdict Research, the median settlement for age cases from 1994 to 2000 was $65,000, $5,000 higher than the median reported for all types of discrimination, age included (Jury Verdict Research, 2002).

6. Complaints grow

If age discrimination had been decreasing throughout the years, even allowing for more people being aware of their right to complain and more older workers proving their mettle to those who question their ability, it would be reasonable to expect the number of complaints to be trending down. Instead, there are more cases. The EEOC logged 19,921 age discrimination complaints in 2002, an increase of 14.5% from the previous year and accounting for 23.6% of all discrimination claims filed with the agency (U.S. Equal Employment Opportunity Commission, ADEA Charges, 2003).

Some EEOC complainants, either uncertain as to the true basis of the discrimination against them or believing there is more than one basis, file multiple charges. EEOC data reveals that instances of ADEA claimants who alleged an additional type of discrimination are declining. The data suggests there is no move on the part of complainants making their case on some other basis of discrimination (gender, race, religion, or national origin) to add age simply in order to bolster the case, even though it was not thought to be the primary or even substantial basis of the discrimination. For the 3-year period of 1997 to 1999, an average of 17.9% of ADEA claimants made an additional charge. From 2000 to 2003, the average percentage dropped to 15.8%. In addition, states Farber, private lawyers are seeing similar increases in age complaints in proportion to race, gender, and disability (Farber, 2003).

Table 2. Age bias charge filings with EEOC nationwide by age group of charging parties fiscal years 1999–2002[a]

Fiscal year/age	Age 40–49	Age 50–59	Age 60–69
1999	3367	5949	3526
2000	3941	6620	4609
2001	3779	7584	4603
2002	4219	8455	5686

Source: EEOC, Office of Communications and Legislative Affairs (2003).
[a] Note: the three age ranges combined do not comprise the total ADEA charge filings with the EEOC per year, as a small number of charges which are not listed are filed by individuals 70 and older.

7. Profile

Overall, the majority of claimants tend to be white males, 55 and older at the middle management level. However, the number of women filing claims has doubled in the last few years, a trend that Eglit estimates will continue as

Table 3. Age discrimination charge filings with EEOC nationwide fiscal years 1998–2002

Year[a]	FY 1998	FY 1999	FY 2000	FY 2001	FY 2002
Discharge	7054	6733	6851	7376	8741
Harassment	1871	1758	1966	2146	2311
Hiring	1953	1647	1990	3116	4889
Layoff	1036	1149	1128	1107	1810
Promotion	1547	1590	1666	1623	1463
Terms of Employment	2510	2357	2610	3440	3181
TOTAL	15,191	14,141	16,008	17,405	19,921

Source: EEOC, Office of Communications and Legislative Affairs (2003).

[a] Fiscal years run from October 1 through September 30.

women earn more, hold more desirable jobs, and can afford to hire counsel. "The ADEA offers two essential remedies: reinstatement and back pay. If you weren't getting much and your job wasn't worth much, why sue? Now, even with the glass ceiling, women have good jobs and can afford to hire an attorney and sue" (Eglit, 2003) (Table 2).

In 2002, 53% of the cases related to job loss; wrongful discharge, 8,741 and involuntary layoff, 1,463. "They're easier to prove," Eglit says. "If you've been working at a place for 20 years, look around and see five other people fired, you have a case." (Eglit, 2003) It happened in the Woolworth's/Footlocker case, says Michelle Le-Moal-Grey, EEOC attorney. "When they were fired, workers spoke by phone and began to see a pattern forming in their store and beyond" (LeMoal-Grey, 2003).

Of the EEOC claimants between ages 40 and 69, 46% were in their fifties, 31% in their 60s and 23% in their 40s. About 25% of claims were based on failure to hire, an increase of 200% since 1999. As these cases are harder to prove and because damages are limited, it is difficult to find a private attorney for hire without having to pay up-front. "If you're not hired, how do you know what the reason was? It's not so easy to figure it out," Eglit observes (Eglit, 2003).

About 12% of the claimants cited harassment; antagonism, or intimidation, creating a hostile work environment; an increase of 31.5% since 1999. Constructive discharge would be an example, says Dorothy Stubblebine, an expert witness for both plaintiffs and defendants, and President of DJS Associates in Mantua, New Jersey. "Tyically, the older person is pushed out by giving him a really hard time. He's given the worst assignments 'til he can't take it any more" (Stubblebine, 2003) (Table 3).

8. Chances for success

Whatever the claim and whomever the claimant, few gamblers would bet on the probability of prevailing in an ADEA suit. EEOC data reveals that for most claimants, the filing with the EEOC is a dead-end. Last year, of the

cases before it, the agency found "reasonable cause" only 4.3% of the time, "no reasonable cause" 52% of the time, and closed cases for "administrative" reasons 33.5% of the time. Only 6.5% of cases were eventually settled. In contrast, for claimants charging all types of discrimination, age included, the EEOC found reasonable cause 7.2% of the time, found no reasonable cause 59.3% of the time, and closed cases for administrative reasons 26% of the time (U.S. Equal Employment Opportunity Commission, 2003) (Tables 4 and Table 5).

For plaintiffs who win at trial, damages are legally limited to reinstatement, loss of pay, or, where there is a finding of willful discrimination, double the lost salary. In contrast, race and gender plaintiffs have the opportunity to be awarded more lucrative punitive damages. "Why shouldn't someone who's old be compensated for pain and suffering just like someone who's fired for their religion, race, or gender?" Miller asks. "There's nothing worse than, after 30 years' service, to be fired at 58" (Miller et al., 2003).

The solution for many attorneys is to bypass the ADEA and, where possible, sue under local or state statutes. "Everybody tries to stay out of Federal Court," Farber says. "Plaintiffs get their audience but they lose before they can get to a jury. It's so bad that a fellow attorney once told me that if I went to Federal Court when there were other options available, I would be guilty of malpractice." Farber says a plaintiff's chances to reach a jury brighten considerably in state or local courts. Virtually everyone on a jury can identify with the plight of an older worker. "Everybody on the jury is getting older and has a mother and father" (Farber, 2003).

If they get to a state or federal jury, Jury Verdict Research in its study, *Employment Practice Liability: Jury Award Trends and Statistics,* reports a 78% success rate overall for age cases in 2000. In Federal District Courts, from 1994 to 2000, the median verdict was $269,350, tops for all types of discrimination. However, the chances of plaintiffs getting there with the EEOC in their corner are limited. The

Table 4.   EEOC resolution of ADEA claims fiscal years 1998–2002

	FY 1998	FY 1999	FY 2000	FY 2001	FY 2002
Total ADEA Claims	15,191.	14,141	16,008	17,405	19,921
Settlements (%)	4.7	5.3	7.9	6.6	6.5
Withdrawals with benefits (%)	3.6	3.7	3.8	3.6	3.6
Administrative closures (%)	26.1	23.3	22.0	26.1	33.5
No reasonable cause (%)	61.7	59.4	58.0	55.3	52.1
Reasonable cause (%)	3.9	8.3	8.2	8.2	4.3

Source: EEOC, Office of Research, Information, and Planning (2003).

Table 5.   EEOC resolution of all discrimination claims fiscal years 1998–2002

	FY 1998	FY 1999	FY 2000	FY 2001	FY 2002
Total Claims	79,591	77,444	79,896	80,840	84,442
Settlements (%)	4.6	6.2	8.5	8.1	8.8
Withdrawals with benefits (%)	3.2	3.7	4.0	4.1	4
Administrative closures (%)	26.7	24.1	20.5	20.7	20.6
No reasonable cause (%)	60.9	59.5	58.3	57.2	59.3
Reasonable cause (%)	4.6	6.6	8.8	9.9	7.2

Source: EEOC, Office of Research, Information, and Planning (2003).

Office of General counsel states that during the 5-year period from 1997 to 2001, the EEOC filed 205 lawsuits based on the ADEA, leaving plaintiffs who push ahead with claims the EEOC determines are without merit with the risk and expense of proceeding toward litigation on their own (Office of General Counsel, 2002). Jury Verdict Research indicates that the median verdict for more numerous privately initiated state cases was about the same (Jury Verdict Research, 2002).

9. Justification

Critics point out that there may be valid reasons for determining that older workers are less desirable employees. There is no question that technological changes have significantly altered the way we work, especially in white-collar jobs, explains Camille Olson, Chair of the Labor and Employment Practice Group, Seyfeith Shaw, in Chicago, Illinois. "Persons in their 20s and 30s who are comfortable with technology are more responsive and more adaptable to change. Can people in their 40s and 50s without this background feel that they belong in the workplace? You feel that time has passed you by. Does that affect your motivation, your ability to do things? It does" (Olson, 2003).

"A lot of people who think they've been screwed over have it wrong," agrees AARP's McCann. "Though I'm an advocate, I'd be the first to admit that when someone gets

fired or doesn't get promoted, they yell foul. An age discrimination claim is the last resort for older white males. "If you're a 55 year old male who's lost your $70,000 job, what do you do? The odds of finding any job, let alone a comparable job, are slim, so you fight" (McCann, 2003).

"If a person has lost a step or two and doesn't project or have the kind of energy to move forward, the fact that he isn't promoted may show that's where he belongs," explains Ed King, Executive Director of the National Senior Citizen Law Center, a former EEOC mediator in Hawaii. "The question is whether the employer is stereotyping or it is legitimate" (King, 2003).

It is undeniable that age has its advantages; plusses that advocates for older workers tend to downplay. "They do better; get paid more. Their employment rates are high and they get cared for in retirement," Neumark observes. However, he says, it is not all roses and caviar for workers in their 50s or 60s. Once they are unemployed, it is hard for them to find work. They are out of work longer, have difficulty finding jobs with comparable responsibilities and wages, and tend to become disheartened and "retire" (Neumark, 2003).

Adding to the debate is the difference of opinion as to whether age 40, which seemed appropriate in the 1960s, should still be the turning point for providing a person with ADEA coverage. Some experts ask, Why not? There needs to be some beginning point, and 40 is reasonable.

Others disagree, arguing that 45 or 50 are more realistic ages when discriminatory treatment is most likely to occur. Whatever the threshold, it has been clear until recently that all people from 40 on up had to be treated similarly, but no longer.

In an opinion issued February 24, 2004, on General Dynamics Land Systems versus Cline, the U.S. Supreme Court held that the ADEA does not prevent an employer from favoring older employees over younger employees. The court upheld an agreement between General Dynamics and the United Auto Workers union that provided for continued retirement health benefits for employees then over 50 years of age but eliminated that benefit for all other employees. The plaintiffs were between the ages of 40 and 50, and were denied the benefits available only to workers over the age of 50.

10. No special treatment

Should an employer invest extra to help support an older worker? Offer more and different training? Provide less stressful assignments? The issue, Olson says, is whether under the ADEA an employer needs to take affirmative efforts to assist individuals who do not naturally have the same skills, while at the same time paying them more. Clearly, Olson says, the law never contemplated affirmative action. The law is there only to make sure older people are not treated differently (Olson, 2003).

"The ADEA is about equal treatment, not about preferential treatment," agrees Lynn Clemens, Attorney, Office of Legal Counsel at EEOC. "There are no affirmative obligations on the employer's part. That notion goes against the act." Regardless, advocates are making the case that there are other benefits to be gained by retaining older workers anyway, although they are paid more and have fewer skills. Olson says she does not buy it unless there is a compelling business case. "The issue is whether you need to invest in targeted training, making older workers more productive because you need them to stick around" (Olson, 2003).

11. Call for action

Meanwhile, William Rothwell, Professor of Workforce Education and Development at Penn State University observes that Bureau of Labor Statistics projections show that while 13 percent of American workers today are 55 and older, that figure will increase to 20% by the year 2015. At the same time, the nation is expected to experience a drop in the percentage of younger workers aged 25 to 44.

With this information in mind, Rothwell says the current economic slump is the calm before the storm. When the economy turns around and there is more demand for products and services, the worker shortage will be the number one issue. "Employers in the U.S. will be forced to go back to their retiree base and deploy it more effectively than ever before. If we can't get labor from anywhere else, we'll look to the most obvious population who knows everything about our business" (Rothwell, 2003).

Unless we get serious about addressing the stereotypes and focus on reducing the alienation that older workers feel, these workers, as well as retirees, may be unreceptive and unprepared to step up when the market finally swings in their favor. Reforming the ADEA is the first step. To better combat age discrimination, we must move quickly to put more teeth into the law. If we do not, when we go to the well, it may just be dry.

References

AARP. (2003). *Staying ahead of the curve.*

Barrington, L. (2003 April 10). Telephone interview. New York, NY.

Beres M. (2003 April 22). Telephone interview. Rockville, MD.

EEOC Press Release. (2002, November 15). *EEOC settles major age bias suit; foot locker to pay $3.5 million to former Woolworth employees.*

Eglit, H. (2003 April 10). Telephone interview. Chicago, IL.

Farber, M. (2003 April 21). Telephone interview. Rockville, MD.

Jury Verdict Research. (2002). *Employment practice liability verdicts and settlements: Jury award trends and statistics.*

King, E. (2003 April 15). Telephone interview. Washington, D.C.

Klingert, A. (2003 May 1). Telephone interview. Bronx, NY.

LeMoal-Grey, M. (2003 April 28). Telephone interview. New York, NY.

Maurer, T. (2003 April 17). Telephone interview. Atlanta, GA.

McCann, L. (2003 April 17). Telephone interview. Washington, D.C.

Miller, Harlan, Principal, Miller, Billips & Ates. (2003). Atlanta, GA. (18 April).

Neumark, D. (2003 April 8). Telephone interview. San Francisco, CA.

Office of General Counsel. (2002, August 13). The U.S. Equal Employment Opportunity Commission. *Study of the litigation program fiscal years 1997–2001*, Table 2.

Olson, C. (2003 April 10). Telephone interview. Chicago, IL.

Rothwell, W. (2003 April 17). Telephone interview. University Park, PA.

Rubin, J. (2003 April 21). Telephone interview. Rockville, MD.

Smith, B. (2003 April 17). Telephone interview. Ithaca, NY.

Stubblebine, D. (2003 April 4). Telephone interview. Mantua, NJ.

Article 15. The under-reported impact of age discrimination and its threat to business vitality

The Age Discrimination in Employment Act of 1967. (1967). Pub. L. 90–202, as amended. Volume 29 of the United States Code beginning at section 621.

The Conference Board. (2002). *Voices of experience: Mature workers in the future workplace.*

United States Supreme Court. (2004, February 24). *General Dynamics Land Systems,* v. cline, No. 02–1080.

U.S. Equal Employment Opportunity Commission. (2003). *Age discrimination in employment act charges,* FY 1992-FY 2002.

UNIT 4

Problems and Potentials of Aging

Unit Selections

Key Points to Consider

- Why do doctors find it so hard to treat older patients?

- How is a recent Supreme Court ruling going to affect an employer's discrimination against older workers?

- What were the problems outlined that were leading to an increase in divorce among older persons?

- Is the downward regression of Alzheimer's patients' mental abilities consistent and predictable or are there periodic fluctuations? Explain.

Student Website

www.mhcls.com/online

Internet References

Further information regarding these websites may be found in this book's preface or online.

Alzheimer's Association
   http://www.alz.org
A.P.T.A. Section on Geriatrics
   http://geriatricspt.org
Caregiver's Handbook
   http://www.acsu.buffalo.edu/~drstall/hndbk0.html
Caregiver Survival Resources
   http://www.caregiver.com
AARP Health Information
   http://www.aarp.org/bulletin
International Food Information Council
   http://www.ific.org/
University of California at Irvine: Institute for Brain Aging and Dementia
   http://www.alz.uci.edu/

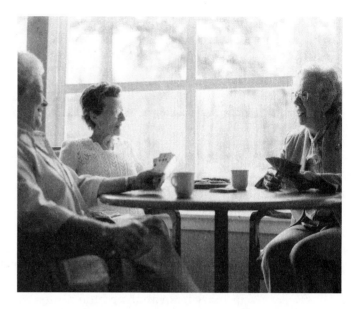

Viewed as part of the life cycle, aging might be considered a period of decline, poor health, increasing dependence, social isolation, and—ultimately—death. It often means retirement, decreased income, chronic health problems, and death of a spouse. In contrast, the first 50 years of life are seen as a period of growth and development.

For a young child, life centers around the home, and then the neighborhood. Later, the community and state become a part of the young person's environment. Finally, as an adult, the person is prepared to consider national and international issues—wars, alliances, changing economic cycles, and world problems.

During the later years, however, life space narrows. Retirement may distance the individual from national and international concerns, although he or she may remain actively involved in community affairs. Later, even community involvement may decrease, and the person may begin to stay close to home and the neighborhood. For some, the final years of life may once again focus on the confines of home, be it an apartment or a nursing home.

Many older Americans try to remain masters of their own destinies for as long as possible. They fear dependence and try to avoid it. Many are successful at maintaining independence and the right to make their own decisions. Others are less successful and must depend on their families for care and to make critical decisions. However, some older people are able to overcome the difficulties of aging and to lead comfortable and enjoyable lives.

In "Primary Care for Elderly People: Why Do Doctors Find It So Hard?" the authors point out that geriatric patients often have multiple and compounding adverse medical events that are much more difficult to diagnose and treat than the single illness that most patients seeking medical attention are experiencing.

In "Breakthrough," David Newman points out that older workers filing a discrimination suit against an employer no longer have to prove that they were singled out for unfair treatment but rather that they were the victim of a policy that caused harm to older workers. Jeffrey Zaslow, in "Will You Still Need Me When I'm...84? More Couples Divorce After Decades," examines the reason for the increase in the number of divorces for couples sixty years of age and older.

Alzheimer's disease destroys brain cells controlling memory, communication, reasoning, and behavior, as well as physical control of the body. In "The Disappearing Mind," Geoffrey Cowley describes the current scientific findings of the causes of Alzheimer's disease and the current state of research on possible cures for the disease. In "Alzheimer's Disease as a 'Trip Back in Time'," the authors develop a model to help caregivers working with Alzheimer's patients to understand their wide variations in mood, memory, and behavior.

Primary Care for Elderly People: Why Do Doctors Find It So Hard?

Wendy L. Adams, MD, MPH,[1] Helen E. McIlvain, PhD,[1] Naomi L. Lacy, PhD,[1] Homa Magsi, MD,[1] Benjamin F. Crabtree, PhD,[2] Sharon K. Yenny, RNP, MS,[3] and Michael A. Sitorious, MD,[1]

Purpose: Many primary care physicians find caring for elderly patients difficult. The goal of this study was to develop a detailed understanding of why physicians find primary care with elderly patients difficult. *Design and Method:* We conducted in-depth interviews with 20 primary care physicians. Using an iterative approach based on grounded theory techniques, a multidisciplinary team analyzed the content of the interviews and developed a conceptual model of the difficulty. *Results:* Three major domains of difficulty emerged: (i) medical complexity and chronicity, (ii) personal and interpersonal challenges, and (iii) administrative burden. The greatest challenge occurred when difficulty in more than one area was present. Contextual conditions, such as the practice environment and the physicians's training and personal values, shaped the experience of providing care and how difficult it seemed. *Implications:* Much of the difficulty participants experienced could be facilitated by changes in the health care delivery system and in medical education. The voices of these physicians and the model resulting from our analysis can inform such change.

Key Words: Primary health care, Health services for the aged

America is in the midst of a major demographic shift that will have repercussions for health care for some time to come (Manton & Vaupel, 1995). Currently, people aged 65 and older account for 30–40% of primary care physician visits (Schappert, 1999; Stafford et al., 1999; U.S. Bureau of the Census, 1996). As the rapid aging of the population continues toward its projected midcentury plateau, general internists and family physicians will be called upon to provide primary care to an increasing volume of elderly patients. At present, many of these physicians are unwilling or unable to do so. Surveys of primary care physicians show that between 30% and 50% limit the number of elderly patients they admit to their practices (AARP, 1995; Cykert, Kissling, Layson, & Hansen, 1995; Damiano, Momany, Willard, & Jogerst, 1997; Geiger & Krol, 1991; Lee & Gillis, 1993; Lee & Gillis, 1994). To meet the primary care needs of the aging population, researchers and policy makers must understand and respond to this phenomenon.

There have been surprisingly few attempts to determine the reasons physicians limit the number of elderly patients in their practices, and results have been inconsistent. Studies have focused on concerns with Medicare fees and documentation requirements, which clearly are sources of frustration for physicians (Cykert et al., 1995; Geiger & Krol, 1991). However, frustration with Medicare seems to explain only a small part of physicians' willingness to provide care to elderly patients. In one survey of primary care physicians, 65% reported that low Medicare fees were a very important problem in their practices, but this did not predict whether or not they limited the number of Medicare patients they accepted (Damiano et al., 1997). Some demographic variables are associated with practice limitation, including primary care specialty (Lee & Gillis, 1993; Lee & Gillis, 1994), urban location (Cykert et al., 1995), and type of practice (solo, single specialty, or multispecialty; Cykert et al., 1995). Studies have generally not measured psychosocial or practice level variables that

Table 1. Characteristics of Participants

Characteristic	Internists (n = 10)	Family Physicians (n = 10)
Age, mean (range)	44.9 (32-69)	49.5 (35-70)
Years since board certification, mean (range)	14.1 (2-37)	14.7 (4-26)
Female, %	60	90
Urban location, %	90	70
Practice 65 or older, mean percent (range)	57 (25-100)	32.8 (15-65)
Size of group	solo practice: 1	solo practice: 2
	2-5 physician group: 5	2-5 physician group: 2
	> 5 physician group: 4	> 5 physician group: 6
Do nursing home practice, %	60	70
Nursing home medical directors, %	40	10

might contribute to physicians' perceived need to limit geriatric practice and no previous qualitative studies have addressed these issues.

Though data are sparse, there are suggestions in the literature that primary care physicians find elderly patients more difficult to treat (Damiano et al., 1997). This may have to do with medical training. In a national survey, only 60% of general and/or family practice physicians and 50% of general internists felt that their formal medical training did a good or excellent job of preparing them to manage care needs for frail elders (Cantor, Baker, & Hughes, 1993). Another survey of primary care physicians in Virginia found that fewer than half thought their current geriatric knowledge was adequate (Perez, Mulligan, & Myers, 1991). Characteristics of the health care system may also contribute to physicians' willingness to provide care to elders. In a survey of Canadian family physicians, respondents endorsed poor reimbursement, time pressure, and inadequate community resources all as sources of frustration in caring for older patients (Pereles & Russell, 1996). Although these studies suggest potential contributors to physicians' limitations on practice with elderly patients, a detailed understanding of the problems physicians encounter in geriatric primary care and a clear direction for change are sorely needed.

Given the paucity of data in this area, a research approach that allows in-depth examination of physicians' perspectives is needed. To gain a deeper, more detailed understanding of the key issues, we conducted a qualitative study that explored how physicians view providing primary care to elderly people. This article focuses on the theme that most consistently pervaded the interviews: the increased difficulty of primary care with elderly patients. We present a conceptual model, developed from these data, which suggests vital areas to be addressed to ensure that primary care of elderly people meets current and future needs.

Methods

Design and Participants

We conducted a qualitative in-depth interview study with a diverse sample of 20 practicing general internists and family physicians. The first two respondents were physicians known by one of the authors to have busy internal medicine practices with a relatively high proportion of elderly patients. Subsequently, we selected physicians practicing in the vicinity of Omaha, Nebraska, from a database maintained in the Chancellor's office at the University of Nebraska Medical Center comprising demographic information about all physicians practicing in the state. We used a maximum variation sampling strategy (Kuzel, 1999), in which we selected physicians from the list by gender, age, and specialty to compile a sample representing both men and women, internists and family practitioners, and a wide age range. We approached physicians by an introductory letter followed up by a telephone call. In all, we contacted 141 physicians to recruit the 20 participants.

Demographic and practice information about participants is shown in Table 1. Of the 20 participants recruited, 19 were White and 1 was Hispanic. Eight were women. Ages ranged from 32 to 70 years. Three respondents limited the number of elderly patients they accept into their practices; all three were busy internists with a high volume of elderly patients. In this article, a code letter has been randomly assigned to identify participants.

Procedure

Two of the authors (W. A. and H. M.), both physicians, conducted in-depth interviews (Crabtree & Miller, 1999) with the participants. The average interview lasted 50 min, with a range from 30 to 120 min. Participants appeared to respond in an equally open and forthcoming way to both interviewers. We examined interview content for systematic differences in responses to the different interviewers and were unable to detect any. We were also unable to detect any systematic differences between the responses of the two participants who were previously acquainted with the interviewer and the others, who were not. The interview questions were broad and open ended. We invited the participants to relate personal narratives regarding experiences with geriatric primary care with the initial "grand tour" question: "Please tell me about some of your experiences taking care of elderly people." We then asked them to relate both satisfying and frustrating experiences. The existing literature suggests certain topics important for physician satisfaction that may relate to their views on care of elderly patients. If these did not come up spontaneously, we asked participants to comment on them. We used such prompts for reimbursement issues (Cykert et al. 1995; Damiano et al., 1997; Lee & Gillis, 1993; Lee & Gillis, 1994), time pressure (Burdi & Baker, 1999; Lewis, Prout, Chalmers, & Leake, 1991; Linn, Yager, Cope, & Leake, 1985; Linzer et al., 2000; Mawardi, 1979), confidence in addressing geriatric syndromes (Cantor, Baker, & Hughes, 1993; Perez, Mulligan & Myers, 1991), community resources for elderly patients (Pereles & Russell, 1996; Siu & Beck, 1990), the doctor–older patient relationship (Adelman, Greene, & Ory, 2000; Bates, Harris, Tierney, & Wolinsky, 1998; Greene, 1993; McMurray et al., 1997; Roter, 1991), and frailty and death (Krakowski, 1982; Morrison, Morrison, & Glickman, 1994). We asked the physicians to describe how the doctor–patient relationship was different with older and younger patients. Other questions did not ask physicians to compare and contrast experiences with older and younger patients, but they frequently made such comparisons when discussing their experiences.

Analysis

We audiotaped and transcribed interviews verbatim. A multidisciplinary team including 2 physicians, a nurse practitioner, a medical anthropologist, a medical sociologist, and a psychologist then analyzed these data. We used a three-stage coding process derived from the sociologic tradition of grounded theory (Strauss & Corbin, 1998). In the initial *open coding* stage, each team member independently read each transcript several times and marked key phrases, terms, or sentences. We then met and discussed the interviews in detail, sharing insights from our various disciplines and assigning topical codes to the text of the interviews. We grouped these codes into categories as it became evident which concepts were emerging as keys to understanding physicians' perspectives on primary care with elderly patients. As the analysis proceeded, we compared the content of each new interview to the existing categories and the coding modified accordingly. In the *axial coding* phase, we developed the categories further and began to define the relationships among them and their possible implications. In the final *selective coding* process, we developed the conceptual model that is presented here.

We used several techniques common to qualitative research to ensure that standards of rigor were met. To maximize the trustworthiness of our data collection and analysis, we continued recruiting participants until no new major themes were emerging (Patton, 1990). In the process of developing codes and interpreting the data, the diversity of the team kept one point of view from dominating and biasing the results (Creswell, 1998; Lincoln & Guba, 1985). We also routinely searched for disconfirming evidence in the interviews, (Patton, 1990). We conducted follow-up interviews, also known as *member checking* (Lincoln & Guba, 1985), with 5 of our participants. In these interviews, we gave participants written descriptions of the categories of difficulty and contextual conditions we had developed in the analysis process. In the last member checking interview, we presented the evolving conceptual model, similar to Figure 1 in this article. We then asked for discussion and feedback. Although not every point of difficulty was important to every physician, all strongly confirmed the importance of the increased difficulty and the appropriateness of the categories of difficulty presented here.

Results

Overview

Most participants enjoyed their interactions with older patients and emphasized that advanced patient age alone was not problematic. All, however, related experiencing increased difficulty in caring for elderly patients, which fell into three major domains: (i) medical complexity and chronicity, especially patients' vulnerability to adverse events; (ii) personal and interpersonal challenges, including time pressure, communication problems, and ethical dilemmas; and (iii) administrative burden, including more telephone calls and paperwork as well as Medicare's documentation requirements. As illustrated in Figure 1, these categories overlap and interact. For example, a medically complex situation may lead to nursing home placement, which challenges the doctor–patient–family relationship and increases administrative burden. Figure 1 also illustrates that the difficulty was experienced in the context of the practice environment and seen in the light of the personal characteristics of the physician. Although

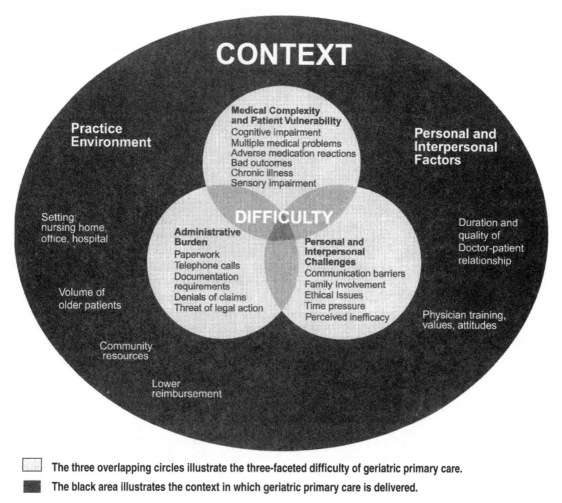

The three overlapping circles illustrate the three-faceted difficulty of geriatric primary care.

The black area illustrates the context in which geriatric primary care is delivered.

Figure 1. The difficulty of primary care for older people and its context.

the nature of the difficulty was similar for physicians with small and large volumes of elderly patients, it had more impact on physicians with a high volume.

The Nature of the Difficulty

Medical Complexity and Vulnerability to Adverse Events. —Elderly patients were seen as medically more difficult to care for than younger people. They had more medical conditions, and their illnesses often presented atypically. They were more likely to become seriously ill and were vulnerable to rapid declines in their condition. Multiple medications and the risk of adverse medication reactions also contributed to the difficulty. Participants described diagnostic and therapeutic uncertainty as well as anxiety about causing unintended harm to patients. An internist who had inherited a large volume of elderly patients from a retiring colleague remarked, "There problems were kind of special compared with the general medical population.... The thing that impressed me the most is, their homeostatic mechanisms didn't leave much room for goof-ups" (Dr. C). Another internist described a patient's adverse drug reaction: "I thought, here is something I have done to hurt this patient by giving him this medicine.... What other things can I do to hurt people?... In a lot of ways you've got to be very careful with things" (Dr. I).

Elderly patients often have chronic conditions with symptoms that are difficult to control. "In general, they have more things wrong with them and in general, they're on way more medication and in general, they don't feel good most of the time and they don't sleep at night and they are deteriorating... " (Dr. P). This can lead to a disinclination to see these patients:

> Every time they come in something's aching or hurting or... "My back's a little sore" or "I'm a little stiff, I don't have the energy I used to," "Well, maybe I'm a little depressed." Sometimes they get to be those people that you look at the list and go, "Ah-h-h-h, doggone, that name again" (Dr. E).

Many participants described frustration at their perceived inability to help with older patients' chronic conditions. One family physician related,

No matter what you do, they hurt. No matter what you do, they get agitated. And no drug exists to stop a cognitively impaired patient from falling. You know, yeah, that's frustrating. You bet it is. But hey, somebody needs to take care of these folks (Dr. I.).

An internist reported,

You know, there are some patients that they're always going to have the same problems year after year after year. They're not going to be fixed. You know, it's their back pain from their osteoporosis and scoliosis and you can't do anything about it, or they may be a little depressed, but they won't take any medicine, and they're chronically constipated and, you know, sometimes those are the most frustrating (Dr. O).

Medical complexity also had a positive side. Several participants enthusiastically told of satisfying experiences in which they had made a difficult diagnosis and helped patients substantially. Regarding a 96-year-old woman with an atypical presentation of ischemic heart disease, a family physician remarked,

I was able to stabilize her in the hospital, get her feeling good and actually took care of her for another two years or so.... She was so grateful that I had been able to find what was wrong with her, and she became a very dear patient to me... so that was a really good experience (Dr. J).

Adjusting to the increased prevalence of chronic illness and the relative infrequency of cures requires a change of outlook on the physician's part. One young internist seemed to be in the midst of this process when she related,

But then I was thinking, I need to think of it in a different frame of mind. More of maybe getting them to understand that this is a chronic problem and what can we do to make them feel better as opposed to fix them. (Dr. O).

This may be an adjustment that not all physicians are able to make. Regarding caring for cognitively impaired patients, Dr. I. said,

I mean in general, there's not a lot that medicine can do about that. Our interventions are somewhat limited, so this just adds to this area of medicine. It takes a special kind of mind set, a special kind of provider to grapple with those on a day-to-day basis.

Personal and Interpersonal Challenges. —Communication barriers, especially those resulting from hearing problems or cognitive impairment, contributed to difficulties with history taking, treatment, and the quality of the relationship. One physician remarked, "[There are] lots of various obstacles to getting the whole story, getting the truth out and sometimes 'cause they don't remember and sometimes they just don't think it's important and sometimes they're just in denial of what's really wrong" (Dr. P). Another commented, "It's sometimes frustrating when you've got an older person who can't hear and won't wear hearing aids and you know, you have to shout so loud that everyone else in the building hears everything you say to them" (Dr. J).

Families often became involved in the care of frail elders. For the physicians we interviewed, this had both positive and negative implications. Involved family members increased the safety of medication use and the home environment. However, their participation increased the length of office visits, the complexity of the doctor–patient relationship, and the difficulty of decision making. Friction with families sometimes arose when it was unclear whose responsibility it was to provide personal care:

You know, I don't mind dealing with it as long as the family is going to deal with it too. If they act like it's all my problem to deal with Mom or Dad and figure out, you know, a solution at home for care and you know, that's what's irritating because that's not my responsibility (Dr. G).

When older patients were unsafe driving or living alone but wished to continue to do so, the need to balance safety and autonomy was sometimes difficult.

It's usually a struggle between the family wanting them to move to a more supervised level of care or out of their home and the... parents not wanting to do that, so it's usually a negotiating process, usually a slow process (Dr. Q).

On the whole, physicians found caring for elderly patients who are dying one of the most important and meaningful aspects of practice. Most, however, had experienced serious conflicts with family members in this area. One related,

The most difficult thing... is just the actual end of life issue when the patient is in the hospital and you have a family there, and the family doesn't get along, and then trying to be a mediator within the family to get some kind of good consensus (Dr. K).

Physicians were challenged to examine their values and balance them with the family's.

When you internally feel like a family member is making decisions on behalf of the patient that are maybe prolonging the patient's misery... then we are kind of put into the awkward position of having to carry out what they want (Dr. L).

These decisions are frequently emotionally charged. "Our culture is so afraid of death, that usually it isn't that peaceful. It's just wrought with being torn apart by just an incredible amount of argument and bickering between family members. It's terrible" (Dr. P).

Time pressure was a major issue for participants with a large volume of elderly patients. "That's probably the biggest problem I have right now, is managing my time with the older individuals" (Dr. A). Medical complexity, family involvement, ethical decision making, and communication barriers all made caring for frail elders more time consuming. History taking was slower, physical examinations took longer, and mobility impairment slowed down the flow of office activities. Medicare's extensive documentation requirements and lengthy claims processing also make heavy demands on the physicians' time, so do paperwork and phone calls from home health agencies and nursing homes. "[If you see 15 elderly people] it takes time. You feel like you've done a big day's work. You can see 15 young people with sore throats and be done in an hour" (Dr. M). In the current health care environment, where efficiency is highly valued, this presents a major difficulty for physicians. "You have to have sheer volume with Medicare patients but Medicare patients also require most of your time because they need so much, so it's a hard situation out there" (Dr. I).

Administrative Burden. —Nearly all of the physicians felt they spent too much time, effort, and worry on Medicare regulations. Claims were often denied for apparently trivial reasons and resubmitting them requried substantial personnel time. In some situations, "The amount of return is less than the effort made in acquiring the reimbursement" (Dr. Q). Medicare regulations seemed particularly frustrating because they did not seem to relate to the quality of care.

> It has nothing to do with the care the patient got.... You go through a whole long physical exam of stuff that is irrelevant really to the problem at hand,... and spend more time on the paperwork than you do taking care of the patient. And so that's extremely frustrating as well as stupid (Dr. M).

The threat of legal action from Medicare adds additional anxiety to geriatric primary care:

> You wake up in the middle of the night in a cold sweat thinking, "Oh my God! The Office of Inspector General showed up at my office today

and wants to go through every file in my charts!" So it's sobering to know what Medicare could do to you and your practice if they chose to. And I'm of the opinion they could probably find improper documentation/coding/billing in every office in this country (Dr. L).

In general, Medicare was seen in an adversarial light, increasing the burden of providing primary care to older patients.

Multifaceted Complexity

In the initial coding process, complexity and difficulty were noted in all 20 interviews. As we returned to the data for the axial coding process, it was evident that participants rarely felt overwhelmed by difficulty in one area alone. In every interview, however, there was a discussion of at least one situation where an elderly patient's medical needs overlapped with psychosocial and/or administrative difficulty. These were the situations in which caring for older patients became seriously problematic. "It's just that you have a number of these things happening all at the same time. Physicians are human. It wears on you" (Dr. N). When considering Figure 1 in a member-checking interview, one participant remarked,

> This helps me understand why these patients are so hard. It's OK if they just have difficulty in one of these areas, but when there's more than one, and especially in that area (pointing to the model) where they have all three, the difficulty is exponential, or logarithmic or something (Dr. B).

Contextual Conditions

The three-faceted difficulty presented above occurred within the context of the practice environment. There was also a context of personal and interpersonal factors. For instance, a complex medical situation that occurred within the context of a long-term doctor–patient relationship was perceived differently from a complex medical situation in the context of a new relationship. Various constellations of these contextual conditions shaped the experience of providing care and how difficult it seemed. In Figure 1, the larger circle represents this context.

Personal and Interpersonal Factors. —All participants found elderly patients more grateful and appreciative than younger patients. Some also enjoyed hearing their stories and experiencing their wisdom. For many, this mitigated the difficulty of their care.

> I enjoy taking care of elderly patients, mostly for the personal interaction with them as opposed to their medical problems. I would look at the med-

ical care of those individuals to be a little more cumbersome than younger people from an operational standpoint. It's harder to do things, more difficult. But the interaction with the individuals is more rewarding I would say (Dr. Q).

When patients are severely cognitively impaired, on the other hand, the limited relationship often made the care seem meaningless. One internist related,

> The very severe cognitively impaired people,... I don't find any particular satisfaction in taking care of them. Whatever was... the essence of their humanity is long since gone and I'm tending to a body, which has no hope of recovery and it's hard for me to get real excited and enthusiastic in that setting (Dr. B).

A family physician said, "You have to tell them the same thing every visit. And they don't remember you. It eliminates some of the camaraderie, if you will, with the patient. That's inevitable" (Dr. L).

Physicians' personal characteristics, values, and training also affected how they viewed geriatric primary care. For instance, older physicians felt closer to their elderly patients:

> I'm not exactly young myself anymore and so I guess I have a fair amount of good feeling towards the elderly. It's easier for me to identify with somebody who is 75 and has lived through some of the things they lived through or the depression, World War II, raising children, than a very young person with an earring in their nose and ear and their lip and I'm not sure I have much in common with that person (Dr. H).

Some participants felt a social obligation to care for nursing home patients, whereas others did not.

> It's not that much fun but I just feel like it's something that I have to do for society, part of my job. I could never do that as a full-time job or even have a larger practice in a nursing home (Dr. G).

The Practice Environment. —Certain aspects of the practice environment facilitated or hindered caring for elderly patients. The volume of older patients in the practice had a major impact on how the difficulty was experienced and whether the participant was limiting or was planning to limit the number of new elderly patients. Physicians with a high volume of older patients found it more difficult to incorporate their complex care into the usual flow of work. One internist who had currently cut back her practice related,

> The patients are so complex and they take so much time sometimes and they have side effects from medications and phone calls, that yeah, you get overwhelmed. It's just not physically, humanly possible. It just isn't. You would need to have a smaller patient population to do a good job (Dr. P).

The roles of office staff members and their relationships with the physician and each other also affected how well they were able to cope with a high volume of elderly patients. One geriatrician remarked, "[Nurses] can make you or break you. I mean, if they left, I'd have to leave" (Dr. A).

Community resources were generally perceived as inadequate. None of our participants had ready access to social workers in the office, so arranging home health care, adult daycare, and other community services added to the difficulty of primary care.

> You know, there's no one place, no one clearing house that you can go for those kind of services. You just have to kind of make a patchwork quilt almost of that. It'd be nice to have someplace where you can have one phone call... and say, here's my patient's needs, what can you provide for us? (Dr. C).

Caring for patients in nursing homes was generally regarded as difficult and unpleasant. Prominent difficulties with nursing home care included the logistics of providing care, communication with nursing home staff, and dysfunctional regulations.

> Their regulations are ridiculous, you know, especially the one where they have to call you if somebody scrapes their elbow. Nursing home visits usually aren't the most stimulating... and you have to sift through charts that you're not familiar with and where anything is and I don't know (Dr G).

Although caring for frail elders is difficult and time consuming, Medicare reimbursement is lower than private insurance. Low fees did not contribute to the difficulty of geriatric primary care, but clearly influenced how physicians responded to it.

> If you told me that I had to run this place on the basis of what I get from Medicare, I would have to tell you I couldn't do it, which is kind of sad, because they claim that they're bankrupt and everything. Where in the hell are they spending their money? They sure ain't giving it to me (Dr. F).

The mismatch between patient needs and the level of reimbursement generates a conflict between the physician's role as healer and his or her role as business person or employee.

> You owe it to your employer to be as productive as you can but you also owe it to your patient to be as helpful as you can and sometimes the two masters can't be served at the same time (Dr. C).

The imbalance between the time required and reimbursement sometimes leads to physicians limiting geriatric practice even if they enjoy it.

> In the real world, communication takes time, whether you're communicating with an elderly person who has a delay between the time that you give them a question and the time they give you an answer, or those that can't understand or deal with complex questions.... It takes longer to take care of patients like that. You superimpose upon this slow reacting patient a worried... family member who has a number of questions.... It adds more time to the office visit and the way Medicare is paying us for office visits. From an economic standpoint it just does not make sense to take care of old people (Dr. C).

Discussion

This study, using face-to-face interviews with practicing physicians, gives an in-depth look at the difficulty involved in providing primary care to elderly patients. The voices of these physicians and the framework we propose for understanding the difficulty they described can inform future efforts to meet the health care needs of our aging population. On the whole, participants enjoyed interactions with their elderly patients, but the high prevalence of multiple medical problems and declining physical and cognitive function among these patients gave rise to interacting medical, interpersonal, and administrative difficulty. Physicians struggled to deal with the difficulty in a practice environment that was not set up to provide the support and resources these patients needed.

We are by no means the first to recognize the mismatch between the chronic care needs of our aging population and the acute orientation of our health care system (Kottke, Brekke, & Solberg, 1993; Wagner, Austin, & Von Korff, 1996). This study vividly demonstrates the real impact of this mismatch on the daily practice of medicine. In so doing, it strongly supports the need for health system change. The recent Institute of Medicine report, *Crossing the Quality Chasm,* calls for efforts to improve health care by approaching it as a "complex adaptive system" (Institute of Medicine, 2001). To effect positive change in such a system, it is essential to recognize which elements can change and which cannot. The three-faceted difficulty at

the center of our model must be regarded as a fixed element of the system. Caring for chronically ill elders is and will remain complex and time consuming. There is great potential for positive change in the context in which care is delivered, however.

Our results suggest potential for change in practice organization, health care policy and medical education. In the area of practice organization, a number of interventions to facilitate primary care of chronically ill elders have been proposed and a few have been studied (Boult, Boult, Morishita, Smith, & Kane, 1998; Leveille et al., 1998; Schraeder, Shelton, & Sager, 2001; Netting & Williams, 2000; Wagner et al., 1996). The participation of nurse case managers in primary care practices, for instance, has shown benefits in elderly patient mortality and physician satisfaction (Schraeder et al., 2001). As yet, however, such interventions have met with very little acceptance by health care organizations or third party payers (Boult, Kane, Pacala, & Wagner, 1999; Wagner, Davis, Schaefer, Von Korff, & Austin, 1999). None of our participants had access to such personnel. Perhaps the greatest interpersonal challenge our participants experienced was the expansion of the doctor–patient relationship to include family members and other caregivers. Programs that facilitate communication between families and staff in the nursing home setting have shown great promise (Pillemer, Hegeman, Albright, & Henderson, 1998; Specht, Kelley, Manion, Maas, Reed, & Rantz, 2000). A similar intervention to enhance doctor–patient–family communication could be extremely helpful in the primary care setting.

Regarding health care policy, participants confirmed that Medicare documentation requirements are onerous and fees too low. Simplification of documentation requirement and increased reimbursement for complex nonprocedural care would clearly facilitate caring for elders. Participants also found the infrastructure of support services inadequate and difficult to access. Policy directed at improving community resources to meet the needs of chronically ill elders would also be extremely beneficial.

Changes in medical education could have important impact on physicians, who are themselves modifiable elements of the health care system. On the whole, participants felt confident managing specific illnesses, but lacked confidence in dealing with geriatric issues, such as vulnerability to adverse medical events and cognitive impairment. They experienced the greatest difficulty when the medical problems overlapped with interpersonal challenges and administrative burden. Despite the long recognition of the demographic imperative, few medical schools have mandatory geriatrics rotations and residencies devote minimal time to geriatrics training (Association of Professors of Medicine, 2001). With additional training, physicians could become more skilled and comfortable with the special needs of elderly patients.

This report has both strengths and limitations to consider. The qualitative format allowed participants' views to be explored in depth, adding important information to our understanding of primary care for elderly patients. Because of its intensive nature, however, a qualitative study can include only a small number of participants. Although we found striking consistency in the main themes, it is possible that our participants were systematically different from nonparticipants or physicians in other locales. Larger quantitative studies will determine the generalizability of our findings.

Although primary care for elderly people is rewarding and enjoyable, it is also complex, difficult, and time-consuming. Physicians alone cannot meet the wide range of needs these people have in the current practice environment. Our findings suggest that changes in practice organization, health policy, and medical education will be needed if primary care physicians are to care for a larger volume of elderly patients effectively.

References

AARP. (1995). *Reforming the health care system: State profiles 1995*. Washington, DC: Public Policy Institute.

Adelman, R., Greene, M., & Ory, M. (2000). Communication between older patients and their physicians. *Clinics in Geriatric Medicine, 16*, 1–24.

Association of Professors of Medicine. (2001). Internal medicine: At the nexus of the health care system in responding to the demographic imperative of an aging population. *The American Journal of Medicine, 110*, 507–513.

Bates, A., Harris, L., Tierney, W., & Wolinsky, F. (1998). Dimensions and correlates of physician work satisfaction in a midwestern city. *Medical Care, 36*, 610–617.

Boult, C., Boult, L., Morishita, L., Smith, S., & Kane, R. (1998). Outpatient geriatric evaluation and management. *Journal of the American Geriatrics Society, 46*, 296–302.

Boult, C., Kane, R., Pacala, J., & Wagner, E. (1999). Innovative healthcare for chronically ill older persons: Results of a national survey. *American Journal of Managed Care, 5*, 1162–1172.

Burdi, M., & Baker, K. (1999). Physicians' perceptions of autonomy and satisfaction in California. *Health Affairs, 18*, 134–145.

Cantor, J., Baker, L., & Hughes, R. (1993). Preparedness for practice. Young physicians' views of their professional education. *Journal of American Medical Association, 270*, 1035–1040.

Crabtree, B., & Miller, W. (1999). *Doing qualitative research*. Thousand Oaks, CA: Sage.

Creswell, J. (1998). Standards of Quality and Verification. In *Qualitative Inquiry and Research Design: Choosing Among Five Traditions* (pp. 193–218). Thousand Oaks, CA: Sage.

Cykert, S., Kissling, G., Layson, R., & Hansen, C. (1995). Health insurance does not guarantee access to primary care: A national study of physicians' acceptance of publicly insured patients. *Journal of General Internal Medicine, 10*, 345–348.

Damiano, P., Momany, E., Willard, J., & Jogerst, G. (1997). Factors affecting primary care physician participation in Medicare. *Medical Care, 35*, 1008–1019.

Geiger, W., & Krol, R. (1991). Physician attitudes and behavior in response to changes in Medicare reimbursement policies. *Journal of Family Practice, 33*, 244–248.

Greene, W. (1993). *Econometric analysis*. New York: Macmillan.

Institute of Medicine. (2001). *Crossing the quality chasm: A new health system for the 21st century*. Washington, DC: National Academy Press.

Kottke, T., Brekke, M., & Solberg, L. (1993). Making "time" for preventive services. *Mayo Clinical Proceedings, 68*, 785–791.

Krakowski, A. (1982). Stress and the practice of medicine: II. Stressors, stresses and strains. *Psychotherapy and Psychosomatics, 38*, 11–23.

Kuzel, A. (1999). Sampling in qualitative inquiry. In B. F. Crabtree & W. Miller, *Doing qualitative research* (pp. 33–46). Thousand Oaks, CA: Sage.

Lee, D., & Gillis, K. (1993). Physician responses to Medicare physician payment reform: Preliminary results on access to care. *Inquiry, 30*, 417–428.

Lee, D., & Gillis, K. (1994). Physician responses to Medicare payment reform: An update on access to care. *Inquiry, 31*, 346–353.

Leveille, S., Wagner, E., Davis, D., Grothaus, L., Wallace, J., LoGerfo, M., et al. (1998). Preventing disability and managing chronic illness in frail older adults: A randomized trial of a community-based partnership with primary care. *Journal of the American Geriatrics Society, 46*, 1191–1198.

Lewis, C., Prout, D., Chalmers, E., & Leake, B. (1991). How satisfying is the practice of internal medicine? *Annals of Internal Medicine, 114*, 1–5.

Lincoln, Y., & Guba, E. (1985). *Naturalistic inquiry*. Newbury Park, CA: Sage.

Linn, L., Yager, J., Cope, D., & Leake, B. (1985). Health status, job satisfaction, job stress, and life satisfaction among academic and clinical faculty. *Journal of the American Medical Association, 254*, 2775–2782.

Linzer, M., Konrad, T., Douglas, J., McMurray, J., Pathman, D., Williams, E., et al. (2000). Managed care, time pressure, and physician job satisfaction: Results from the physician work-life study. *Journal of General Internal Medicine, 15*, 441–450.

Manton, K., & Vaupel, J. (1995). Survival after the age of 80 in the United States, Sweden, France, England, and Japan. *The New England Journal of Medicine, 333*, 1232–1235.

Mawardi, B. (1979). Satisfaction, dissatisfaction, and causes of stress in medical practice. *Journal of the American Medical Association, 241*, 1483–1486.

McMurray, J., Williams, E., Schwartz, M., Douglas, J., Van Kirk, J., Konrad, R., et al. (1997). Physician job satisfaction: Developing a model using qualitative data. *Journal of General Internal Medicine, 12*, 711–714.

Morrison, R., Morrison, E., & Glickman, D. (1994). Physician reluctance to discuss advance directives. *Archives of Internal Medicine, 154*, 2311–2318.

Netting, F., & Williams, F. (2000). Expanding the boundaries of primary care for elderly people. *Health and Social Work, 25*, 233–242.

Patton, M. (1990). *Qualitative evaluation and research methods*. Newbury Park, CA: Sage.

Pereles, L., & Russell, M. (1996). Needs for CME in geriatrics, part 2: Physician priorities and perceptions of community representatives. *Canadian Family Physician, 42*, 632–640.

Perez, E., Mulligan, T., & Meyers, M. (1991). Interest in geriatrics education among family practitioners and internists in Virginia. *Academic Medicine, 66*, 558–559.

Pillemer, K., Hegeman, C., Albright, B., & Henderson, C. (1998). Building bridges between families and nursing home staff: The partners in caregiving program. *The Gerontologist, 38*, 499–503.

Roter, D. (1991). Elderly patient-physician communication: A descriptive study of content and affect during the medical encounter. *Advances in Health Education, 3*, 15–23.

Schappert, S. (1999). Ambulatory care visits to physician offices, hospital outpatient departments, and emergency departments: United States, 1997. *Vital Health Statistics, 13* (143), 1–39.

Schraeder, C., Shelton, P., & Sager, M. (2001). The effects of a collaborative model of primary care on the mortality and hospital use of community-dwelling older adults. *Journal of Gerontology: Medical Sciences, 56A,* M106–M112.

Siu, A., & Beck, J. (1990). Physician satisfaction with career choices in geriatrics. *The Gerontologist, 30,* 529–534.

Specht, J., Kelley, L., Manion, P., Maas, M., Reed, D., & Rantz, M. (2000). Who's the boss? Family/staff partnership in care of persons with dementia. *Nursing Administrator Quarterly, 24,* 64–77.

Stafford, R., Saglam, D., Causino, N., Starfield, B., Culpepper, L., Marder, W., et al. (1999). Trends in adult visits to primary care physicians in the United States. *Archives of Family Medicine, 8,* 26–32.

Strauss, A., & Corbin, J. (1998). *Basics of qualitative research: Grounded theory procedures and techniques.* Newbury Park, CA: Sage.

U.S. Bureau of the Census. (1996). Current population reports, special studies, P23-190, 65 + in the United States. *Current Population Reports.* Washington, DC: U.S. Government Printing Office.

Wagner, E., Austin, B., & Von Korff, M. (1996). Organizing care for patients with chronic illness. *Milbank Quarterly, 74,* 511–544.

Wagner, E., Davis, C., Schaefer, J., Von Korff, M., & Austin, B. (1999). A survey of leading chronic disease management programs: Are they consistent with the literature? *Managed Care Quarterly, 7,* 56–66.

We are most grateful to all the physicians who donated their time for the interviews. We also thank Jeff Susman, MD, Kurt Stange, MD, and Lynn Meadows, PhD, for their helpful critiques of earlier drafts of this article; John Creswell, PhD, for methodologic advice; and Linda Ferring for manuscript preparation. This study was approved by the Institutional Review Board at the University of Nebraska Medical Center.

Address correspondence to Wendy L. Adams, MD, MPH, Department of Family Medicine, University of Nebraska Medical Center, 983075 Nebraska Medical Center, Omaha, NE 68198-3075. E-mail: Wadams@ unmc.edu

[1]Department of Family Medicine, University of Nebraska Medical Center, Omaha.

[2]Department of Family Medicine, Robert Wood Johnson Medical School, University of Medicine and Dentistry of New Jersey, New Brunswick.

[3]VA Nebraska–Western Iowa Health Care System, Omaha, NE.

Breakthrough

A landmark Supreme Court decision is being hailed as 'the Emancipation Proclamation for older workers'

David Newman

The U.S. Supreme Court struck a major blow for age equality in the workplace when it declared last month that a bulwark of civil rights laws against race and sex discrimination should also protect employees who bring suits in federal court under the Age Discrimination in Employment Act (ADEA). Plaintiffs can now bypass what is often the hardest-to-prove aspect of their cases—showing that their employer's discrimination was deliberate—by arguing instead that they were victims of a policy that caused harm to older workers and went beyond "reasonable" business considerations.

Just as important as the practical benefits of the result, which AARP supported in a friend-of-the-court brief, is the long-term effect that the decision, *Smith v. City of Jackson, Miss.*, will have in elevating age discrimination legally closer to the level of race or gender bias. After years of standing on the sidelines, says Washington lawyer Richard Seymour, a former chair of the Employment Rights Division at the American Trial Lawyers Association, the Supreme Court has finally sent a message that age discrimination is a serious problem that must be attacked when it is unintentional as well as when it is intentional. Seymour goes so far as to call the decision "the Emancipation Proclamation for older workers."

"We were thrilled with the decision," says Laurie McCann, an AARP senior attorney. "We were losing this battle in the federal courts, so the victory was somewhat unexpected."

The justices' reasoning for the *Smith* decision is steeped in references to a race discrimination case from 1971 that represents a high-water mark in employment discrimination law. In *Griggs v. Duke Power Co.* the Supreme Court found that even a seemingly neutral job requirement (the case was about making employment conditional on having a high school diploma) counted as discrimination, since its effect was to keep a disproportionate number of qualified black applicants from getting hired, a so-called disparate impact.

The scope of discrimination based on age will be narrower because the ADEA, while generally modeled on race and sex discrimination laws, allows employers to treat older workers differently as long as they do so based on "reasonable factors other than age."

The effect of this provision is apparent in the result in *Smith* itself, a case about whether the city of Jackson could restructure its salaries for police officers in a way that gave the bulk of a new raise package to more junior officers. The plaintiffs—older officers—contended that this kind of pay-raise system, even if devised in good faith, amounted to illegal age discrimination because it worked mostly to the benefit of officers who tended to be younger.

Reversing two lower courts, the Supreme Court agreed that, in theory, a case could go forward even if the city did not intend to discriminate against older officers. (This step is what opens the door to a new standard in future cases.) However, the court went on to say that the city's justifi-

cation for its policy—that it wanted to make its entry-level salaries competitive with those offered in neighboring towns—was "reasonable" and justified the discrepancy. Even applying the new standard, in other words, the court found that the *Smith* case should be dismissed.

Because *Smith* and similar age discrimination cases focus on broad policies affecting large numbers of workers, they mostly involve big businesses and other employers (like governments) that make employment decisions using objective formulas. That means the Supreme Court's latest decision gives victims of age discrimination a powerful new weapon, McCann says. If they can tell a story with statistics, they no longer need to have a "smoking gun," such as a memo showing hostility to older workers, to persuade a judge to move their case forward to the evidence-gathering phase.

Merely getting to that point is often tantamount to victory. It is during this pretrial phase that a plaintiff's lawyer can force the other side to produce additional evidence—and gain additional leverage to settle—by subpoenaing documents, taking depositions and preparing witnesses.

With most defendants limited to large employers, Seymour says, the number of lawsuits filed may never be overwhelming. But he is also "as confident that we will catch companies doing wrong as I am that the sun will rise tomorrow," predicting there will soon be at least one major suit against a nationwide employer.

That would jibe with what's going on in Minnesota, Michigan and Ohio, which already have disparate impact standards in place at the state level. In Michigan, for example, AARP attorneys joined a suit that alleged bias against older workers in Ford Motor Company's employee ranking system.

Ford had implemented an A-B-C letter system for ranking its 18,000 employees, which it used to justify terminations and salary increases. "The statistics were just staggering," McCann says. "If you were over 40, the chances of getting a C ranking and not getting a raise were much higher. I don't think Ford wanted to defend a disparate impact case given those numbers."

In the end, Ford paid $10.6 million in a settlement with older workers who had brought the suit.

With the matter of proving intent settled, many experts agree the latest decision fails to give lower courts sufficient guidance about what is "reasonable" and "unreasonable" when it comes to issues like salary and experience, factors that are often correlated with age and can figure prominently in employer calculations. That will be the focus in the next wave of litigation. "AARP plans to be very active by filing friend-of-the-court briefs to make sure 'reasonable' isn't drawn too broadly," McCann says.

Paul Mollica, a partner in a Chicago-based firm that specializes in discrimination cases, believes that in the near term the latest decision will allow lawyers to go after "capricious, arbitrary" policies. It remains to be seen, however, what effect the decision will have on employers that have carefully considered their policies and the alternatives.

"We don't yet know what it means for an employer to have made a 'reasonable' business decision," says Tom Goldstein, an appellate court litigator who represented the veteran Jackson police officers at the Supreme Court.

Part of the tangle is trying to reconcile *Smith* with the court's previous rulings in discrimination cases. In 1993 a unanimous Supreme Court rejected the age discrimination claim of a 62-year-old worker who alleged he had been fired by his employer because he was about to become eligible for a pension. Intentional discrimination, the court stated, "captures the essence of what Congress sought to prohibit in the ADEA." Although March's opinion seems to push back against that kind of reasoning, the court notably did not go so far as to overrule it—and in fact took pains to stress that "age, unlike race or [sex] classifications … not uncommonly has relevance to an individual's capacity to engage in certain types of employment."

In *Smith*, Justice Antonin Scalia cast the deciding vote. While emphasizing that he didn't agree with all of the reasoning of the concurring justices, Scalia said he could reach the same result because the Equal Employment Opportunity Commission, the federal agency that has the job of enforcing the ADEA, had already endorsed the position. "This is an absolutely classic case for deference to agency interpretation," Scalia wrote.

When it comes to age, Scalia has given himself room to break away from the other four justices in future cases that ask the court to say more about what kind of discrimination is "reasonable." Scalia's thinking also indicates that he might be willing to shift his position if the EEOC were to shift its interpretation of the statute.

The EEOC is already under fire for a controversial regulation it issued in the age discrimination context (see Retirees Win on EEOC's Benefits Rule), and McCann cautions that "it would be a horrible PR move for them to try to undermine this Supreme Court decision."

David Newman *is a contributing editor to* Legal Affairs *magazine.*

Will You Still Need Me When I'm ... 84? More Couples Divorce After Decades

By JEFFREY ZASLOW

John and Francis Thomas of Guthrie, Okla., did not make it to their golden wedding anniversary. In 2001, after five children and 49 years of marriage, John, a minister, filed for divorce, saying he couldn't handle the nagging and fighting. He says he was tired of being told, "You made me do it, but I won't do it again."

"We were both in a state of depression and not giving each other what we needed," admits Mrs. Thomas, 71 years old. She longs for reconciliation. "I've been sending him e-mails saying I love him so much."

Mr. Thomas, 72, still calls his ex-wife "dear," but insists he won't return. Due to the stress of his marriage, he says, "I was constantly fighting health problems. Now, they have virtually disappeared."

As divorce has become more accepted in the U.S., older couples are often seen as models of how the institution of marriage is supposed to work. We assume couples that survive the first few decades have accepted their spouse's quirks and problems, and are more apt to live out their lives together.

But that notion is now being shattered. Like Mr. Thomas, more and more people in their 60s, 70s and 80s are seeking divorce as a way to find health, happiness and a new start. In 1990, 6% of senior citizens were divorced or separated. By 2001, that figure had jumped to 10%, with a total of 2.2 million people divorced, according to U.S. Census data. That surge will continue as divorce-prone baby boomers age, lawyers say.

These divorces are being fueled by longevity, economics and self-awareness. Seniors are healthier now, and don't want to waste two or three decades of the golden years with someone they can no longer stand. More than in previous generations, older women today had careers and now have their own pensions, so they're less dependent on husbands. Meanwhile, Viagra may be giving older men new incentives to rediscover passion elsewhere.

The Gray Divorcee

Some factors in the boom in breakups among seniors:

- Lack of a common purpose: No more kids to raise, interests diverge.

- Boredom: Retired for decades, couples blame each other for tedium.

- Sexual woes: One partner is uninterested in sex, or can't perform.

- Longevity: Healthy couples see long life ahead, so why live it with someone they no longer love?

- Times have changed: Older women, fed up with being selfless servants, are putting their foot down.

The late anthropologist Margaret Mead saw it all coming. She argued that marriage was designed for earlier eras, when parents raised children and then died in their 40s or 50s. Now, as people live longer, they're tied to marriages for decades of empty-nesting. "I don't think marriage was contemplated to last

50 years. A lot of people grow in different directions," says Constance Putzel, an attorney in Towson, Md., who wrote the American Bar Association's book "Representing the Older Client in Divorce."

One telling statistic: A full 65% of the people who have passed age 50 in the history of mankind are still walking the earth today. Marriage is a longer-term commitment than it ever has been—too long for a growing number of seniors.

That doesn't mean exit strategies are easy. For divorcing seniors, a breakup can be agonizing and complex, especially when there are issues involving long-term care and inheritances. Because Medicaid doesn't take effect until a couple's assets are depleted, people who delay a divorce can wind up paying for it financially. Also, splitting up assets for heirs gets hairier if it's a second or third marriage being dissolved and there are children from previous marriages.

Attorneys warn seniors to insist that all divorce settlements address health and life insurance, as well as retirement benefits. Under the Employees Retirement Income Security Act, if your spouse has a qualified Erisa pension, you're entitled to share it. But you lose that right once you're divorced, unless there's an agreement or court order. Before negotiating a trade-off of assets to compensate for a pension, it's crucial to get a qualified actuary to value the pension.

Some seniors say such financial nuts and bolts are incidental. They just want out. Don Benjamin, 71, of Morehead City, N.C., was married 30 years, but the final decade was devoid of intimacy, he says. "I felt like I was living with my sister. Emotionally, my life was slowly being extinguished." After getting divorced in 1998 and remarrying, he now says older divorced people are reveling in rediscovered sexuality, "even if it takes all night to do what we used to do all night."

Such scenarios are hard for many adult children of seniors to contemplate. There's an old joke in which a couple married 75 years visits a divorce attorney, who asks why they waited so long. They reply: "We wanted to wait until the children were dead."

In seminars given by Leslie Fram, author of "How to Marry a Divorced Man," older women complain that a large part of the courtship process is dedicated to winning the thumbs up from a divorced man's adult children. "I liken this to an updated version of yesteryear, when teenage boys had to impress their prom dates' fathers before whisking them off to the dance," says Ms. Fram.

Meanwhile, some seniors are remarrying too quickly, leading to a second wave of divorces. That's why divorce attorneys are advising altar-bound seniors to write prenuptial agreements, and to include a separate affidavit from a doctor, signifying their competency to make such decisions.

In Boca Raton, Fla., psychologist Felicia Romeo says that divorced or widowed clients in her geriatric practice often jump into new marriages out of fear and loneliness. Some are pushed along by adult children "who want mom to find someone so she's not dependent on them," she says.

But in Oklahoma, Mrs. Thomas is not looking for a new man. Vowing to do "anything in my power" to reunite with her ex-husband, she's living the sadder side of the senior divorce equation. "It comes across to me like it was time for John to spread his wings," she says, "and for me to take my lumps."

The Disappearing Mind

By the year 2050, as many as 14 million Americans could be suffering from Alzheimer's disease. Scientists are now using imaging technology to diagnose the condition at its earliest stages—and racing to develop new treatments that can stop its terrifying progression. Will they succeed?

BY GEOFFREY COWLEY

Do SENIOR MOMENTS SCARE YOU? Eight years ago Nancy Levitt had one that would unsettle anyone. She was in her mid-40s at the time, and watching her father drift into the late stages of Alzheimer's disease (several aunts and uncles had suffered similar fates). Levitt's son was about to graduate from high school, so she called a mail-order company to order fluorescent-light sticks for him and his friends to wear around their necks at a party. When her package arrived in the next day's mail, the receipt and postmark knocked her flat. She had ordered the same gift a few days earlier—and lost all recollection of it. "I just freaked," she says. Suddenly, every forgotten name, misplaced pencil and misspelled word became a prophecy of doom. Was she getting Alzheimer's herself?

When Levitt sought testing at UCLA, researchers gave her the usual cognitive tests—name some simple objects, repeat a list of words—and assured her she was fine. But the occasional lapses continued, so she returned to the same clinic several years later and enrolled in a study aimed at distinguishing early Alzheimer's from run-of-the-mill forgetfulness. This time the researchers didn't just talk to her. They placed her under a scanner and recorded detailed images of her brain, both at work and at rest. Alzheimer's disease has traditionally been diagnosed by exclusion. If you lagged significantly on a memory test—and your troubles couldn't be blamed on strokes, tumors or drug toxicity—you were given a tentative diagnosis and sent on your way. To find out for sure, you had to die and have your brain dissected by a pathologist. Levitt didn't have to do any of that. By looking at the images on his video screen, Dr. Gary Small was able to give her some reassuring news. She didn't have Alzheimer's disease—and the odds were less than 5 percent that she would develop it any time soon. Levitt calls the images "the most wonderful thing I've ever seen."

"Without a good method of early detection, the best Alzheimer's treatment would be worthless."
—DR. FERENC JOLESZ

Technology is changing all of medicine, but it is positively transforming our understanding of Alzheimer's. Armed with state-of-the-art PET scanners and MRI machines, specialists are learning to spot and track the disease in people who have yet to suffer symptoms. It's one thing to chronicle the brain's disintegration, quite another to stop it, but many experts are predicting success on both fronts. Drugmakers now have two dozen treatments in development. And unlike today's medications, which offer only a brief respite from symptoms, many of the new ones are intended to stall progression of the disease. As Alzheimer's runs its decades-long course, it replaces the brain's exquisite circuitry with mounds of sticky plaque and expanses of dead, twisted neurons. No drug will repair that kind of damage. But if the new treatments work as anticipated, they'll enable us to stop or slow the destruction while our minds are still intact. A decade from now, says Dr. Dennis Selkoe of Harvard Medical School and Boston's Brigham and Women's Hospital, physicians may monitor our brain health as closely as our cholesterol levels—and stave off Alzheimer's with a wave of the prescription pad.

Until we can control this awful illness, early detection may seem a fool's errand. "With diagnostics ahead of therapeutics,

A-BETA FORMATION
Disease stage: APP is a normal protein housed in the outer membranes of brain cells. When APP is snipped by scissorlike enzymes called beta and gamma secretase, a fragment called A-beta is released. If the brain does not clear A-beta, it builds up and causes trouble.

Neuron
Outer membrane
Neuron APP
Secretase
A-beta protein
A-beta cluster (plaque)

Attack strategy: Secretase inhibitors may stall A-beta production by disabling the scissorlike enzymes. Such drugs are in animal testing.

there's a lot of potential for harm," says University of Pennsylvania ethicist Arthur Caplan. He worries that entrepreneurs will peddle testing without counseling, leaving patients devastated by the findings. He wonders, too, whether employers and insurers will abandon people whose scans show signs of trouble. Advocates counter that early detection can help patients make the most of today's treatments while giving them time to adjust their plans and expectations. With so many people at risk, they say, anything is better than nothing. Some 4 million Americans have Alzheimer's today, but the number could hit 14 million by 2050 as the elderly population expands.

> ## "There are a lot of people who could benefit from today's treatments, but they aren't getting help."
> ### –DR. GARY SMALL

The diagnostic revolution began during the 1990s, as researchers learned to monitor neurons with an imaging technique called PET, or positron-emission tomography. Unlike an X-ray or CT imaging, PET records brain activity by homing in on the glucose that fuels it. And as Small's team has discovered, it can spot significant pathology in people who are still functioning normally. Instead of glowing with activity, the middle sections of their brains appear dim and torpid. And because Alzheimer's is progressive, abnormal scans tend to become more so with time. In a study published last fall, UCLA researchers scanned 284 people who had suffered only minor memory problems. The images predicted, with 95 percent accuracy, which people would experience dementia within three and a half years.

PET scanning has yet to transform patient care; few clinics have the machines, and Medicare doesn't cover their use. But scientists are now using the technique to see whether drugs already on the market (such as the anti-inflammatory ibuprofen) can slow the brain's decline. And PET is just one of several potential strategies for tracking preclinical Alzheimer's. San Diego researchers have found that seniors who score inconsistently on different mental tests are at increased risk of dementia— even if their scores are generally high. And in a study published this spring, research-

ers at the Oregon Health Sciences University hit upon three signs of imminent decline in octogenarians. The 108 participants were all healthy at the start of the study, but nearly half were demented six years later. As it turned out, they had entered the study with certain traits in common. They walked more slowly than their peers, requiring nearly two extra seconds for a 30-foot stroll. They lagged slightly on memory tests. And their MRI scans revealed a slight shrinkage of the hippocampus, a small, seahorse-shaped brain structure that is critical to memory processing. The changes were subtle, says Dr. Jeffrey Kaye, the neurologist who directed the study, but they presaged changes that were catastrophic.

Powerful as they are, today's tests show only that the brain is losing steam. The ideal test would reveal the underlying pathology, letting a specialist determine how much healthy tissue has been replaced by the plaques and tangles of Alzheimer's. It's not hard to fashion a molecule that will highlight the wreckage. Unfortunately, it's almost impossible to get such a probe through the ultrafine screen that separates the brain from the bloodstream. If a probe is complex enough to pick out plaques and tangles, chances are it's too large to pass from the bloodstream into the brain. At UCLA and the University of Pittsburgh, researchers have developed probes that are small enough to get through, yet selective enough to provide at least a rough measure of a person's plaque burden. At Brigham and Women's Hospital, meanwhile, radiologist Ferenc Jolesz is trying to open the barrier to bigger, better probes. His technique employs tiny lipid bubbles that gather at the gateway to the brain when injected into the bloodstream. The bubbles burst when zapped with ultrasound, loosening the mesh of that ultrafine screen and allowing the amyloid probe to enter. Lab tests suggest the screen will repair itself within a day, but no one yet knows whether it's safe to leave it open that long.

One way or another, many of us now seem destined to learn we have Alzheimer's disease while we're still of sound mind. The question is whether we'll be able to do anything more constructive than setting our affairs in order and taking a drug like Aricept to ease the early symptoms. Fortunately the possibilities for therapy are changing almost as fast as the diagnostic arts. Experts now think of Alzheimer's not as a sudden calamity but as a decades-long process involving at least a half-dozen steps—each of which

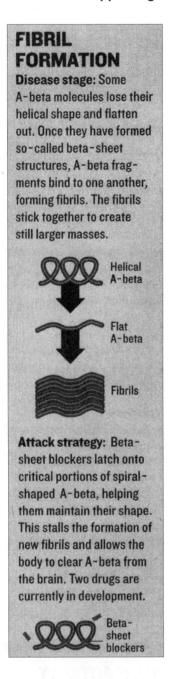

FIBRIL FORMATION

Disease stage: Some A-beta molecules lose their helical shape and flatten out. Once they have formed so-called beta-sheet structures, A-beta fragments bind to one another, forming fibrils. The fibrils stick together to create still larger masses.

Helical A-beta

Flat A-beta

Fibrils

Attack strategy: Beta-sheet blockers latch onto critical portions of spiral-shaped A-beta, helping them maintain their shape. This stalls the formation of new fibrils and allows the body to clear A-beta from the brain. Two drugs are currently in development.

Beta-sheet blockers

provides a target for intervention. Slowing the disease may require four or five drugs rather than one. But as AIDS specialists have shown, the right combination can sometimes turn a killer into a mere menace.

THOUGH EXPERTS STILL QUARREL ABOUT the ultimate cause of Alzheimer's, many agree that the trouble starts with a scrap of junk protein called amyloid beta (A-beta for short). Each of us produces the stuff, and small amounts are harmless. But as A-beta builds up in the brain, it sets off a destructive cascade, replacing healthy tissue with the plaques seen in Alzheimer's suf-

Brain Spotting

For the first time, PET scans can spot plaque in the brains of Alzheimer's patients. The advance will allow for confident early detection of the disease.

PLAQUE BUILDUP Red areas in the brain scan of an Alzheimer's patient show plaque accumulation. The healthy brain shows none.

Alzheimer's brain

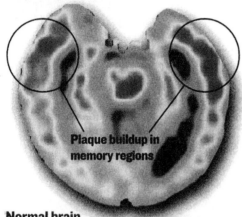

Plaque buildup in memory regions

Normal brain

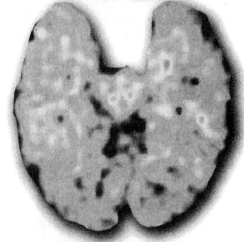

BRAIN ACTIVITY Blue areas in the Alzheimer's patient's memory regions indicate reduced activity caused by the plaque.

Alzheimer's brain   **Normal brain**

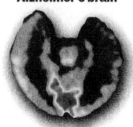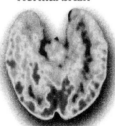

Leading causes of death in the U.S., all ages, 1999

Heart disease	725,192
Malignant tumors	549,838
Vascular disease	167,366
Respiratory disease	124,181
Accidents	97,860
Diabetes	68,399
Pneumonia/flu	63,730
Alzheimer's	**44,536**
Kidney disease	35,525
Blood disease	30,680

Projected cases in the U.S.*

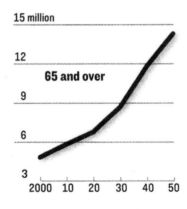

15 million

12

65 and over

9

6

3

2000 10 20 30 40 50

Projected cases by age group*

10 million

8

6   2050

4

2   2000

2

0

65-74   75-84   85+

PLAQUE FORMATION

Disease stage: A-beta fibrils bind with proteins like SAP. The SAP reinforces the fibrils, making them less soluble and harder for the body to clear. Fibrils bind with other fibrils and grow into plaques.

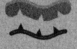

SAP

A-beta fibril

A-beta bound to SAP

Attack strategy: Specially designed chemicals bind SAP before it can link to fibrils. This helps prevent fibril accumulation. A few drugs are in early trials.

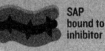

SAP

SAP inhibitor

SAP

SAP bound to inhibitor

SOURCES: GARY W. SMALL, M.D., UCLA; DENIS EVANS, M.D., CDC

ferers. No one knew where this pesky filament came from until 1987, when researchers discovered it was part of a larger molecule they dubbed the amyloid-precursor protein (APP). Thanks to more recent discoveries, they now know exactly how the parent molecule spawns its malevolent offspring.

proteins faster than others, but after seven or eight decades of service, even the healthiest brain carries an amyloid burden. When it reaches a certain threshold, the brain can no longer function. That's why Alzheimer's dementia is so rampant among the elderly. Given enough time, anyone would develop it.

cell development, damaging bone marrow and digestive tissues. A few companies are still pursuing gamma blockers, but beta secretase now looks like a safer target for therapy. More than a half-dozen drugmakers are now working on beta inhibitors. "In the industry," says Dr. Ivan Lieberburg of Elan, "we're hoping that the beta-secretase inhibitors will have as much therapeutic potential as the statins." Those, of course, are the cholesterol-lowering medicines for which 35 million Americans are now candidates.

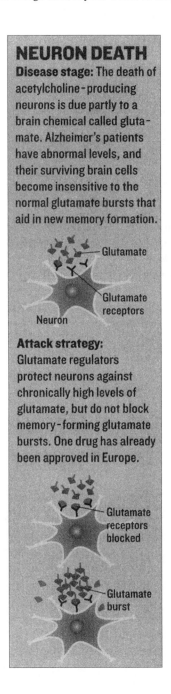

PLAQUE BUILDUP

Disease stage: As Alzheimer's progresses, more and more healthy brain tissue is displaced by tough, insoluble plaque. In the process, the brain loses the ability to produce acetylcholine, a neurotransmitter critical to memory and cognition.

Antibody

Plaque buildup

Attack strategy: Antibodies targeted to plaques can mark them for destruction by the immune system. Antibodies can improve memory in mice.

Macrophage

NEURON DEATH

Disease stage: The death of acetylcholine-producing neurons is due partly to a brain chemical called glutamate. Alzheimer's patients have abnormal levels, and their surviving brain cells become insensitive to the normal glutamate bursts that aid in new memory formation.

Glutamate

Glutamate receptors

Neuron

Attack strategy: Glutamate regulators protect neurons against chronically high levels of glutamate, but do not block memory-forming glutamate bursts. One drug has already been approved in Europe.

Glutamate receptors blocked

Glutamate burst

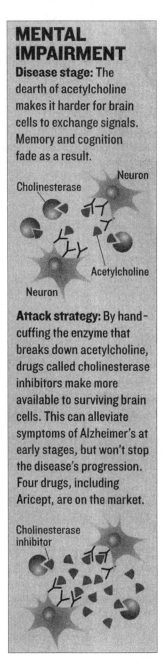

MENTAL IMPAIRMENT

Disease stage: The dearth of acetylcholine makes it harder for brain cells to exchange signals. Memory and cognition fade as a result.

Cholinesterase

Neuron

Acetylcholine

Neuron

Attack strategy: By handcuffing the enzyme that breaks down acetylcholine, drugs called cholinesterase inhibitors make more available to surviving brain cells. This can alleviate symptoms of Alzheimer's at early stages, but won't stop the disease's progression. Four drugs, including Aricept, are on the market.

Cholinesterase inhibitor

APP is a normal protein that hangs from a neuron's outer membrane like a worm with its head in an apple. While performing its duties in and around the cell, it gets chopped up by enzymes called secretases, leaving residues that dissolve in the brain's watery recesses. Occasionally, however, a pair of enzymes called beta and gamma secretase cleave APP in just the wrong places, leaving behind an insoluble A-beta fragment. Some people produce these junk

The ideal Alzheimer's remedy would simply slow the production of A-beta—by disabling the enzymes that fabricate it. Elan Corp. was the first drugmaker to try this tack. During the mid-'90s its scientists developed several gamma-secretase blockers and tested them in animals—only to find that they sometimes derailed normal

Secretase inhibitors may be our best hope of warding off Alzheimer's, but they're not the only hope. As scientists learn more about the behavior of A-beta, they're seeing opportunities to disarm it before it causes harm. One thing that makes A-beta fragments dangerous is their tendency to bind with one another to form tough, stringy fibrils, which then stick together to create still larger masses. Three companies are now testing compounds designed to keep A-beta from forming fibrils—and at least two other firms are working to keep fibrils from aggregating to create plaque. All of their experimental drugs have helped reduce amyloid buildup in plaque-prone mice, suggesting they might help people as well. But human studies are just now getting underway.

Suppose for a moment that all these strategies fail, and that amyloid buildup is simply part of the human condition. As Selkoe likes to say, there's more than one way to keep a bathtub from overflowing. If you can't turn down the faucet, you can always try opening the drain. Recognizing that most of the people now threatened by Alzheimer's have already spent their lives under open amyloid faucets, researchers are pursuing several strategies for clearing deposits from the brain. One elegant idea is to mobilize the immune system. Three years ago Elan wowed the world by showing that animals given an antiamyloid vaccine mounted fierce attacks on their plaques. Vaccinated mice reduced their amyloid burdens by an astounding 96 percent in just three months. The vaccine proved toxic in people, triggering attacks on normal tissue as well as plaque, but the dream isn't dead. Both Elan and Eli Lilly are now developing ready-made antibodies that, if successful, will target amyloid for removal from the brain without triggering broader attacks by the immune system.

Even later interventions may be possible. As a person's amyloid burden rises, so does the concentration of glutamate in the brain. This neurotransmitter helps lock in memories when it's released in short bursts, but it kills neurons when chronically elevated. At least two teams are now betting they can rescue cells surrounded by amyloid, simply by shielding them from glutamate. One possible life jacket is a drug called Memantine, which is already approved in Europe. It covers a receptor that lets glutamate flow freely into neurons, but without blocking the glutamate bursts needed for learning and memory. New York's Forest Laboratories is now launching an American trial of the drug, and hoping for approval by next year.

If even half these treatments fulfill their promise, old age may prove more pleasant than today's projections suggest. For now, the best we can expect is an early warning and perhaps a year or two of symptomatic relief. That may seem a paltry offering, but it's a far cry from nothing. As Small argues in a forthcoming book called "The Memory Bible," people at early stages of Alzheimer's can do a lot to improve their lives, but few of them get the chance. Three out of four are already past the "moderate" stage by the time their conditions are recognized. Some may find solace in ignorance. But the case for vigilance is getting stronger every day.

**With ANNE UNDERWOOD and
ANDREW MURR**

Alzheimer's disease as a "trip back in time"

Christopher J. Johnson, PhD
Roxanna H. Johnson, MS, CTRS

Abstract

Persons with Alzheimer's disease (AD) seem to vary from day to day in their recall of loved ones' names and faces. Such erratic fluctuating and regressive cognition is often puzzling and stressful to caregivers. This paper explores the possibility of conceptualizing AD as a "trip back in time" to help caregivers understand the variation in an AD person's memory, behavior, and physical abilities. Clinical observations suggest that these individuals experience a cognitive, emotional, social, physical and functional regression with AD. The "trip back in time" paradigm uses aspects of Piaget's theory of adult development in reverse, Reisberg and associates FAST and GDS, and other cognitive, behavioral, and affective research on AD. Using past research to indicate how patients tend to lose many of their functions, the conceptualization goes further to advance a non-linear regression model of AD. This paradigm of AD as a "trip back in time" uses connecting loops spiraling downward to depict the fluctuating regression. Previous theoretical frameworks have tended to rely solely on fixed stage regression models of AD. The insight this model provides will hopefully increase gerontologist/caregivers' understanding and provide new ways to develop strategies to enhance future caregiving techniques.

Introduction

The purpose of this paper is to propose a new theoretical conceptualization and model of Alzheimer's disease (AD) as a "trip back in time." This model offers a new approach to understanding the cognitive, emotional, social, physical and functional journey of an AD victim. The "trip back in time" was developed as a non-linear model to explain the variations in functioning throughout the course of AD. The paradigm builds on the linear theory of development of Piaget in reverse and the seven stage AD

model of Reisberg and Associates as is seen in their Functional Assessment Staging (FAST Scale) as well as their Global Deterioration Scale (GDS) research.[1-8] The "trip back in time" uses a downward spiral with connecting loops to demonstrate the fluctuating non-linear, but progressive regression of the disease. The "trip back in time" model can account for the AD victim's ability to fluctuate in both memory and/recognition of family members as they travel back through time. The primary benefit of this model is a sensitive provision and explanation of AD for caregivers as well as a theoretical and clinical tool for the regression of AD. This theoretical paradigm can also serve as an insightful pedagogical aide for both clinicians and caregivers.

Alzheimer's disease: A brief overview

Alzheimer's disease (AD) has been called the disease of the century, and is more likely to occur as a person ages. About 10 percent of those over age 65, and 47 percent of those past age 85 are estimated to have AD.[9] The literature suggests that over half of all causes of dementia is the result of AD.[10,11] Furthermore, demographic trends and age-related rates of AD suggest that it will become increasingly prevalent in the United States as we move into the new millennium.[12,13] Dementia is believed to affect 50 to 60 percent of the 1.3 million individuals in long term care facilities and may account for greater than half of the $26 billion spent annually on institutionalization.[14]

AD is characterized by failing memory, intellectual deterioration, functional decline and frequent behavioral disturbances. The result of this decline can be seen in the steadily diminishing mental capacity coupled with a shortened life expectancy. There have been reports suggesting that the age of onset determines the severity of illness.[15] The youngest documented age of an AD victim is about age 28.[16] Ironically, with the exception of the very old (85 or older) who have other maladies, the young patients seem to die sooner.[17] It has been asserted that early onset (under age 65) cases may progress more rapidly and move through the stages of the disease more quickly than late onset cases.[18] Yet, scientists do not clearly understand why this happens. The decline of cognitive abilities in AD typically begins with short term memory loss and progresses at varying rates to a state in which virtually no cognitive abilities are spared.[19]

With the progressive nature of AD-related intellectual deterioration, caregivers often assign unrealistic behavioral expectations to their AD loved ones. This frequently happens by either over estimating or under estimating the AD person's potential for understanding, ability and cooperation. Due to the fact that AD patients' abilities are erratic and are often misunderstood, caregiver expectations are often unrealistic. What makes the situation worse is that some caregivers believe that the AD person is in a particular stage where only regression is possible. These expectations and subsequent reactions may trigger the person with AD to react adversely by exhibiting frustration, anxiety or a catastrophic reaction.[20-22]

Linear models

Scientists have a goal of increasing scholarly understanding and prediction of decrements in cognitive functioning. The pathological process of deteriorating has a profound effect on the biological age of individuals, such that the chronological age is no longer a valid and reliable indicator of the age of the individual.[23] The key issues in addressing order in theories of adult development pertain to:

- Concepts regarding the theoretical and clinical basis for universally invariant sequences of achievement;
- Concepts concerning the rate people progress along developmental sequences.[24]

The first issue is not often addressed and when addressed, is usually rapidly answered by outlining innate organismic processes which occur. The second issue is more frequently addressed in a normative fashion, thereby creating the impression that chronological age is not correlated with, but is a causal determinant of, individual progress. However, several lines of evidence suggest the need to disassociate the notion of developmental sequence from chronological age.[25,26]

Over the duration of AD, there appears to be deterioration in mental function that is developmentally reversed and hierarchically consistent. Thirty years ago, de Ajuriaguerra demonstrated that the functional decline in those suffering from Ad closely resembles Piaget's developmental stages in reverse.[27] The description of AD patients' behaviors as childlike make it seem logical that Piaget's theory could be utilized to examine the performance of AD patients on "typical" developmental tasks. This theoretical insight has facilitated further understanding of the disease process. Moreover, it provided some guidelines for the organization of scientific studies to substantiate the observations of immature or childlike behaviors that are often associated with AD patients.[28] In fact, some studies have used Piaget's model to chart the regressive course of AD persons traveling cognitively back from adulthood to childhood.[29-31] Thornbury showed how the use of Piaget's theory in reversal could even be applied to aid in caregiving techniques with AD persons. Such linear stage models of AD have helped caregivers learn to progressively take on more responsibility in providing care and planning for the future as the AD victim loses abilities.

For over a decade, Reisberg's seven-stage model of AD has provided clinicians with a means to describe the anticipated time course and progression of the disease. The clinical findings support a theory that the stages in AD appear to reverse normal human functional development. Reisberg's[32] protocol tool was based on:

- The definable consistency of AD.
- The idea that dementing processes associated with other causes progress differently than AD;
- The notion that functional decrements can be described in universal terms.

The FAST stages of AD were numbered to correspond with the Global Deterioration Scale's (GDS) stages of normal aging to facilitate comparison.[33] Reisberg's FAST has very defined deficits that AD patients experience as they go through each of the seven stages. This is an advancement over the shorter stage theories that dominated the 1970s and 1980s.

Although the FAST, GDS and Piaget's adult development in reverse have been extremely useful clinical tools—they have limitations. The linearity of these stage theories fail to account for the day to day and month to month fluctuations in behavior, memory and recall that occur with AD persons throughout the course of the disease (See Table 1).

In 1962, Thomas Kuhn presented an argument that challenged a linear view about scientific activity and progress. Based on historical studies of the physical sciences, Kuhn wrote that scientific knowledge advances in two ways:

- First by gradual elaboration of fundamental understandings through the testing of particular hypothesis and the refinement of research technology; and
- Second by alterations in fundamental understandings that provide new frameworks for interpreting old and emergent facts.

FAST stage	Characteristics	Clinical DX	Estimated duration in AD*	Approximate age at which function is acquired**
	Table 1. Correspondence of functional assessment stages in AD to normal human development			
1	No decrement	Normal adult	50 years	Adult
2	Subjective deficit in word finding	Normal aged adult	15 years	Adult
3	Deficits noted in demanding employment settings	Compatible with incipient AD	7 years	Young adult
4	Requires assistance in complex tasks, such as handling finances, planning dinner parties	Mild AD	2 years	8 years to adolescence
5	Requires assistance in choosing proper attire	Moderate AD	18 months	5 to 7 years
6	a. Requires assistance dressing	Moderately severe AD	5 months	5 years†
	b. Requires assistance bathing properly		5 months	4 years†
	c. Requires assistance with mechanics of toileting (e.g., flushing, wiping)		5 months	48 months‡
	d. Urinary incontinence		4 months	36 to 54 months§
	e. Fecal incontinence		10 months	24 to 36 months†‡§
7	a. Speech ability limited to about a half-dozen intelligible words	Severe AD	12 months	15 months†‡
	b. Intelligible vocabulary limited to a single word		18 months	12 months†‡
	c. Ambulatory ability lost		12 months	12 months†‡
	d. Ability to sit up lost		12 months	24 to 40 weeks†‡
	e. Ability to smile lost		18 months	8 to 16 weeks†‡
	f. Ability to hold up head lost		Not applicable	4 to 12 weeks†‡

* In subjects who survive and progress to the subsequent deterioration stage; ** Similar to Piaget's stages of adult development;
† Eisenberg[19], ‡ Vaughn[20], § Pierce[21]

Kuhn called the first concept normal science and the second one scientific revolution.[34] This paper provides a revolutionary new framework or paradigm for conceptualizing the course of AD as a "trip back in time." The attempt here is to alter the current view of the course of AD from fixed stage models to that of a fluid, non-linear model.

So far, research has tended to adopt either linear or fixed stage models, as with Reisberg, et al, and Piaget to describe the course of AD.[35,36] Linear models are based on the assumption that decline tends to be uniform, in fixed stages showing only incremental variations throughout the course of the disease. Unfortunately, studies indicated over a decade ago that the decline in individual mental functions with AD is far from uniform.[37]

Individuals vary tremendously in the rate and progression of AD which make it difficult to predict time tables and fixed regression paths for the course of the disease.[38-40] In addition, based upon age of onset and other variables, not all people with AD exhibit the same pattern of cognitive, physical and functional deficits. Therefore, it is improbable that a single developmental pattern of decline can actually portray the course of the disease.[41]

The "trip back in time"

The concept of the "trip back in time" offers a new theoretical model of the course of AD. It uses a downward spiral with connecting loops to demonstrate the fluctuat-

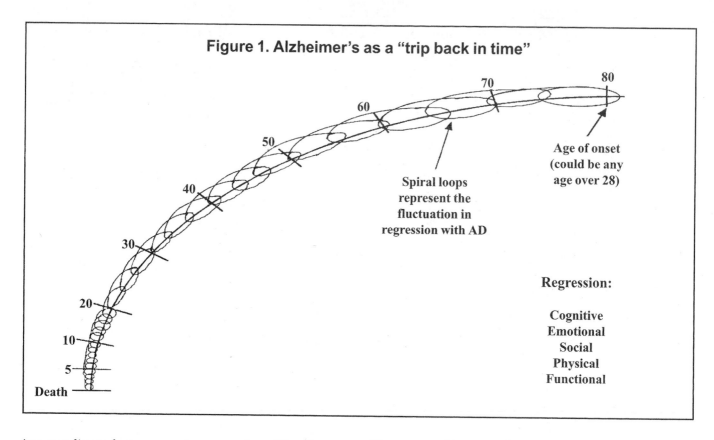

Figure 1. Alzheimer's as a "trip back in time"

Spiral loops represent the fluctuation in regression with AD

Age of onset (could be any age over 28)

Regression:

Cognitive
Emotional
Social
Physical
Functional

Death

ing, non-linear, but progressive regression of the disease. This regression is both fluid and fluctuating while the AD person travels from the age of onset of the disease back through time to his or her earliest years. The "trip back in time" model can account for the AD victim's ability to fluctuate in both memory and/recognition of family members as they travel back through time.

The use of the downward spiral diagram with loops (see Figure 1) suggests that the loops are all connected allowing for cognitive flow and fluctuation. The capabilities of the AD person are going to change throughout the course of the disease, beginning with short term memory loss followed by long term memory loss. The AD person's physical regression goes from normal to super human strength, then to problems with ambulation, and finally to the fetal position in a bedridden state similar to an infant in the womb.

The connecting "loops" progress downward which accounts for the adult development in reverse aspect of AD as delineated by Reisberg and others. However, this new theoretical model accounts for the non-linear variances on a daily basis through time, with both recall and functional abilities. The connected loops explain how an AD person's memory can make small or quantum leaps springing back up from the past to the distant present for brief time spans. Although until now it has not been labeled, past studies have suggested that a theoretical "trip back in time," involves a cognitive, emotional, social, physical and functional regression back to infancy (see Table 2).

The case of Mrs. Park

Through clinical observations, Mrs. Park, an 89-year-old grandmother has cognitively regressed back approximately to age 59 and will typically not recognize her grandchildren at that point. Yet Mrs. Park frequently experiences lucid moments where she cognitively returns back up to age 89, clearly recognizing her grandchildren again. What accounts for this extreme variation in Mrs. Park's memory? For most people, normal brain function allows for good days and bad, with some variation in mental acuity. However, for the cognitively impaired persons, these variations can be exaggerated. Eventually, decline is inevitable and the 89-year-old grandmother will continue on a downward spiraling path, fluctuating back and forth, while she cognitively travels back to infancy. AD persons rarely return to the present time but on a few occasions can, as will be pointed out later. How much variation (*e.g.*, a decade or two decades?) either downward or upward, will require future research?

As the AD person regresses back and forth in time vortexing downward toward infancy, these variations in functioning make it extremely frustrating for caregivers. They often do not understand this aspect of the disease, because one day the grandchildren are recognized and the next day they are not. This may make caregivers think that the person with AD is playing a game or not trying hard enough to remember. For example, one of the co-authors clinically observed a confused nursing home resident respond one day to being called Ms. Jones (her first

Table 2. The multifaceted regressions of Alzheimer's disease	
Cognitive regression	Short term memory loss is followed by long term memory loss. As they travel back to different ages through their life, they remember details specific to that time frame that can be positive or negative. Concomitantly, the AD person often goes through a regressive personality change in a "trip back in time" from adulthood to infancy.
Emotional regression	Rational thinking is lost, but the person actually becomes more in touch with their emotions. Child psychologists paradoxically suggest that infants are more emotionally in touch and honest than adults.
Social regression	Past self, people, places, and things have meaning whether positive or negative based upon where they are on their "trip back in time." Reality orientation may frustrate them versus validation which legitimates their cognitive world.
Physical regression	At first, they have normal physical strength that typically turns into super physical strength which is followed much later by psychomotor retardation with falling, swallowing difficulties, and choking. Eventually the person with AD is no longer able to ambulate, and is finally curled up into a fetal position in a metamorphic womb-like state in bed.
Functional regression	Activities of daily living change through time restricting independence. Movement from verbal to non-verbal communication is the norm. Hence, communication patterns are lost in a similar way in which they are gained from infancy to adulthood.

* There is typically no upward movement physically as opposed to the other areas.

husband's name), and the next day to Ms. Davis (her second husband's name), and then back to Ms. Jones again. This example describes her fluctuating regression downward on a path through time headed toward her family of origin where eventually only her maiden name would be remembered. At other times, we have observed that the AD person may mistake their children for a sibling one day and the next day not recognize them at all.

This model (Figure 1) suggests that the person with AD is on a "trip back in time" to earlier ages or time periods where the person with AD is making short time shifts reliving positive, negative and sometimes traumatic experiences of their life again. Studies show that the younger the dementia victim is, the quicker they regress through the course of the disease to death.[42] Perhaps the "trip back in time" may shed some light on why younger Alzheimer's patients die sooner than the norm. Maybe it is because younger victims have a shorter journey to infancy than the older patients who typically live longer with AD.

The case of Mr. Joe

Currently it is not clear why on certain occasions victims may make brief mega-shifts in memory moving upward through three or four decades for retrieval of information (recall). In the final bedridden state, the AD person becomes more rigid with extra pyramidal symptoms and primitive reflexes. Other primitive release signs (sucking and grasping reflexes) paralleling infancy occur and weight loss is often severe.[43] We have clinically ob-

served a patient in a nursing home who was bedridden and in a semi-fetal position. This patient had not spoken in full sentences for over a year and was basically non-verbal. One day however, as his daughter entered his room, Joe said, "Susan, your new hair style looks nice." Using a linear model discussed earlier, this interaction would not be explainable or plausible. However, the "trip back in time" model with connecting loops offers some explanation to this erratic cognition that is often puzzling and stressful to caregiver perceptions. Toward the end of the journey of AD, these patients cannot ambulate, suffer from psychomotor retardation, are non-verbal and typically only recognize pictures of their family of origin. In addition, the bedridden victims who have cognitively time travelled back to their childhood years, do not recognize or even respond to any of their nuclear family unless they resemble an extended family member. Nevertheless, at any given time the AD person can make tremendous cognitive shifts upward to the present. Such phenomena as in the above case, indicate that AD persons not only vary from day to day in their recall of loved ones' names and faces, but may be capable of making brief quantum leaps in memory. Hence, the use of the "trip back in time" model can help caregivers understand the presence of variation that can occur no matter how short the time period is.

Summary

The fluctuation of cognition in AD is often puzzling and stressful to caregivers. The conceptualization of AD as a "trip back in time" with connected loops on a downward spiral offers caregivers new insights into the unpredictable variation their AD loved ones may experience. The paradigm of the "trip back in time" may increase gerontologist and caregiver understanding by using a non-linear model versus a fixed stage regression of AD. This explanation of the course of AD provides a paradigm shift referred to by Thomas Kuhn as scientific revolution offering a new approach to enhance future caregiving techniques. Therefore, it is suggested that instead of conceptualizing steady predictable linear stages, future theory and research should take into account the non-linear spiral effect of connecting loops or varying shifts in the AD victim's trip back in time.

As Carrie Knowles so eloquently stated in her book, *Alzheimer's: The last childhood*:

> "It is not always easy to understand what is happening. Alzheimer's does not come on full blown, nor does it attack in a clean clear cut manner. It is often muddied by a family's history. It is camouflaged by the quirks of aging and all those rough edges you don't want, or just plain refuse, to see in someone you love."[44]

By utilizing this "trip back in time" model as a basis for competency-based care, researchers may in turn caution against overestimating or underestimating the capacities of AD patients. Then perhaps, caregivers and health care providers would be less likely to inappropriately assign the AD person a fixed deficit and reinforce dependency and exaggerated helplessness.

References

1. Reisberg B: Stages of cognitive decline. *American Journal of Nursing*. 1984; 2: 225–228.
2. Reisberg B: Dementia: A systematic approach to identifying reversible causes. *Geriatrics*. 1986; 41: 30–46 (39).
3. Reisberg B, Ferris S, Franssen E: Functional degenerative stages in dementia of the Alzheimer's type appear to reverse normal human development. *Biological Psychiatry*. 1986; 1319–1321.
4. Reisberg B, Ferris S, de Leon M, *et al*: Stage-specific behavioral, cognitive, and in vivo changes in community residing subjects with age-associated memory impairment and primary degenerative dementia of the Alzheimer's type. *Drug Development Research*. 1988; 15: 101–114.
5. Reisberg B, Ferris S, de Leon M, Crook T: Global Deterioration Scale. *Pharmacology Bulletin*. 1988; 24(4): 661–663.
6. Reisberg B: Memory dysfunction and dementia: Diagnostic considerations. In second ed. Carl Salzman (Ed) *Clinical Geriatric Psycho-Pharmacology*. Baltimore: Williams & Wilkins, 1992: 225–276.
7. Auer S, Sclan S, Yaffee R. Reisberg B: The neglected half of Alzheimer's disease: Cognitive and functional concomitants of severe dementia. *Journal of American Geriatrics*. 1994; 42(12): 1266–1272.
8. Souren L, Franssen E, Reisberg B: Contractures and loss of function in patients with Alzheimer's disease. *Journal of American Geriatrics*. 1995; 43(6): 650–655.
9. Andersen G: *Caring for People with Alzheimer's Disease: A training manual for direct care providers*. Baltimore: Health Professional Press, 1995.
10. Beck C, Heacock P, Mercer S, *et al*: The impact of cognitive skills remediation training of persons with Alzheimer's disease or mixed dementia. *Journal of Geriatric Psychiatry*. 1988; 21: 73–78.
11. Gwyther L: *Care of Alzheimer's Patients: A Manual for Nursing Home Staff*. American Health Care & Alzheimer's Disease and Related Disorders Association, 1985.
12. Dastoor DP, Cole MG: The course of Alzheimer's disease: an uncontrolled longitudinal study. *Journal of Clinical and Experimental Gerontology*. 1985; 74: 289–99.
13. Sloane PD, Mathew LJ (eds.): *Dementia Units in Long-Term Care*. The Johns Hopkins University Press, 1991.
14. Office of Technology Assessment: Special Care Units for People with Alzheimer's and Other Dementias: Consumer education, research, regulatory, and reimbursement issues. Congress of the United States, 1992.
15. Dastoor DP, Cole MG: The course of Alzheimer's disease: An uncontrolled longitudinal study. *Journal of Clinical and Experimental Gerontology*. 1985; 74: 289–299.
16. Andersen G: *Caring for People with Alzheimer's Disease: A training manual for direct care providers*. Baltimore: Health Professional Press, 1995.
17. Heyman A, Wilkinson WE, Hurwitz BJ, *et al*: Early-onset Alzheimer's disease: Clinical predictors of institutionalization and death. *Neurology*. 1987: 37: 980–984.
18. Dastoor DP, Cole M: Age-related patterns of decline in dementia as measured by the Hierarchic Dementia Scale. *American Journal of Alzheimer's Care and Related Disorders Research*. 1988; 3: 29–35.
19. Brooks JO, Kraemer HC, Tanke ED, Yesavage JA: The methodology of studying decline in Alzheimer's disease. *Journal of the American Geriatrics Society*. 1993; 41: 623–28.
20. Oliver R. Bock F: *Coping with Alzheimer's: A caregiver's emotional survival guide*. North Hollywood: Wilshire Book Co., 1987.
21. Thornbury JM: Cognitive performance in Piagetian tasks by Alzheimer's disease patients. *Research in Nursing and Health*. 1992; 15: 11–18.
22. Thornbury JM: The use of Piaget's theory in Alzheimer's disease. *The American Journal of Alzheimer's Care and Related Disorders Research*. 1993; 8(4): 16–21.
23. Emery OB: Language and aging. *Experimental Aging Research*. 1985; 11(1): 3–60.
24. Schulz R., Ewen RB: *Adult Development and Aging: Myths and Emerging Realities*. New York: Macmillan Publishing Co., 1993.
25. Uzgiris IC, Hunt JM: *Assessment in Infancy: Ordinal Scales of Psychological-Development*. Chicago: University of Illinois Press, 1975.
26. Dworetzky JP: *Introduction to Child Development*. Minneapolis: West Publishing Co., 1993.
27. Dastoor DP, Cole M: Age-related patterns of decline in dementia as measured by the Hierarchic Dementia Scale. *American Journal of Alzeimer's Care and Related Disorders Research*. 1988; 3: 29–35.
28. Thornbury JM: The use of Piaget's theory in Alzheimer's disease. *The American Journal of Alzheimer's Care and Related Disorders Research*. 1993; 8(4): 16–21.
29. Thornbury JM: The use of Piaget's theory in Alzheimer's disease. *The American Journal of Alzheimer's Care and Related Disorders Research*. 1993; 8(4): 16–21.
30. Bailey C, Haight BK: The use of visual cues in mid-stage Alzheimer's disease. *The American Journal of Alzheimer's Care and Related Disorders Research*. 1994; 9(4): 23–29.

31. Houlthaus J: I-FAAD (Instrument for affirming Alzheimer's Disease): Understanding & affirming stage specific cognitive decline as it correlates to early childhood development. *The American Journal of Alzheimer's Disease*. 1997; 12(4): 167–170.

32. Reisberg B: Dementia: A systematic approach to identifying reversible causes. *Geriatrics*. 1986; 41: 30–46 (39).

33. Reisberg B, Ferris S, de Leon M, Crook T: The global deterioration scale for assessment of primary degenerative dementia. *American Journal of Psychiatry*. 1982; 139: 1136–9.

34. Gubrium JF: *Oldtimers and Alzheimer's: The Descriptive Organization of Senility*. Greenwich: JAI Press, 1986, pg. 201.

35. Gwyther L: *Care of Alzheimer's Patients: A Manual for Nursing Home Staff*. American Health Care & Alzheimer's Disease and Related Disorders Association. 1985.

36. Reisberg B: Dementia: A systematic approach to identifying reversible causes. *Geriatrics*. 1986; 41:30–46 (39).

37. Dastoor DP, Cole M: Age-related patterns of decline in dementia as measured by the Hierarchic Dementia Scale. *American Journal of Alzheimer's Care and Related Disorders Research*. 1988; 3: 29–35.

38. Johnson CJ: Sociological Interventions through developing low stimulus Alzheimer's wings in nursing homes. *The American Journal of Alzheimer's Care and Related Disorders Research*. 1989; 4(2): 33–41.

39. Moore RH: The use of symbolic interaction in the management of Alzheimer's disease: A review of the literature. *The American Journal of Alzheimer's Care and Related Disorders Research*. 1991; 6(5): 28–33.

40. Lucca U, Comelli M, Tettamanti M, *et al:* Rate of progression and prognostic factors in Alzheimer's disease: a prospective study. *Journal of the American Geriatrics Society*. 1993; 41: 45–49.

41. Brooks JO, Kraemer HC, Tanke ED, Yesavage JA: The methodology of studying decline in Alzheimer's disease. *Journal of the American Geriatrics Society*. 1993; 41: 623–28.

42. Heyman A, Wilkinson WE, Hurwitz BJ, *et al:* Early-onset Alzheimer's disease: Clinical predictors of institutionalization and death. *Neurology*. 1987; 37: 980–984.

43. Kovach CR: *Late-Stage Dementia Care, A Basic Guide*. Washington, DC: Taylor & Francis, 1997.

44. Knowles C: *Alzheimer's: The last childhood*. Fuquay-Varina, NC: Research Triangle Publishing Co., 1997: 85.

Christopher J. Johnson, PhD, Professor of Gerontology, Institute of Gerontology, University of Louisiana at Monroe, Monroe, Louisiana. Roxanna H. Johnson, MS, CTRS, President, Aging Consultants Inc., Monroe, Louisiana.

Reprinted from the *American Journal of Alzheimer's Disease,* March/April 2000, pp. 87-93. © 2000 by the American Journal of Alzheimer's Disease. Reprinted with permission.

UNIT 5

Retirement: American Dream or Dilemma?

Unit Selections

Key Points to Consider

- What are some of the individual adjustment problems older people often face during their first year of retirement?

- Upon arriving at retirement age, why do some workers choose to continue to work either full-time or part-time?

- What are the advantages to the employers of retaining older employees on a full-time or part-time basis?

- What factors lead older people to retire early?

- Given different choices of lifestyles between work and retirement, which older Americans are most satisfied during their later years?

- What incentives could employers develop to keep older persons working longer?

- Is the retirement of older workers more prevalent in rural or industrialized countries? Why?

Student Website
www.mhcls.com/online

Internet References
Further information regarding these websites may be found in this book's preface or online.

American Association of Retired People
http://www.aarp.org

Health and Retirement Study (HRS)
http://www.umich.edu/~hrswww/

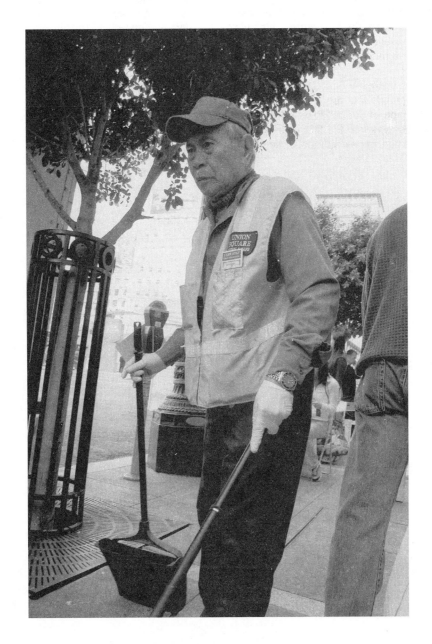

Since 1900, the number of people in America who are age 65 years and over has been increasing steadily, but a decreasing proportion of that age group remains in the workforce. In 1900 nearly two-thirds of those over the age of 65 worked outside the home. By 1947 this figure had declined to about 48 percent (less than half), and in 1975 about 22 percent of men 65 and older were still in the workforce. The long-range trend indicates that fewer and fewer people are employed beyond the age of 65. Some people choose to retire at age 65 or earlier; for others, retirement is mandatory. A recent change in the law, however, allows individuals to work as long as they want with no mandatory retirement age.

Gordon Strieb and Clement Schneider (Retirement in American Society, 1971) observed that for retirement to become an institutionalized social pattern in any society, certain conditions must be present. A large group of people must live long enough to retire; the economy must be productive enough to support people who are not in the workforce; and there must be pensions or insurance programs to support retirees.

Retirement is a rite of passage. People can consider it either as the culmination of the American Dream or as a serious problem. Those who have ample incomes, interesting things to do, and friends to associate with often find the freedom of time and choice that retirement offers very rewarding. For others, however, retirement brings problems and personal losses. Often, these individuals find their incomes decreased, they miss the status, privilege, and power associated with holding a position in the occupational hierarchy. They may feel socially isolated if they do not find new activities to replace their previous work-related ones. Additionally, they might have to cope with the death of a spouse and/or their own failing health.

Older persons approach retirement with considerable concern about financial and personal problems. Will they have enough retirement income to maintain their current lifestyle? Will their income remain adequate as long as they live? Given the current state of health, how much longer can they continue to work?

The next articles deal with changing Social Security regulations and changing labor demands that are encouraging older persons to work beyond the age of 65. In "How to Survive the First Year," Kelly Greene observes that the first year of retirement is the most difficult transition for new retirees. Critical questions that each prospective retiree should address are outlined. In "Reshaping Retirement: Scenarios and Options," the authors examine whether retirement in the future will be restructured to mix part-time work with free time to give older workers a more satisfying later life. In "Old. Smart. Productive." the author points out the reasons why he believes a significant number of the baby boom generation will work beyond age 65. Kinsella and Phillips in "Work, Retirement, and Well-Being" discuss the labor force participation rate and different pension plans utilized in countries throughout the world. In "Work/Retirement Choices and Lifestyle Patterns of Older Americans," the authors examine six different work, retirement, and leisure patterns that older people may choose to determine which is most satisfying to the individual.

"How to Survive the First Year"

BY KELLY GREENE

PATRICIA BREAKSTONE, age 63, remembers her first year of retirement from her 38-year career as a state-government analyst in San Diego as a "terrible transition period."

Shortly after leaving her job last spring, she started a long-awaited kitchen renovation, which turned her condo upside-down right when she was starting to spend her days at home for the first time in her adult life. Then her dog was struck by kidney disease, and Ms. Breakstone wound up spending $7,000 in veterinary bills over two months as she tried in vain to nurse her pet back to health.

As the months wore on, "I didn't want to get up in the morning," she says. Finally, a friend goaded her into applying for a part-time job at a bakery near her home, which helped her regain some structure in her days—along with providing a social outlet. "Retirement," she says now, "is a real balancing act."

For all its allure, for all the time that people spend planning and daydreaming about it, the actual act of retiring can turn out to be a wrenching experience. That's what we learned from canvassing dozens of people across the country about their first year outside the office. We wanted to find out—at a time when the 50-plus crowd, in particular, is apprehensive about its future and finances—just how satisfying, or scary, those first 12 months can be.

Among the questions we asked: Did the transition prove to be easy or difficult? If people did any planning beforehand, had it paid off? Did they find themselves spending more or less money than they had anticipated? Had they gone back to work? What did they miss most about their jobs? What was the biggest surprise?

The answers showed that while some people clearly enjoyed leaving work behind, many were disoriented. Just like college freshmen, first-year retirees often change their "majors." Even people who start out

with a road map rarely wind up following it the way they expected. And rare is the retiree who spends significantly less money than when he or she was working full time.

But as the first year winds down, many retirees start settling into Plan B—or C, or D, for that matter. That's when post-work life finally starts to get comfortable.

"There doesn't seem to be the big hole that I expected after all those years working," says Steve Holt, age 63, who retired from General Electric Co. in Seattle in late 2001, and moved to Tucson, Ariz., the following May. "I was surprised that it was so easy to find things to do and become involved."

In hopes of providing a shortcut for people contemplating retirement—or retirees still struggling to make it work—here are the first-year lessons we heard most often.

■ BE CHOOSY WITH YOUR TIME

You might expect to have an empty calendar during your early days of retirement. But whether you find that prospect frightening or appealing, your schedule could fill up quickly if you aren't careful—and with things you may not really want to be doing.

Debbie Lynch, for example, was asked to stay on for several months as director of communications and head of an educational foundation at the Aurora, Colo., school system after she officially retired, in November 2001. As the school year drew to a close, she was offered two consulting jobs that would start the following fall, one in fund raising for the local community college, the other helping to set up a foundation for the local chamber of commerce.

"I initially thought, every job that comes along, I have to take," says Ms. Lynch, 54 years old. Despite the fact that she and her husband both have secure pensions, "every once in a while, I think, 'Who will take care of me when I'm old?' I don't have any children." Plus, she wanted to

stay connected with the professional friends she had made through the years.

But last summer, between the old job and new consulting work, "I discovered there are a lot of things you can do during daylight hours. It was a real treat to go to the grocery store at 10 a.m.," she says. "It was the first time in years and years that I had that much time. I played a little golf, walked every day, did some long-term cleaning I probably should have done 25 years ago. I just piddled."

When it came time to begin the consulting job, "I started thinking, 'Why did I agree to do this?'" Ms. Lynch recalls. "It was one of the biggest surprises I had. I wasn't ready to get back into being responsible on a regular basis." Although she enjoys her community ties, she regrets the fact that work eats up four days a week. "I really think I would prefer in the long run to do more project-based things that have a beginning and an end. I'm less interested in being tied down to certain days and hours."

Part of the initial temptation to fill up the calendar stems from the fear "that if you say no, nobody's ever going to ask you to do something again," says Bob Atchley, a Boulder, Colo., gerontologist who has studied retirees since 1963. As a result, retirees can be victimized by time poachers who volunteer them for tasks they might not necessarily want to do but may feel guilty turning down.

"You have to learn the lesson of how to say 'no,' whether it's to the kids saying, 'Oh, you can baby-sit, can't you?' Or someone saying, 'You can co-chair this project. What else do you have to do?'" advises Jeri Sedlar, a New York retirement-transition counselor.

Robert Carpenter, 64, who participates in a "Reinventing Retirement" class at Emory University's Academy for Retired Professionals in Atlanta, says many of his friends are "activity addicted." It's a trap

ON YOUR MARK, GET SET...

Are you ready to retire? In their book "Don't Retire, Rewire," authors Jeri Sedlar and Rick Miners offer the following questions, developed by Tessa Albert Warschaw, to help people gauge where they stand in their preparations:

TAKING STOCK

- Have you thought about restructuring or reinventing yourself?

- Have you spent time asking yourself, "What's next?"

- Are you aware of the loss you may feel (i.e., loss of position, power, the game, the deal, a place to go, schedule, agenda, assistants, secretary, etc.)?

- Have you considered whether you will miss the travel and entertainment perks?

- Have you thought about how you will feel doing your own paperwork?

- Have you considered how you will feel?

- Have you thought about whether you will miss all those problems to solve?

- Have you anticipated whether you will miss the triumphs and approvals?

- Have you considered whether you will miss your title?

- Have you thought about whether your spouse will miss your title?

FAMILY DYNAMICS

- Have you considered the changes in your family dynamic?

- Will your being home more affect your partner?

- Will your family see you as less powerful?

- Will you consider yourself less powerful?

- Will you transfer your "work style" to your home?

- Do you see yourself setting up a command post at home-issuing directives, responsibilities and orders?

- Do you see yourself taking on household duties, running family errands, cooking, etc.)?

- Do you see yourself assisting younger family members or "baby-sitting" the grandchildren or elder parents?

- Will you feel resentment for your partner who hasn't retired and continued to work inside and/or outside the home?

Source: "Don't Retire, Rewire," © 2002, Alpha Books-Penguin Group, USA

---

he found himself falling into during his retirement from Georgia Power Co., before he started making a conscious effort to clear time on his calendar.

"I found myself filling up my calendar with 'good' things, which was the enemy of the 'best' things when they came up." For example, when he decided to skip an enrichment course on a recent weekday, he and his wife seized on the sunny weather to check out a nearby lakeside resort for lunch. And after they cleared from their schedules an annual golf tournament that they usually attend, it freed them up to accept an invitation to their granddaughter's fifth birthday party. "That's something we would have rather done anyway," he says.

■ IT'S OK TO SLOW DOWN

Taking time for yourself can change your outlook on what you want to do with all your newfound free time, as Ms. Lynch in Colorado and many others have found.

"Drift time" is something that many retirees rediscover, says Joel Savishinsky, an anthropologist at Ithaca College in New York, who has studied people during their first year in retirement. One couple he watched would take long bike rides "presumably to go from Point A to Point B in their community, and they rarely made it to Point B. In retirement, if you allow yourself, you have the luxury to be diverted, to digress, to slow down, to change directions. To get off the bike."

And as you're making the adjustment to retirement, that can be especially important. Mary Roberson, who retired as an elementary-school librarian in Dallas last spring, recommends taking some initial time "to just veg." For most people, she says, "those last couple of months before retirement are nonstop. It was incredible how many things had to be done before I turned the library over to the next person."

"I didn't take on any new projects," says Ms. Roberson, 61. "I gave myself time to work in the yard and feel better about the flower beds. I cleaned out a few closets. I sat and had a second cup of cof-

fee and read the whole paper. I needed a couple of unwinding months before I did anything else."

Now, she's starting to take on short-term projects. She recently wrapped up five weeks of work at her son's law firm as he scrambled to prepare for a big trial, "and five weeks is as long as I want to commit to anything," she says.

By all means, try new things and challenge yourself—but don't get stressed out about it. Ed Susank, 58, a retired health-care benefits consultant with Mercer Human Resource Consulting, says he initially made a list of things he wanted to do after he retired, including "becoming more proficient in a foreign language." But he isn't rushing to cross things off. "I like to have a few pegs around which the rest of it can kind of drape casually."

That's an approach that Dr. Atchley, the gerontologist, considers healthy. "In our world, most people push themselves beyond anything that's good for them physically and mentally," Dr. Atchley says. "So the idea that people actually could cut back quite a bit on the complexity and the level of activity that they're involved in after they retire and still be at the level any full-time person ought to be has a lot to recommend it."

■ WORK OUT THE GROUND RULES

If you have a partner, chances are you'll be spending a lot more time together under one roof when you retire. That could lead to some stomping (albeit unintentional) on each other's toes.

Ken Schumann says that within two months of his retirement last year as director of the North American agriculture business for Ciba Special Chemicals AG, his wife, Patty, came up with three rules for him: "No. 1, I cannot fall asleep in front of the TV from Monday to Friday. No. 2, I cannot follow Patty around and ask what she's doing next. No. 3 is, since I traveled so much and she wasn't used to cooking seven days a week, we needed an outside life, including dinners out. I now have a 3A. I must answer the telephone because the calls are for me for a change."

Mr. Schumann, who is 59 years old and lives in suburban Atlanta, talked about his new rules at a recent meeting of the same Emory class that Mr. Carpenter attends. Their classmates agree that negotiating personal space with your partner is one of the biggest hurdles in the first year.

Among their recommendations: Shell out the bucks for separate phone lines, computers and e-mail addresses. Stake out space in your home that is yours alone. Mr. Carpenter says he has a "cave" with his own TV, computer, and recliner. Also, negotiate the time you spend together—and apart. Derek Moore, 64, a retired aerospace executive with Lockheed Martin Corp. in Marietta, Ga., had planned on selling antiquarian books as a new career, with help from his wife. That pastime ended after five months, because they each realized the project was keeping them from individual interests they considered important. Mr. Moore, for his part, wanted more time to pursue the arts, and he has since taken up painting.

■ BE PREPARED TO SWITCH GEARS

Jim Matheson was always bothered by the litter he saw along the road during his 10-mile commute to Worcester, Mass., as an insurance executive. "I swore that when I retired, I was going to get a little pickup trailer, and in the course of a year, I was going to pick up the trash on all 116 miles of roads in our town," he recalls.

Mr. Matheson retired in January 2002, shortly after he turned 55 and could take an early-retirement package. A few months later, he visited the local police department to explain his plan "before someone reported that there was this vagrant along the side of the road." While he was there, the chief told him the department could use some help with its roadside radar-information unit (responsible for the signs that say, "Slow Down, Your Speed Is . . .").

"I said, 'Wait a minute. You're telling me I get to drive the cruiser, right?'" Mr. Matheson recalls. What started out as an effort to pick up bottles and cans evolved into what Mr. Matheson considers the chance of a lifetime: getting behind the wheel of a police car—even if it's only to haul the signs around. The first time he drove the vehicle on a major highway, "traffic backed up for miles behind me," he says. "What a feeling of power."

Sometimes, your retirement plans don't work out the way you envisioned, as with Mr. Moore's book-dealing business. In that case, "if you've tried it and you don't like it, discard it," says Ms. Sedlar, the counselor. She steers many people to volunteer-match.org, a Web site that matches your interests and location to community needs.

But make sure you give a retirement plan, whether it's volunteer or for pay, a fair shake before you move on, Ms. Sedlar adds. She recalls a woman in New York who tried volunteering with a political group. In her first days there, not surprisingly, the woman was assigned several humdrum tasks, including licking envelopes. But rather than giving her new position a chance, the woman quickly "called up and got her old job back," Ms. Sedlar says. "That's the road of least resistance."

Another reason to stay flexible: Sometimes, the retirement gig you were counting on doesn't materialize. Malcolm McNeill took early retirement as a 55-year-old manager with General Electric's GE Capital unit in Cincinnati last year, and then moved to Fort Collins, Colo., planning to teach graduate business courses at Colorado State University, as he had done in the past at other colleges.

"But they are going through the same budget downturn as everyone else," he says, and as a result, he wasn't hired. "That was disappointing. I don't know if colleges know it, but they could hire people like me almost for free."

Mr. McNeill found a way to teach after all. He has volunteered to lead personal-enrichment courses in photography through the Front Range Forum, a retirement-learning institute where "everyone is there because they want to be there."

■ A ROLE MODEL OR TWO CAN HELP

Mark Feinknopf, a 66-year-old retired architect, was laid off about a year ago from his job as an urban planner for the Metropolitan Atlanta Rapid Transit Authority. A year earlier, he had started interviewing his mentors, most of them in their 70s and 80s, to find out how they had handled later-life transitions, including retirement and the premature deaths of spouses.

One of those role models, Josiah Blackmore, is a retired president of Capital University in Columbus, Ohio, who now spends his days in the countryside as an alpaca farmer. He and his wife have even opened a retail store on their farm where they're having trouble keeping enough alpaca fiber in stock.

Mr. Feinknopf hasn't decided what he wants to do yet with his own retirement, but talking to more-experienced retirees helped him settle on a goal: "I'm spending the second year trying to . . . find an opportunity to build something of value with other people."

Many retirees seek out role models without even realizing it, says Dr. Savishinsky, the anthropologist. In his studies, he notes, people's thoughts about retirement were "partly based on what they had learned from watching other people go through it," most often their parents and older co-workers. The recent retirees he followed were more likely to fixate on negative role models than positive ones. "Many retirees seem to be concerned with not blowing it," he says. "It was almost more important to know what not to do than it was to have a clear idea of what they wanted to do, which provided a very helpful road map of the people and places or pursuits to avoid."

Indeed, Mr. Matheson thinks many people are afraid to retire early because "they superimpose themselves on their parents and say, 'My father, when he retired, sat in the living room, drank beer and watched TV.' I think we [baby boomers] break that mold. If you can shake yourself loose, you see there's a big bad world out there, and there's a lot of fun stuff to do."

■ FINDING FRIENDS CAN TAKE MORE WORK

Mr. McNeill, the retired GE manager, made an unpleasant discovery when he and his wife moved to Colorado: Making friends their own age was more difficult than he had imagined.

"The thing that's been a little tough for us, and we probably should have foreseen, is most retirees are older than us, and most people's lives revolve around work," he says today. "That's where you make most of your friends."

In the McNeills' case, the solution has come through strong interests they have had for many years. He has immersed himself in photography, making frequent expeditions to Arches National Park near Moab, Utah; she plays the tuba and cello in community music groups.

Mr. Susank and his wife moved to Alexandria, Va., a few years before he retired from Mercer in late 2001, after living in Los Angeles for most of their lives. A big part of their relocation strategy was buying a townhouse in a new complex where everyone would be getting to know one another at the same time. That way, they reasoned, it would be easier to make friends with neighbors than if they moved into an established development where everybody else already had found their barbecuing buddies.

They got lucky, too. "The lady who is right next door to us had a husband in the Navy for many years," says Mr. Susank. "She's done a lot of traveling, and she has introduced us to many people."

Finding friends the same age isn't just a matter of dinner-table company, says Dr. Atchley. "All of the doubts and funny stuff you do yourself that are connected to the transition become a little more obvious when you talk about it. It's funnier when you see it in your friends, too," he says. "You begin to laugh at your own foibles, and that's a good thing. A sense of humor is adaptive."

■ DON'T EXPECT SPENDING TO FALL

When Mr. Schumann, the former Ciba executive, began thinking about expenses in later life, he used a familiar benchmark. "Everything you read says you spend 20% less in retirement, so I [factored] that in my monthly budget." But he never realized how much of his entertainment expenses—for meals, trips and the like—actually were tied to business and reimbursed by his company.

Today, he says, "I think I'm spending a little bit more in retirement than I was when I was working."

Other retirees mention the loss of similar job-related extras leading to increased retirement spending: company cars, frequent-flier miles—even technical assistance for their home computers.

Then there's the whopper: health insurance. If you're lucky enough to get any coverage at all from your former employer, the premiums and deductibles are likely to rise steeply in coming years. A study of 56 retiree health plans last year by Watson Wyatt Worldwide, a human-resources consulting firm in Washington, found that 17% require retirees to pay the full premiums. And 20% have eliminated such plans altogether for new hires.

When Fred Hattman retired from Milford, Conn., to Nags Head, N.C., two years ago, he took a job delivering the local Coastal Times newspaper three times a week. That way, Mr. Hattman, 64, can pay his share of his health-insurance premiums. It's a sizable expense—$550 a month—even though he's able to piggy-back on his wife's coverage through her full-time job at a local bank. "I knew I had to get some money somewhere to pay for the medical," he says, adding that the cost is "pretty scary, when you consider I'm pretty healthy."

Even for people who have turned in their time cards for good, the reduced costs of business suits, gasoline for the commute, dry cleaning, lunches and other expenses are often offset by the cost of new interests, says Wicke Chambers, a retired communications consultant in Atlanta who teaches the Emory course.

"You suddenly become a gardener," she says. "Or you become a golfer and you take more lessons, and you buy more balls, and you get a new bag."

Not only that, but being around the house more can make people "project-happy," she says. "You decide to redo the kitchen," for instance. "So the spending goes from a lot less in clothes and cleaning and things like that to the 'impulse itch.'"

■ RETIRING CAN BE TOUGH IF YOUR SPOUSE STILL WORKS

After a one-year trial, some people find that they still haven't eased into retirement, so they dust off their resumes and go back to work. Often, the people who wrestle with their newfound leisure time are those with spouses still on the job.

Marla Church, 60, a lawyer who took a buyout a year ago from Elan Corp. in Atlanta, says her husband "leaves at 6:45 in the morning and comes home at 4:30 in the afternoon. I need to find something productive to do in this period." Especially because her Elan stock has plummeted in value, she says, "I feel guilty if I do watercolors during the day."

At the moment, she's doing consulting work with Elan and is patent attorney of counsel with a local law firm. But she's also exploring the idea of doing "something entirely different," perhaps in the field of archaeology. She's taking a course in geology through the Emory program, at the moment, among other classes. Still, "it's hard to start over again without going back to school for years," she says. "My husband loves his work, and here I am floundering. It's a tough situation."

Myrna Weiss, a retired marketing executive in New York, had started doing many of the activities while she was working that people typically look forward to in retirement. She already was spending at least 10 hours a week volunteering and has gone to the opera and ballet regularly for years. "I don't feel like I've denied myself," she says.

But her spouse, too, still heads for the office each day. "My husband is going to work until he's disabled or horizontal," Ms. Weiss says. "He's happy as a clam."

When she first retired, Ms. Weiss pursued consulting work, but soon found it old hat since she had done a similar stint in the 1980s. Now, to scratch her entrepreneurial itch, she's exploring the chance to invest in and work with a group planning to buy and restructure an existing financial business.

"I'm looking for a niche that is going to keep the adrenaline going," she says. "It's just a matter of my being patient to alight on something that I want to do, versus getting antsy enough to choose anything."

Ms. GREENE is a staff reporter in The Wall Street Journal's Atlanta bureau. She can be reached at encore@wsj.com.

RESHAPING RETIREMENT

SCENARIOS AND OPTIONS

Retirement may disappear altogether in the future as aging workers outlive their savings and as pension systems are stretched beyond their capacities. A new report looks at what policy makers need to do now to help ensure rewarding lives for older persons in the next 20 years.

BY MICHAEL MOYNAGH AND RICHARD WORSLEY

The pensions crisis and longer life expectancy are forcing policy makers and employers throughout the world to rethink retirement. Policy makers in Britain and other industrialized countries over the next 20 years must assume that people will need to work until they are older. Will retirement as we know it be postponed for a few years? Or will retirement be reshaped, to become less age-related and more fulfilling?

In the recent study *Reshaping Retirement*, Britain's Tomorrow Project addressed a wide range of topics about the future of people's lives in Britain over the next two decades. The study focused not just on particular drivers of change, such as demographic, economic, and social developments, but also on issues that will have a decisive impact on retirement in the next two decades, such as what will happen to the labor market for older people, to government pensions, and to lifetime savings for retirement.

The key issue for retirement is how to square the triangle of longer life expectancy adequate retirement incomes, and younger workers' desire to increase their current living standards. Our starting point is that people will resolve this conundrum by working till they are older. The recent reversal of the trend toward early retirement will continue, and growing numbers will work beyond the state pension age.

As this happens, three questions will have to be tackled. How will the transition out of employment be managed? Given that Britain's labor market is likely to re-main highly polarized in both skills and income, will the state pension system prevent those at the lower earnings level from slipping into old age poverty? What will be done to encourage people to increase their long-term savings?

Linking these issues is an overarching theme: How will old age be experienced in the future? Will it remain much as it is now, but just start at an older age? Or will retirement be reshaped so that many more older people mix part-time work with extended leisure, and have higher incomes with which to enjoy their old age, bringing about a much more positive view, in society of the aging process?

UP FOR GRABS:
RETIREMENT ON THE AGENDA

Retirement is a relatively modern concept. Until recently, there has been a trend toward longer retirement (i.e., leaving the workforce at younger ages), but longer retirements are now being questioned because lower fertility rates will reduce the size of the working population, making it harder to fund government pensions and other benefits for older people. Later retirement is an obvious part of the solution. People are working for fewer years but retiring for longer periods, which is financially untenable; again, later retirement is an obvious answer.

Tackling poverty among older people has become a political priority, but the current solution—means testing—is unpopu-lar. Later retirement in return for a higher state pension for all is the most realistic alternative. Many people will not have saved enough for their retirement if it lasts for as long as it does now; they may have to postpone retirement instead. The government is starting to make it easier for people to stay on at work by encouraging phased retirement and introducing (from 2006) a ban on age discrimination.

We also have an opportunity to transform how we think about retirement and to improve the quality of life for older people. Instead of personal life being divided up on the basis of age, many people are making transitions between work and learning or leisure at many different ages.

A key difference is that individuals have greater choice over these transitions. Traditional retirement might be replaced by greatly expanded choice and by a dramatic shift in how old age is viewed—as a period of human flourishing before a final stage of dependency.

FETTERED OR FREED?
WORK IN LATER LIFE

The economic pressure on workers to retire later will mount, but it remains unclear how employers will respond. One possibility is that they will simply postpone workers' eligibility for retirement, forcing older people to work till they drop. Alternatively, they might introduce more flexible forms of employment, tailor-made to the needs of older workers.

Change will not be easy. Today's concept of retirement is deeply entrenched and will not transform overnight. Many people still see retirement as both a reward for hard work and a right to an extended period of leisure. This view is reinforced by the experience of many older workers, who often find jobs stressful and exhausting—an experience that is likely to persist.

Encouraging more-flexible employment, with work lasting till later in life, may be seen as chipping away the right to retirement and damaging to older people's health—an outcome strongly to be resisted. At the same time, age discrimination against older workers by employers could further entrench current patterns of employment by older workers. However, employers will also have to respond to several pressures driving change in the labor market.

Legislation is due in the United Kingdom by 2006 for equal treatment in employment on grounds of age, including the likelihood that compulsory retirement ages (at least up to age 70) will be outlawed. The form of the legislation and the manner of its implementation will help to determine whether retirement will be postponed or reshaped. Pressure may build within the European Union for further legislation to encourage employment by older workers.

Skill shortages, which loom in many U.K. sectors, may be a second spur to a different view of retirement, as parts of the economy become more labor intensive rather than less, technology slices away fewer jobs than expected, the demand for skills rises, the supply of young people entering the workforce begins to tail off, and skill mismatches persist. Employers may respond by investing in labor-saving equipment or by recruiting more immigrant workers, but the recruitment of older workers will be their main strategy. How well will employers respond to older workers' needs?

The aspirations of older workers will be important. They will be influenced by the continued expansion of choice (not only for the better-off, but also for those on lower incomes as living standards rise), by caring commitments to relatives, and by the likelihood that older workers will want employment that is less demanding but still worthwhile.

Commercial constraints may make it difficult to create high-quality flexible employment. These will include the size and location of the business, increasing

consumer demands, and heavy competitive pressures on costs. Attracting older workers will either be seen as costly and difficult or as vital for competing in tighter labor markets.

TWO SCENARIOS FOR WORKERS FACING RETIREMENT

1. Retirement Postponed. In this scenario, employers respond with "more of the same" over the next 20 years. They meet the growing economic need for people to work into their late 60s by effectively postponing retirement rather than reshaping it. Older workers acquiesce, despite their health concerns, because they need the money.

The public retains its deep-seated attachment to retirement as a right. Age discrimination at work remains deeply entrenched. Most employers remain cautious and unimaginative. Older workers continue working full time in good-quality jobs, if they have them, or trading down to part-time, more marginal employment, which narrows the opportunities for lower-paid workers. Retirement is still broadly age-related, though at a later age, and the routes into it remain inflexible.

2. Retirement Reshaped. In this scenario, retirement is not postponed but transformed, so that it is far less age-related. Routes out of work are more flexible—driven by a generation of older workers who demand more flexibility in retirement so that they can continue work but without feeling too stressed and worn out. Skill shortages have become so acute that employers are clamoring for older workers. Employers respond by creating more flexible patterns of work.

By 2025, the traditional concept of retirement has begun to change. Retirement is becoming less age-related, and the pathways out of employment are more varied. Although a substantial proportion of people still leave work in their late 60s, a growing minority continue working into their early 70s—and some even later.

PATCHING UP OR LASTING REFORM?

Britain's government pension system makes a statement about the nature of retirement. It gives younger people a rough idea of when they can expect to retire, and by being strongly age-related it

props up a traditional view of retirement. But the present national pension system is under challenge from many quarters. It is criticized for being too complex, for containing disincentives to save, for failing to address poverty adequately, for being ill-attuned to longer life expectancy, and for being costly to the taxpayer. There is widespread agreement that the system will have to be overhauled at some stage.

"Encourage more-flexible employment, with work lasting till later in life, may be seen as chipping away the right to retirement."

Yet there are strong political constraints in the way. These include the long-term costs of improving state pensions when set against other demands on the public purse, fears that the benefits of improvement would go to those who need it least, opposition on health grounds to requiring older people to work longer in return for pension reform, and a lack of consensus over the desired nature of reform.

TWO SCENARIOS FOR THE STATE PENSION

1. More of the Same. In this scenario, the British government tries to make the current system work. Elements of the state pension system are improved and indexed to earnings. These steps lift many pensioners off means-tested benefits.

Government meets the additional costs from savings elsewhere and by phasing in an increase in the state pension age to 67, starting in the early 2030s.

Lack of consensus drives government to a minimalist approach, designed to keep intact as much of the present system as possible. No additional steps are taken to make state pensions more flexible as a further encouragement to phased retirement.

2. A Flexible State Pension. This scenario is more radical, though it is presented as the further evolution of the current plans.

A new "Flexible State Pension" is phased in from 2030 and indexed to earnings. It is paid to everyone, irrespective of contribution record, on a residency basis and at a flat rate, set just

AGING AND RETIREMENT TRENDS: CAUSES AND OBJECTIVES

Several nations in the European Union are addressing the challenges posed by aging, focusing on the key causes and common objectives.

CAUSES OF DEMOGRAPHIC AGING:

- The baby-boom generation will reach retirement age within the next 10 to 15 years.
- The weak birthrate of recent decades.
- Life expectancy continues to rise.

COMMON OBJECTIVES:

- Preventing social exclusion of elderly people.
- Allowing retired persons to maintain their standard of living.
- Promoting solidarity among and within generations.
- Increasing employment rates.
- Prolonging the professional life span.

- Guaranteeing viable pensions within a context of healthy public finance.
- Adjusting benefits and contributions so as to distribute in a fair manner among generations the financial consequences of an aging population.
- Ensuring that private pension plans are financially healthy.
- Adapting pension plans to new, more flexible employment and career schemes.
- Responding to the aspirations of more equality between women and men.
- Making pension plans more transparent and proving their capacity to overcome the challenges by systematically informing stakeholders.

Source: EUROPA, portal for the European Union, europa.eu.int.

above the poverty line. Eventually, when all pensioners are covered, the Flexible Pension makes means-tested benefits for this age group largely redundant.

Individuals have increased choice over when they start to receive their Flexible Pension. They can take it any time between ages 60 and 80. The value of the pension is adjusted downward if taken before age 70 and upward if taken later. Those who settle for a reduced pension require an annuity (or equivalent), which will guarantee that their retirement income, including the state pension, remains at the level of the Flexible Pension or higher.

The substantial net costs of the Flexible Pension are met by raising the pension age to 70, phased in over a 10-year period starting in the mid-2030s. People whose lifetime earnings average out at close to the poverty line receive a slightly higher pension.

The age at which the full Flexible Pension becomes payable is adjusted automatically to reflect changes in life expectancy, with those affected notified well in advance of the date at which the full pension becomes payable.

The new Flexible State Pension supports the reshaping of retirement. It further erodes the notion that older people enter a stage of life that is strongly age determined. It embodies the principles of choice and flexibility. It lifts the incomes

of the poor, helping them have a more fulfilled old age.

WITH OR AGAINST THE GRAIN? THE FUTURE OF LIFETIME SAVINGS

The government hopes that there will be a strong shift to saving for retirement through an occupational or personal pension scheme. But this seems unlikely under present arrangements.

Among the reasons many workers will remain reluctant to save is that a good number are still too poor to do so. Those on middle to higher incomes who can afford to save for retirement may not save enough; many are not doing so now.

In the future, savings by middle earners will be curtailed by breaks in full-time employment (for example, to look after children), by additional financial commitments (notably paying more for higher education and other government services), by the costs for some of family breakdown (living on your own is a lot more expensive than with another person), by the strong allure of day-to-day consumption, and by longer life expectancy, which makes it harder for young people to imagine their old age and plan for it.

Defined contribution schemes will be unattractive to many people and will gradually wither away. Mistrust is widespread following a succession of scandals

and recent collapses in the financial services industry, and they are seen as too costly and risky for employers. Equity-based pensions involve considerable risks for the individual, even if investments are moved into bonds as retirement approaches. Also, the huge range of pension products, complicated charging structures; and complex tax treatments leave consumers confused.

Alternatives to pensions may become more attractive, such as equity release schemes through which people raise income on their homes (called reverse mortgages in the United States), and inheritance.

TWO SCENARIOS FOR LIFETIME SAVINGS

1. Compulsion Plus. In this scenario, employers are obliged to contribute a minimum of 5% of each worker's earnings to his or her pension. To encourage workers to save more, employers are required to match the contributions of individuals up to a total of 9%. So if you put 5%–9% of your salary into a pension, your employers would have to match it.

Despite this new incentive, workers remain reluctant to increase their savings substantially. So in 2011, as part of the reform of state pensions, compulsion is extended to individuals (and retained for employers). The state pension age is raised to 67. Private pensions follow suit, giving individuals more time to save.

Compulsion removes the need for tax relief on contributions to private pensions, which is phased out. The abolition of tax relief funds a substantial cut in income tax, making compulsion politically acceptable. Compulsion rather than choice becomes a key feature of the pensions regime.

2. Lifelong Savings Account. This scenario adopts a more flexible approach to lifetime savings—a different way of thinking about savings altogether. The Lifelong Savings Account bundles together various current savings schemes that attract government support.

This new approach to savings is designed around the life cycle rather than around retirement alone, as currently with pensions. It encourages people to travel through life with a Lifelong Savings Account, into which they put contributions when they can and from which they can make withdrawals to purchase three types of assets: property, work-related learning that will push-up their income, or a pension. These purchases attract government financial support up to a ceiling, replacing the support that is given to other current forms of savings. They also attract (compulsory) employer support, again replacing employer contributions to pensions.

The Lifelong Savings Account is kick-started with a much-enhanced "baby bond," financed by receipts from inheritance tax. An annual savings forecast is a further feature.

To qualify for matching contributions, the Lifelong Savings Account is held in a designated bank or building society account, but only with banks and building societies that offer financial advice independent of the sale of financial products.

The scenario responds to reservations about a one-size-fits-all approach to savings. It works with rather than against the short-termism of consumer behavior, it encourages savers to spread risks, and it enshrines the values of choice and flexibility needed for the reshaping of retirement.

TWO FINAL SCENARIOS

We can now pull together the previous sets of scenarios into two final scenarios that provide alternative maps for policies on retirement, the state pension, and savings for old age.

1. Putting It Off. Retirement remains much as we know it today, but it starts later. The beginning of retirement remains age-related, but the age is merely postponed. The financial preparation for retirement is squeezed into a one-size-fits-all straitjacket, which ignores the fluidity and diversity of many people's experiences. This inflexibility leads to inadequate incomes for many people and jeopardizes their ability to lead healthy and fulfilling lives in old age.

Employers are reluctant to devote management time and other resources to creating flexible work for older people. A relatively tepid approach to pension reform reinforces existing views of retirement. Inflexible savings are still the road to inflexible retirement.

2. Liquid Lives. This scenario looks very different. Its foundations are laid during the first quarter of the century, although its main features are not fully apparent till some 25 years later.

"Flexible work for older people would influence the terms and conditions of younger workers."

Retirement is no longer a distinct phase of life. People can mix and match work and more-extended leisure, with more numerous routes out of full-time employment. Indeed, the distinction between working life and retirement becomes so blurred for many people that eventually the notion of retirement itself comes into question. The financial preparation for retirement is released from its traditional straitjacket. Individuals have more savings options, backed by state and employer financial support. They can tread a more flexible financial path to a more flexible old age.

The need to encourage flexible employment becomes a policy priority. The Flexible Pension cuts pensioner poverty, enabling those on low income to enjoy a somewhat more fulfilling old age. Lifelong Savings Accounts embody the values of choice and flexibility to reshape lifetime savings, so that people are more willing to save, can acquire more assets, and are able to use these assets to support their old age.

THE PREFERRED FUTURE FOR RETIREMENT

The Liquid Lives scenario would reduce the dominant role of age in retirement arrangements. It would offer older people more choice and flexibility and more opportunities for fulfillment and self-improvement. It would transform the experience of old age and have a "ripple down" effect on younger age groups—not least by making their work more flexible. Flexible work for older people would influence the terms and conditions of younger workers.

Even if few active steps were taken to reshape retirement, social forces may bring it about in any case. Surely it would be better to work with the grain of those forces. Many of the milestones along the Liquid Lives route are in place already.

Retirement and the financial preparation for old age could be reshaped bit by bit over the next two decades, so that by 2025 the foundation would have been laid for a very different approach to later life and a more flexible, fulfilling, and rewarding old age.

About the Authors

Michael Moynagh is an ordained priest in the Church of England and co-director of the Tomorrow Project, a U.K. charity researching the future of people's lives.

Richard Worsley formerly headed the personnel function in British Aerospace and British Telecom and is co-director of the Tomorrow Project.

Moynagh and Worsley founded the Tomorrow Project in 1996 and are the coauthors of several books on the future of people's lives in addition to their individual publications.

This article summarizes their latest report, *The Opportunity of a Lifetime: Reshaping Retirement*, which was the result of a two-year project involving a series of consultations, interviews, and focus groups. Copies of the report (2004, £20) may be ordered from The Tomorrow Project, P.O. Box 160, Burnham Norton, King's Lynn, Norfolk PE31 8GA, United Kingdom. Web site www.tomorrowproject.net.

OLD. SMART. PRODUCTIVE.

Surprise! The graying of the workforce is better news than you think

Peter Coy

EMMA SHULMAN IS A DYNAMO. THE VETERAN SOCIAL WORKER WORKS up to 50 hours a week recruiting people for treatment at an Alzheimer's clinic at New York University School of Medicine. Her boss, psychiatrist Steven H. Ferris, dreads the day she decides to retire: "We'd definitely have to hire two or three people to replace her," he says. Complains Shulman: "One of my problems is excess energy, which drives me nuts."

Oh, one more thing about Emma Shulman. She's nearly 93 years old.

Shulman is more than one amazing woman. She just might be a harbinger of things to come as the leading edge of the 78 million-strong Baby Boom generation approaches its golden years. Of course, nobody's predicting that boomers will routinely work into their 90s. But Shulman—and better-known oldsters like investor Kirk Kerkorian, 87, and Federal Reserve Chairman Alan Greenspan, 79—are proof that productive, paying work does not have to end at 55, 60, or even 65.

Old. Smart. Productive. Rather than being an economic deadweight, the next generation of older Americans is likely to make a much bigger contribution to the economy than many of today's forecasts predict. Sure, most people slow down as they get older. But new research suggests that boomers will have the ability—and the desire—to work productively and innovatively well beyond today's normal retirement age. If society can tap their talents, employers will benefit, living standards will be higher, and the financing problems of Social Security and Medicare will be easier to solve. The logic is so powerful that it is likely to sweep aside many of the legal barriers and corporate practices that today keep older workers from achieving their full productive potential.

INTERNET MEMORY TOOLS

In coming years, more Americans reaching their 60s and 70s are going to want to work, at least part-time. Researchers are finding that far from wearing people down, work can actually help keep them mentally and physically fit. Many highly educated and well-paid workers—lawyers, physicians, architects—already work to advanced ages because their skills are valued. Boomers, with more education than any generation in history, are likely to follow that pattern. And today's rapid obsolescence

of knowledge can actually play to older workers' advantage: It used to be considered wasteful to train people near retirement. But if training has to be refreshed every year, then companies might as well retrain old employees as young ones.

"One of my problems is excess energy, which drives me nuts"

Equally important, high-level work is getting easier for the old. Thanks to medical advances, people are staying healthy, enabling them to work longer than before. Fewer jobs require physically demanding tasks such as heavy lifting. And technology—from memory-enhancing drugs to Internet search engines that serve as auxiliary memories—will help senior workers compensate for the effects of aging. "Assuming that the improved health trends continue, boomers should be able to work productively into their late 70s" if they choose to, says Elizabeth Zelinski, dean of the Leonard Davis School of Gerontology at the University of Southern California.

But realizing that potential requires that government and business discard the outdated rules, practices, and prejudices that prematurely retire people who would prefer to keep working. In many corporations, there's an unspoken assumption that older workers are much less capable than their younger counterparts. So in addition to ensuring older workers get their fair share of training, CEOs may also need to directly confront unintended age discrimination.

Society will also have to grapple with the tricky question of how to change the Social Security system to suit an aging but healthier population. A balanced approach might be to increase the Social Security retirement age at a more rapid clip while beefing up the Social Security disability program—which now covers 8 million disabled workers and dependents.

This optimistic vision of aging in America stands in sharp contrast to the conventional wisdom, which looks ahead with dread to the 60th birthday parties of the first boomers in 2006. Pessimistic pundits expect that boomers will retire in droves soon after hitting 60, as their predecessors did, while those who do keep working will dial back to less challenging and less productive jobs. The fear is that boomers will finally heed Timothy

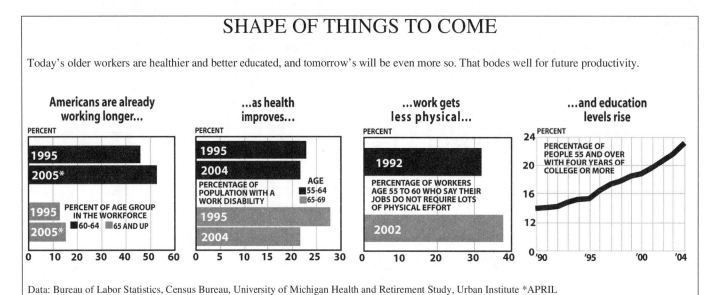

SHAPE OF THINGS TO COME

Today's older workers are healthier and better educated, and tomorrow's will be even more so. That bodes well for future productivity.

Data: Bureau of Labor Statistics, Census Bureau, University of Michigan Health and Retirement Study, Urban Institute *APRIL

Leary's call, dropping out (of the workforce) and turning on (the TV). "This explosion in the number of elderly Americans will place an unprecedented economic burden on working-age adults," investment banker Peter G. Peterson wrote last year in his latest book, *Running on Empty*.

But the burden won't be nearly so heavy if people's productive careers stretch out in synch with their extended lifetimes. How much could the economy benefit from people working longer and better?

An analysis by *BusinessWeek* finds that increased productivity of older Americans and higher labor-force participation could add 9% to gross domestic product by 2045, on top of what it otherwise would have been. (This assumes, for example, that over the next 40 years better health and technology reduce the productivity gap between older workers and their younger counterparts.) This 9% increase in gross domestic product would add more than $3 trillion a year, in today's dollars, to economic output.

The added growth would be a pure win for government finances, since a bigger economy with more productive workers yields higher tax revenues. And there's little doubt that encouraging people to work longer in step with longer life spans would do much to guarantee the solvency of Social Security.

The idea that citizens of a wealthy nation such as the U.S. would choose to work extra years is still a little new. For most of the 20th century, retirement ages fell as life spans grew. The trend seemed unstoppable: While in 1950, 46% of men 65 and older were in the labor force, by 1985 the fraction had plummeted to 16%. An influx of women into the labor force only partially offset the overall decline.

But starting in the mid-1980s, something highly unexpected began to happen: The trend reversed, and more older Americans chose to keep working. The upsurge accelerated even in the weak labor markets of recent years. The share of men 65 and over in the labor force is back up to almost 20%—the highest since the 1970s.

In part, of course, the latest uptick in working ages can be blamed on the stock market's drop from its 2000 peak, which

dented retirement savings. Also, fewer workers have good defined-benefit pension plans, which would allow them to retire young. But financial need can't be the whole reason older Americans are working more. Federal Reserve surveys show that older families have been getting richer, not poorer. The average net worth of families headed by 55- to 64-year-olds soared by 74% from 1992 to 2001, after adjusting for inflation, and likely has gone up since then.

At least as important is that many institutional barriers to working longer have been removed. In 1986, in the name of equal rights, Congress banned mandatory retirement for all but a handful of workers, such as airline pilots. And 401(k) plans, which are gradually replacing defined-benefit plans, don't induce people to retire at a certain age.

YOUNG AS YOU FEEL

Better yet, work doesn't feel like a burden to today's fit, older Americans. Many people over 60 don't think of themselves as old. A good example is Theodora Emiko "Teddy" Yoshikami, 61, who organizes cultural programs at New York's American Museum of Natural History. In her spare time, she whacks big drums in a Japanese percussion group. "People are always surprised to hear how old I am," says the former dancer.

The Baby Boom generation is even fitter for its age and more determined to stay active. Two-thirds of the people surveyed last year by the Employee Benefit Research Institute, a company-backed organization, said they expect to work for pay in retirement. A survey of boomers by AARP in January found that two in five workers age 50 to 65 were interested in a gradual, "phased" retirement instead of an abrupt cessation of work—and nearly 80% of those said that availability of phased retirement programs at work would encourage them to keep working longer. While it's likely that many boomers won't stick to those brave resolutions, the trend in work is clearly up.

Good health will help. The share of 65- to 69-year-olds with a disability affecting their ability to work fell from nearly 28% in 1995 to less than 22% last year. Advances in medicine are curing many of the problems that once forced older workers into retirement. For example, Genentech Inc. announced on May 23 that a drug undergoing trials for treatment of macular generation improves eyesight in the elderly. And better health is coinciding with less strenuous work, thanks to automation and the shrinkage of manufacturing. The share of workers 55 to 60 who said their jobs did not require lots of physical effort rose from 32% in 1992 to 38% in 2002, according to an Urban Institute study.

TRIAL AND ERROR

Mental health appears to be improving as well. USC's Zelinski has discovered that heart disease, hypertension, and diabetes directly impair brain functioning—and she sees evidence that modern medicine is getting a better handle on those diseases. As a result, memory and other functions are improving among the elderly. Emma Shulman's boss at NYU Medical Center, Steven Ferris, expects further gains for older workers from the spreading use of memory-enhancing drugs and technological aids such as personal digital assistants and search engines. Says Ferris: "I remember my father with little scraps of paper to remember things. People don't have to do that anymore."

"Once I got gray hair, people actually listened to me. This is working really well"

Older workers who thrive tend to have skills that are prized in the workplace, even if they can't easily be measured by standard tests. What matters most, according to psychologist Regina Colonia-Willner, president of consultancy Practical Intelligence at Work Inc. in Boca Raton, Fla., is the ability to solve ill-defined business problems using rules of thumb that can't be put down on paper. Example: how to deal with a difficult boss. In a study of 200 banking executives, she found that the ones who exhibited the highest "practical intelligence" were as likely to be old as young—and the older among them excelled even though their scores on traditional intelligence tests were no better than average for their age. "Practical intelligence stays with you," says Colonia-Willner. "You don't lose it when you get older."

The rap that older workers are inflexible and uncreative is also overstated. Research by economists David W. Galenson of the University of Chicago and Bruce A. Weinberg of Ohio State University finds that the innovations of older people are more likely to be "experimental," vs. the break-the-mold "conceptual" innovations of younger types. The conceptual types tend to have a bolt from the blue, whereas the experimenters build new ideas from a lifetime of observation, trial, and error. Among the "experimental" innovators who produced some of their best work later in life: painters Henri Matisse and Paul Cézanne, author Fyodor Dostoevsky, and architect Frank Lloyd Wright.

Some enlightened companies are catching on to all of this. They're hiring or retaining older workers with flexible work schedules and ample training. United Technologies Corp. spends more than $60 million a year on its Employee Scholar Program, which pays the costs of workers of any age who study in their spare time. At UTC's Hamilton Sundstrand facility in Miramar, Fla., 61-year-old lead mechanic Ed Perez is working on a bachelor's degree in legal studies. He finished an associate's degree in aviation-maintenance management two years ago and hopes to go to law school. "If I don't run out of time and UTC doesn't run out of money, I'll keep going," he says.

UTC Chairman and Chief Executive George David, at 63 a candidate himself for discounted movie tickets, argues that an educated worker like Perez is a better worker, regardless of age or area of study. What's more, the free education incentive tends to appeal to UTC's most skilled and motivated employees, so it's a way for the company to retain the people it most wants. Retention rates among "employee scholars" are about 20% higher than for regular U.S. workers.

OLDER AND WISER

Businesses often act as if older workers are a liability in an economy that prizes productivity, flexibility, and innovation. But research suggests that they are underestimating these employees.

TWO KINDS OF INNOVATION

Creativity isn't just for the young. Economist David Galenson of the University of Chicago has identified two types of innovators. Break-the-mold **"conceptual" innovators** (like Vietnam Veterans Memorial designer Maya Lin), **do their best work when young.** In contrast, **"experimental" innovators** (novelist Fyodor Dostoevsky, sculptor Auguste Rodin) **do their best work at older ages,** drawing on a lifetime of observation, trial, and error.

SOUND BODIES

University of Southern California gerontologist Elizabeth Zelinski has found that ailments such as **high blood pressure, diabetes, and heart disease are key factors depressing brain function among the elderly**. The ease with which we can treat these conditions now helps reduce the apparent cognitive handicap of older workers. In short, medicine is postponing mental decline.

PROBLEM SOLVING

Conventional measures of mental function don't capture abilities important in business, such as accumulated knowledge or judgment. Psychologist Regina Colonia-Willner of Practical Intelligence at Work Inc. found that **managers who are successful at older ages are masters at solving ill-defined problems,** even though they do no better than other older workers on standard psychometric tests.

COMPENSATION

Speed, reasoning, and memory decline steadily after age 20, while vocabulary increases to age 50. University of Virginia psychologist Timothy Salthouse found that **older workers make up for their shortfalls with clever coping strategies.** For example, older typists gain an edge by looking farther ahead in to-be-typed text during pauses, presumably to compensate for the slowdown in their ability to type words as read. **Data:** *Business Week*

HOLDING ON TO EXPERIENCE

Consolidated Edison Inc., a New York power company with an aging workforce, is trying to hang on to its valuable older workers with benefits like an elder-care referral service and career-long training. It wants to retain the experience of workers like Frederick R. Simms, 67, an emergency field manager who has seen just about everything in his 49 years with the company, from water main breaks to the collapse of the World Trade Center. In a job where trust and rapport are vital, Simms is on a first-name basis with Fire Dept. officials and other emergency workers all over Manhattan. Con Ed recently sent him for a two-day "working people-smart" class. "I don't have the zip I used to have, but I'm good enough to work 16 hours if I had to today," says Simms, adding: "I know the company likes having me around."

It's common these days to find older workers on the sales floor of retailers like Home Depot Inc. and CVS Corp., but what's new is the growing presence of older workers in high-pay, high-productivity careers. MITRE Corp., a research and development outfit in Bedford, Mass., is worried about losing its expertise in fields such as radar, which is something of a lost art for young engineers. So it brings back retirees on what it calls a "part-time, on-call" basis. The Energy Dept.'s National Energy Technology Laboratory in Morgantown, W. Va., also recognizes the value of older workers with technical expertise. It has clung to chemical engineer Hugh D. Guthrie, 86, as a full-time technical adviser in part because he has ideas that younger engineers might never think of. Says Guthrie: "My experience gives me a perspective on questions, which may not always be right but nearly always will be different. The greatest service I provide is in stimulating the thinking of people involved in a project."

Unfortunately, many other companies haven't gotten the message. The Society for Human Resource Management, an association of personnel execs, says 59% of members surveyed don't actively recruit older workers and 65% don't do anything specific to retain older workers. The Bureau of Labor Statistics found in 1995, the last time it looked, that workers age 55 and up got only one-third as many hours of formal training as workers 45 to 54. Marian Stoltz-Loike, CEO of SeniorThinking LLC, a consultancy, says executives often aren't even aware that older workers are getting a subtle message that training isn't for them.

Economists have found that businesses are missing an opportunity by giving less training to their older workers. Research shows that they tend to operate information technology more slowly but with fewer errors. Research on displaced workers who got retraining in community colleges in Washington State found that the pay gains were just as big for older workers who took training as for younger ones—indicating that the training they got took hold.

Will longer-working boomers block the advancement of younger workers? Maybe. But what worries employers more is the opposite—labor shortages that could emerge if boomers retire en masse and there aren't enough people to take their place. The Congressional Budget Office is forecasting that labor-force growth will slow by almost half over the next 10 years.

The U.S. takes better advantage of the potential of its older citizens than does most of Europe, where extremely early retirement is routine because of rich retirement benefits. Six in 10 Americans are still working at ages 55 to 64, vs. just four in 10 in the European Union.

Smart policy choices, such as the abolition of most mandatory retirement rules, have helped put the U.S. in a position to tap the ability and energy of older people. Since 2000, Social Security recipients have been allowed to receive their full benefits no matter how much they earn from working after age 65. The Internal Revenue Service has proposed rules, starting next year, to allow people 59½ and older to receive part of their pensions even while they are still working. Because people would not have to retire outright to get a pension, more are likely to remain on the job, experts predict. The proposed rules are a step in the right direction, although employer groups are complaining that there's too much red tape involved.

CREATING INCENTIVES

What more can be done to tap the productivity potential of older workers? The goal is to introduce more flexibility into pay and retirement systems, to create more options as workers age. Consultant Ken Dychtwald, author of **Age Wave,** recommends the example of Deloitte Consulting LLC, which lures highly valued older employees to stay by designating them "senior leaders" and giving them incentives such as flexible hours and work location, special projects, and opportunities for mentoring and research.

Another possibility is to allow companies to convert traditional defined-benefit pensions, which encourage retirement as early as age 55, to cash-balance plans, which have no built-in incentives to retire. Such conversions have been frozen since 1999 over legitimate age-discrimination concerns, though the Bush Administration has proposed legislation that would break the logjam. It's prudent to make sure that switching to cash-balance plans doesn't harm older workers, but such caution is also preserving a system that lures people into retiring when they still have much to contribute in the working world.

Perhaps the most controversial idea is to break the typical link between pay and seniority. As more people work into their late 60s and 70s, pay should be adjusted to match how much people work and what they accomplish on the job.

It's also critical to rethink the role of Social Security in an economy where incomes—and life spans—are rising. In theory, Social Security should provide a secure safety net for those who are truly too old to work and lack savings, while encouraging the huge boomer generation to stay employed and productive for the good of themselves and the economy.

"The greatest service I provide is in stimulating the thinking of people involved in a project."

The logical conclusion: raise Social Security's normal retirement age incrementally to 70. From then on, peg further increases to gains in longevity. It's also essential to increase the age, now 62, at which people can first choose to take early retirement. Research suggests that many take the official early retirement age as a signal that it's O.K. to drop out of the workforce, even though they will get much smaller checks for the rest of their lifetimes. Raising the early retirement age would signal that 62 is too young for most people to quit in an era of marathon-running septuagenarians.

Increasing Social Security's early retirement age would be hard on workers with health problems, or whose jobs require more physical exertion. A possible solution is to liberalize the qualifications for Social Security's disability insurance program. The extra expense of disability payments to aging laborers would be far outweighed by the savings from raising the normal and early retirement ages in tandem.

There's no dispute that America is graying. But the solution to the demographic shift is staring us in the face. As Urban Institute senior fellow C. Eugene Steuerle told the House Ways & Means Committee in May: "People in their late 50s, 60s, and 70s have now become the largest underutilized pool of human resources in the economy." By working longer—and more productively—boomers will help the U.S. economy thrive even as their personal odometers keep clicking forward.

—*With Diane Brady in New York*

Work, Retirement, and Well-Being

No set of issues has galvanized public discourse about aging more than those surrounding work, retirement, and economic security in old age. In eastern Europe's transitional economies, and indeed in much of the less developed world, governments increasingly seek to define a balance between public and private social security systems. The precariousness of old-age security can be seen in stagnant and declining real pensions in transitional economies, in the dire fate of pensioners during the collapse of Argentina's economy in 2001, in the surprisingly high poverty rates among older Japanese, and perhaps most vividly in the lack of social safety nets for a majority of older people in Africa and Asia.

Labor Force Participation

Labor force participation declines with age, especially after age 50, but work patterns for older people vary among and within countries (see Box). Older people in more developed countries are generally less likely to work than those in less developed countries. Only 2 percent of men age 65 or older participate in the labor force in some more developed countries, whereas more than one-half are economically active in certain less developed countries. National differences in labor force activity are associated with societal wealth: Wealthier countries tend to have much lower labor force participation rates among older residents than do low-income countries.

> *Wealthier countries tend to have much lower labor force participation among older residents.*

Labor force participation rates for older men declined in more developed countries in recent decades. One compilation of data for 16 nations showed especially pro-nounced declines in participation for men in their early 60s. In the early 1970s, well over half of men ages 60 to 64 were still working in a majority of countries. By the late 1990s, only four of the 16 countries—Japan, New Zealand, Sweden, and the United States—had male participation rates over 50 percent in this age group. Labor force participation rates fell below 10 percent among the 65-and older age group in most of the countries. Financial incentives for early retirement have enabled many older workers to leave the labor force. Also, new technologies have increased the value of a recently trained labor force relative to older workers. And in countries with persistently high unemployment, older workers may be pressured to leave the labor force to make room for younger workers.

The decline in labor force participation among older workers may have halted. A report from the Organisation for Economic Cooperation and Development (OECD) found a slight increase in employment rates for men in their late 50s and early 60s in the late 1990s in the United States and the Netherlands, and a cessation of the long-term decline in several other OECD countries. The report suggests that the increase was related to an economic upturn in the late 1990s.

Older women have had different labor force patterns than older men. In many industrialized countries, female participation rates have increased for almost all adult age groups up to age 60. The increase was sharp in some countries. In New Zealand, for example, 60 percent of women ages 55 to 59 were economically active in 1998, up from 28 percent in 1971. While female participation was increasing at younger ages, nearly all more developed countries saw a decrease among older women between the early 1970s and the late 1990s. Small propor-tions (typically 4 percent or less) of older women are economically active in more developed nations.

Older men and women in less developed countries are much more likely to work than those in industrialized nations. Older people in predominantly rural agrarian societies often work out of necessity—retirement may be a luxury reserved for urban elites. In nations as diverse as Bangladesh, Indonesia, Jamaica, Mexico, Pakistan, and Zimbabwe, more than 50 percent of all older men are considered economically active. The economic activity of women tends to be under-reported, particularly in less developed countries where much of the work that women engage in is not captured in censuses and labor force surveys, or is not considered economic activity. Older women in less developed societies, for example, often are involved in subsistence agriculture or household industries, neither of which is well documented by conventional data collection methods.

Most older workers in less developed countries work in agriculture. Agriculture remains a major employer of older people, even in many more-developed countries. In 1995 in Japan, one-third of all older workers were engaged in agriculture. Data for 23 OECD countries show that the ratio of workers age 55 or older to workers below age 55 is generally much higher in agriculture, hunting, and forestry than in any other goods-producing or service sector.

Retirement Systems

Public pension systems developed largely because families found it increasingly difficult to support their older and infirm relatives. Just 33 countries had old age, disability, and survivors programs in 1940, compared with more than 165 countries in 2000. In response to general economic conditions, changes in welfare

The Transition to Retirement

In more developed countries, retirement from the workforce occurred almost exclusively at a regulated age until the 1950s; older workers had little possibility of receiving a pension prior to the designated retirement age. Since then, countries have adopted a wide range of approaches to providing old age security, and people have a wider array of routes to retirement.

Part-time work is one option that appeals to many older workers because it enables them to remain active in the labor force while pursuing leisure activities. But the opportunities for part-time work vary tremendously among countries. In nine more developed countries, the prevalence of part-time employment among working men ages 60 to 64 ranged from less than 8 percent in Italy and Germany to more than 35 percent in Sweden and the Netherlands.[1]

Older working women are much more likely than older men to be involved in part-time work. In Australia, three-fourths of women ages 65 and older who were economically active in 1999 worked part-time, compared with fewer than half of economically active older men. A study of 15 European Union countries showed that 41 percent of working women ages 55 to 64 were in part-time positions in 1998, compared with just 8 percent of working men in that age group.[2] The rate of part-time work for people nearing retirement generally was increasing in the 1990s. However, part-time workers often represent a small fraction of the older population.

Disability programs have provided another path to retirement for older workers. Economic recessions and high unemployment in Europe in recent decades led some governments (including Germany, the Netherlands, and Sweden) to enable early retirement via relaxed disability criteria and generous long-term sickness benefits. Wide variations in national programs produced enormous differences in retirement patterns;

among 16 European countries in the mid-1990s, the percentage of older retired men who retired because of illness or disability ranged from 2 percent in Portugal to 29 percent in Switzerland.

Unemployment also has been seen as a bridge to retirement. Older workers typically have low levels of unemployment compared with younger workers, but if older workers become unemployed, they tend to remain unemployed longer than younger workers. OECD data for several wealthy countries show that well over half of unemployed people age 55 or older were unemployed for more than one year. Many enter the ranks of "discouraged workers," people who are no longer looking for work because they think there is no work available or because they do not know where to look. In some countries, older workers may feel excluded from the labor force because of changes in occupational structure and the need for a more-educated workforce that favors younger workers.

One comparison of 13 countries indicated that people ages 55 to 64 accounted for a disproportionate share of discouraged workers, especially in the United Kingdom, where more than two-thirds of all discouraged male workers were ages 55 to 64. In countries with trend data, discouraged older workers were more numerous in the 1990s than in the 1980s. Because of the difficulties older people face in obtaining a new job, discouragement often becomes a transition from unemployment to retirement.

References

1. Organisation for Economic Cooperation and Development (OECD), *Reforms for an Ageing Society* (Paris: OECD, 2000).
2. Statistical Office of the European Communities (EUROSTAT), *The Social Situation in the European Union 2000* (Luxembourg: EUROSTAT, 2000).

philosophy, and private pension trends over the past several decades, many industrialized nations lowered the age at which people become fully entitled to public pension benefits. The proliferation of early retirement schemes has increased the number and usually the proportion of older workers who take advantage of such programs.

Coverage

Mandatory old-age pension plans now cover more than 90 percent of the labor force in most industrialized countries. Governments are responsible for mandating, financing, managing, and insuring public pensions. Public pension plans usually offer benefits that are not tied to individual contribu-

tions, but are financed by payroll taxes. This arrangement is commonly referred to as a "pay-as-you-go" system because taxes on working adults finance the pension payments of people who are retired.

Most pay-as-you-go systems in industrialized countries initially promised generous benefits. When first established, these programs were based on a small number of pensioners relative to a large number of contributors (workers). As systems matured, ratios of pensioners to contributors grew and in some countries became unsustainable, particularly during periods of economic stagnation. One result was the development of private pension systems to complement public systems. Other measures implemented

or considered have included increasing worker contribution rates, restructuring or reducing benefits, and raising the minimum age of retirement.

In less developed countries, public pension systems typically cover a much smaller fraction of workers. Even economically vibrant societies such as Malaysia and Thailand offer no publicly supported, comprehensive retirement pension scheme. Governments that do offer coverage often restrict it to certain workers such as civil servants, military personnel, and employees in the formal economic sector. Rural, predominantly agricultural workers have little or no pension coverage in much of the less developed world, although some governments have taken steps to address this situation. Each state in India, for example, has implemented an old-age pension scheme for destitute people with no source of income and no family support. In addition to these state schemes, the Indian government has developed a means-tested National Social Assistance Programme that seeks to provide uniformly available social protection throughout the country. While pension amounts are minimal and coverage far from universal, the system provides a foundation on which to expand future coverage.

Informal (usually family) systems provide the bulk of social support for older individuals in many countries, particularly in Africa and South Asia. As economies expand and nations urbanize, informal support systems, such as extended family care and mutual aid societies, have tended to weaken. Expanding the older population served by formal systems while maintaining the existing informal support mechanisms has become a major challenge for governments in less developed nations.

Pension Reform

A number of factors have converged to make pension reform a contentious political issue. Increased longevity and early retirement mean that demographic change alone could double retiree–worker ratios in many countries over the next 30 years. Economists have expressed concerns about declining savings rates, while politicians and the general public have been reluctant to embrace increased payroll taxes and higher retirement ages. With the cost of public pensions absorbing upwards of 15 percent of GDP in some countries, there is an emerging consensus that pension systems should be revamped to rely less on traditional public-benefit formulas and to require more from private accounts and individual-worker savings. During the last decade, dozens of books and monographs have debated the often-complex fiscal pros and cons of privatization. There also are strong philosophical (some would say ethical) aspects to the debate. Proponents of privatization seek to promote individual responsibility and reduce the role of government. Other analysts stress that traditional public pension systems are social insurance programs based on the notion of collective responsibility. Beyond the rhetoric, two facts stand out: First, traditional public programs are not set in stone and are periodically reformed to resolve legislated financing problems. Second, there is nevertheless a clear trend toward privatizing public systems. Approximately 30 nations have privatized at least a portion of their public systems, and privatization has been more common in countries with well-developed public systems that cover a large percentage of workers.

Privatization of pensions can take many forms, and it can coexist with strong public programs. One progressive idea, developed by the Switzerland-based Geneva Association, promotes the concept of Four Pillars of Support. In many countries, pension funding rests on two or three pillars: a public pension based on pay-as-you-go funding; a supplemental or mandatory occupational pension (common in some European nations) that often is fully funded; and individual savings, which may include personal investments and life insurance. The Geneva Association proposes a fourth pillar based on a new design for retirement that encourages continued economic activity (either full-time or part-time) by older people, and incorporates the concept of gradual retirement instead of early retirement. Crossnational research on labor force participation at older ages has shown that levels of participation are a consequence (intended or unintended) of retirement provisions and/or tax policy. The financial structure of national social security systems may reward early retirement, and attempts to encourage increased labor force participation at older ages may be largely contingent upon politically difficult changes in these systems.

WORK/RETIREMENT CHOICES AND LIFESTYLE PATTERNS OF OLDER AMERICANS

Harold Cox *Indiana State University*

Terrance Parks *Indiana State University*

Andre Hammonds *Indiana State University*

Gurmeet Sekhon *Indiana State University*

This study examined the work, retirement, and lifestyle choices of a sample of older Indiana residents. The six lifestyles examined in this study were:

1. *to continue to work full-time;*
2. *to continue to work part-time;*
3. *retire from work and become engaged in a variety of volunteer activities;*
4. *to retire from work and become involved in a variety of recreational and leisure activities;*
5. *to retire from work and later return to work part-time; and*
6. *to retire from work and later return to work full-time*

These findings indicate that health was not a critical factor in the older person's retirement decision, and that those who retired and engaged in volunteer or recreational activities were significantly more satisfied with their lives than those who continue to work. Those who retired and engaged in volunteer or recreational activities scored significantly higher on life satisfaction than those who had returned to work full or part-time. There was no significant difference between those who had retired and those who had continued working in terms of how they were viewed by their peers. Of those who retired and then returned to work, the most satisfied with their lives were the ones who returned to work in order to feel productive. Those least satisfied with their lives were the ones that returned to work because they needed money.

INTRODUCTION

There are basically six different choices of lifestyles from which older Americans choose when they reach retirement age. The can (1) continue to work full-time, (2) reduce work commitments but continue to work part-time, (3) retire from work and become engaged in a variety of volunteer activities that provide needed services but for which they will receive no economic compensation or (4) retire from work and become involved in a variety of recreational and leisure activities, (5) retire from work and later return to work part-time, (6) retire from work and return to work full-time.

There are a multitude of life experiences and retirement patterns that may ultimately lead older persons to choose among the diverse ways of occupying themselves during their later years. Some enjoy their work as well as the income, status, privilege, and power that go with full-time employment and never intend to retire. Some retire intending to engage in recreational and leisure activities on a full-time basis only to find this lifestyle less satisfying than they imagined and ultimately return to work. The need to feel productive and actively involved in life is often a critical factor inducing some retirees to return to work. Some retirees who have become widowed, divorced, or never married find themselves too socially isolated in retirement. They return to work either full-time or part-time because their job brings them into contact with a variety of people, and therefore they are less isolated. Thus, there are a variety of reasons why older persons may continue to work or to become active volunteers during their later years. On the other hand, many persons retire, dedicate themselves to recreation and leisure activities, and are most satisfied doing so.

The purpose of this study was to determine which of these six groups were better off in terms of their health, life satisfaction, retirement adjustment and the respect they received from their peers.

A second factor, which will be examined in this study, is the advisability for both government and industry of encouraging older workers to remain in the labor force longer. Changes in Social Security regulations after the year 2000 are going to gradually increase the age of eligibility for Social Security payment from 62 to 64 for early retirement and from 65 to 67 for full retirement benefits. Will changes in the age of eligibility for retirement income derived from Social Security regulations be good or bad for older Americans?

REVIEW OF LITERATURE

Work

The meanings of such diverse activities as work, leisure, and retirement to a member of a social system are often quite complex. Paradoxically, the relevance of work and leisure activities for an individual is often intertwined in his or her thinking. Consequently, the concept of work or occupation has been difficult for sociologists to precisely define.

For some time sociologists have struggled to come up with an adequate definition of work. Dubin (1956), for example, defined work as continuous employment in the production of goods and services for remuneration. This definition ignores the fact that there are necessary tasks in society carried out by persons who receive no immediate pay. Mothers, fathers, housewives, and students do not receive pay for their valued activities.

Hall (1975) attempts to incorporate both the economic and social aspects of work in his definition: "An occupation is the social role performed by adult members of society that directly and/or indirectly yields social and financial consequences and that constitutes a major focus in the life of an adult." Similarly Bryant (1972) tries to include both the economic and social aspects of work life in his definition of labor: "Labor is any socially integrating activity which is connected with human subsistence." By *integrating activity* Bryant means sanctioned activity that presupposes, creates, and recreates social relationships. The last two definitions seem to take a broader view of work in the individual's total life. Moreover, they could include the work done by mothers, fathers, housewives, and students. The advantage of definitions that attach strong importance to the meaning and social aspects of a work role is that they recognize the importance of roles for which there is no, or very little, economic reward. The homemaker, while not receiving pay, may contribute considerably to a spouse's career and success. College students in the period of anticipatory socialization and preparation for an occupational role may not be receiving any economic benefits, but their efforts are crucial to their future career.

The most appropriate definitions of work, therefore, seem to be those that emphasize the social and role aspects of an occupation, which an individual reacts to and is shaped by, whether or not he or she is financially rewarded for assuming these roles. From the perspective of sociology, one's work life and the roles one assumes during the workday will, in time, shape one's self-concept, identity, and feelings about oneself, and therefore strongly affect one's personality and behavior. Moreover, from this perspective, the individual's choice of occupations is probably strongly affected by the desire to establish, maintain, and display a desired identity.

Individual Motivation to Work

Vroom (1964) has attempted to delineate the components of work motivation. The first component is wages and all the economic rewards associated with the fringe benefits of the job. People desire these rewards, which therefore serve as a strong incentive to work. Iams (1985), in a study of the post-retirement work patterns of women, found that unmarried women were very likely to work at least part-time after retirement if their monthly income was below $500. Hardy (1991) found that 80 percent of the retirees who later re-entered the labor force stated that money was the main reason they returned to work. The economic inducement to work is apparently a strong one.

A second inducement to work is the expenditure of physical and mental energy. People seem to need to expend energy in some meaningful way, and work provides this opportunity. Vroom (1964) notes that animals will often engage in spontaneous activity as a consequence of activity deprivation.

A third motivation, according to Vroom, is the production of goods and services. This inducement is directly related to the intrinsic satisfaction the individual derives from successful manipulation of the environment.

A fourth motivation is social interaction. Most work roles involve interaction with customers, clients, or members of identifiable work groups as part of the expected behavior of their occupants.

The final motivation Vroom mentions is social status. An individual's occupation is perhaps the best single determinant of his or her status in the community.

These various motivations for work undoubtedly assume different configurations for different people and occupational groups. Social interaction may be the most important for some, while economic considerations may be most important for others. For still others the intrinsic satisfaction derived from the production of goods and services may be all-important. Thus, the research by industrial sociologists has indicated that there are diverse reasons why individuals are motivated to work.

The critical questions for gerontologists is whether the same psychological and social factors that thrust people into work patterns for the major part of their adult life can channel them into leisure activities during their retirement years. Can people find the same satisfaction, feeling of worth, and identity in leisure activities that they did in work-related activities? Streib and Schneider (1971) think they can. They argue that the husband, wife, grandmother, and grandfather's roles may expand and become more salient in the retirement years. Simultaneously, public service and community roles become possible because of the flexibility of the retiree's time. They believe that the changing activities and roles, which accompany retirement, need not lead to a loss of self-respect or active involvement in the mainstream of life.

Retirement Trends

Demographic and economic trends in American society have resulted in an ever-increasing number of retired Americans. Streib and Schneider (1971) observed that for retirement to become an institutionalized social pattern in any society, certain conditions must be met. There must be a large group of people who live long enough to retire, the economy must be sufficiently productive to support segments of the population that are not included in the work force, and there must be some well-established forms of pension or insurance programs to support people during their retirement years.

There has been a rapid growth in both the number and percentage of the American population 65 and above since 1900. In 1900, there were 3.1 million Americans 65 and over, which constituted four percent of the population. Currently, approximately 31 million Americans are in this age category, which makes up 12.5 percent of the population. While the number and proportion of the population over 65 have been increasing steadily, the proportion of those who remain in the work force has decreased steadily. In 1900, nearly two thirds of those 65 worked. Sammartino (1979) reports that by 1947 this figure had declined to 47.8 percent. By 1987 only 16.5 percent of those 65 and older were still in the work force. In the past 20 years the decline in labor force participation in later years has extended into the 55–64 year old age group. Clark (1988) observed that between 1960 and 1970 the labor force participation of men (55–64) dropped from 86.8% to 83%. By 1990 the labor force participation rate of men in this age group (55–64) had dropped to 65.1% (see Table 1). Table 1 indicates that the labor force participation rates of women 55–64 rose from 27% to 43% from 1950 to 1970 but has remained relatively stable since 1970. Thus, while the labor force participation rate of 55-years and -older women has remained relatively stable since 1970, the labor force participation rate of women 45–54 has grown from 54.4% in 1970 to 69% in 1990. It would appear from these figures that, while younger women are in increasing numbers entering the labor force, women 55 and above are following the same path as their male counterparts and choosing to retire early.

TABLE 1.
Civilian Labor Force Participation Rates:
Actual and Projected*

	Men			Women		
Year	45–54	55–64	65 and over	45–54	55–64	65 and over
1950	95.8	86.9	45.8	37.9	27.0	9.7
1960	95.7	86.8	33.1	49.8	32.2	10.8
1970	94.2	83.0	26.8	54.4	43.0	9.7
1980	91.2	72.3	19.1	59.9	41.5	8.1
1986	91.0	67.3	16.0	65.9	42.3	7.4
1990*	90.7	65.1	14.1	69.0	42.8	7.0
2000*	90.1	63.2	9.9	75.4	45.8	5.4

SOURCE: For the rates from 1950–1970: U. S. Department of Labor (1980:224). For the rates from 1980–2000: Bureau of Labor Statistics (unpublished data).

*Values are projections from the Bureau of Labor Statistics middle growth path.

Similarly, there appears to be a somewhat greater convergence in the work and retirement patterns of men and women when comparing 1900 with 1970. The earlier pattern of work histories seemed to be for men to enter the work force earlier and retire later; women tended to enter later and retire earlier. Current trends indicate that women are entering the work force earlier and working longer.

Men, on the other hand, enter the work force later and retire earlier. Thus, the work histories of men and women are becoming very similar, although men as a group still have longer work histories than women. Today, more women are both entering the labor force and also remaining in the labor force throughout their adult lives.

The trend for both men and women for the past 30 years has been for larger numbers to choose to claim Social Security benefits prior to age 65. Allen and Brotman (1981) point out that in 1968, 48 percent of all new Social Security payment awards to men were to claimants under 65; by 1978 this figure had increased to 61 percent. In 1968, 65 percent of all new Social Security awards to women were to claimants under 65; in 1978, the figure was 72 percent.

Simultaneously, fewer persons are choosing to remain in the labor force beyond the age of 65. Soldo and Agree (1988) report that 62 percent of the men and 72 percent of the women who received Social Security benefits in 1986 had retired prior to age 65 and therefore were receiving reduced benefits. The General Accounting Office reports that almost two-thirds of those receiving private retirement benefits in 1985 stopped working prior to age 65. Of those who do remain in the labor force after age 65, Soldo and Agree (1988) report that 47 percent of the men and 59 percent of the women held part-time positions.

Quinn and Burkhauser (1990) report that probably the most critical factor in the decision to retire early is adequate retirement income. They found that between 1975 and 1990 the proportion of workers covered by two pension plans had risen from 21 percent to 40 percent. Moreover, Gall, Evans, and Howard (1997) report a number of studies that found that those with higher incomes, or at least adequate finances, were more satisfied with their life in retirement (Fillenbau, George, and Palmore 1985; Seccombe and Lee 1986; Crowley 1990; Dorfman 1992).

There is a multiplicity of problems confronting the individual at retirement: the lowering of income; the loss of status, privilege, and power associated with one's position in the occupational hierarchy; a major reorganization of life activities, since the nine-to-five workday becomes meaningless; a changing definition of self, since most individuals over time shape their identity and personality in line with the demands of their major occupational roles; considerable social isolation if new activities are not found to replace work-related activities; and a search for a new identity, new meaning, and new values in one's life. Obviously, the major reorganization of one's life that must take place at retirement is a potential source of adjustment problems. Critical to the adjustment is the degree to which one's identity and personality structure was attached to the work role. For those individuals whose work identity is central to their self-concept and gives them the greatest satisfaction, retirement will represent somewhat of a crisis. For others, retirement should not represent a serious problem.

Work and Retirement Patterns in Later Life

Beck (1983) identified three different work and retirement patterns of older persons which include:

1. the fully retired
2. the partially retired
3. the formerly retired

What could be added to Beck's pattern are "the never retired."

There are a number of different studies and authors who have attempted to identify the critical factor determining who will or will not work during their later years. Beck (1983) found that individuals with high job autonomy and high demand jobs were most likely to return to work after formal retirement. Those with the greatest financial need—service workers and laborers—were less likely to return to work despite financial limitations. Beck concludes that income was the critical factor in the motivation of workers who were very poor to return to work. Those in other income categories were less likely to return to work because of actual financial benefits as much as for other factors.

A number of other studies tended to support Beck's analysis of work and retirement patterns. Tillenbaum (1971) found that those with higher levels of education were more likely to continue working beyond age 65 or to return to work after retiring if they chose to do so. Quinn (1980) found the self-employed were much more likely to work beyond retirement age. Streib and Schneider (1971) found that white collar workers were significantly more likely than blue collar workers to return to work. They found no relationship between income and post-retirement work. Howell (1988) reports that those who formally retire and engage in no substantial work during the next three years are more likely to have been unemployed before retirement and to have lower incomes after retirement. They are also more likely to be nonwhite urban dwellers in poor health.

The past research has indicated then that those who either continue to work after retirement age or return to work after retiring are most likely to:

1. have stable employment patterns throughout their adult life;
2. be in white collar occupations;
3. have higher incomes;
4. have a higher number of years of education;
5. be self-employed.

Those least likely to either work after retirement age or return to work after retirement age:

1. those who experienced periods of unemployment throughout their adult life;
2. those in blue collar occupations;
3. those with low incomes;
4. those who have a lower number of years of education;
5. those who are of minority status (Tillenbaum 1971; Quinn 1980; Howell 1988).

These findings support the idea that many people who continue to work after retirement do so for other than financial reasons. If work was stable and both social and psychologically meaningful to the individual, he/she is much more likely to be found working during the retirement years.

As a rule, retirees do not return to jobs with low autonomy, poor working conditions, and difficult physical labor. Those who most need to continue working during the retirement years for financial reasons are least likely to be able to do so. This is most probably related to their inability to find gainful employment.

Volunteer Work in Retirement

Social integration refers to the individual being actively involved in a variety of groups and organization and thus integrated into the web of community activity. The active older person is likely to be involved in a variety of groups ranging from family to social clubs to church and community organizations. While work and career often place the individual in disparate groups and organizations throughout much of his/her adult life, active engagement in voluntary organizations is likely to keep the individual socially involved during their retirement years.

Moen, Dempster-McClain, and Williams (1992) report that studies as early as 1956 reporting that older persons participating in volunteer work on an intermittent basis and belonging to clubs and organizations were positively related to various measures of health. They concluded that occupying multiple roles in the community was positively related to good health.

A number of studies have found a positive relationship between social integration (in the form of multiple roles) and health in later life (Berkman and Breslow 1983; House, Landes, and Umberson 1988; Moen et al.; Williams 1992).

The researchers were unable to determine if multiple roles lead to improved health or if healthy people were more likely to engage in multiple roles. Moen et al. (1992), however, once again found that being a member of a club or organization appeared to be a critical factor in the current health of the individual, after previous health had been controlled. Paid work over the life course, while positively related to multiple roles in later life, was negatively related to measures of health. However, any volunteer activity at any time during adult life appears to promote multiple role occupancy, social integration, and health in later life.

Mobert (1983) observes that church affiliation itself was not considered a volunteer group or activity; however, membership in groups sponsored by the church such as choir, Old Timers, etc. was considered a volunteer activity. Moreover, church members generally remain active participants in church-related activities long after dropping participation from other voluntary associations (Gray and Moberg 1977). Markides (1983) and Ortega, Crutchfield, and Rusling (1983) argue that the church serves as a focal point for individual and community integration of the elderly and that this is crucial to their sense of well-being. Both of these studies found that church attendance was significantly correlated with life satisfaction.

Productivity in Later Life

Older workers who remain in the work force have been found to be just as productive as younger workers. An industrial survey conducted by Parker (1982) found that older workers were most often regarded as superior to younger workers. Adjectives used by employers to describe older workers were responsible, reliable, conscientious, tolerant, reasonable, and loyal. Older workers have greater stability, they miss work less frequently, change jobs less frequently, and are more dedicated and loyal to the employing organization. Welford (1988) found that performance on production jobs tends to increase with age. While this is true, employers generally offer incentive plans to encourage older workers to retire early. Older workers are generally higher on salary schedules, have accumulated more vacation time and fringe benefits. Thus, many employers see younger workers as cheaper. The fact that they are untested does not seem critical to the employer.

Fyock in discussing the early retirement policies of the 1970's states that:

> *Employers liked it because it enabled them to hire and promote younger, more recently trained and lower paid workers. The public liked it because it didn't appear to cost anything and because at age 62 or earlier they could expect to retire; older workers for obvious reasons loved it. (Fyock 1991:422)*

Fyock (1991) warns however that we currently have an aging work force and that in the near future employers may find it to their advantage to encourage older workers to remain in the work force longer. She believes that employers often find that retirement appeals to their best, instead of the most expendable, employee.

Projected job growth coupled with a declining number of younger workers has raised concern about possible labor shortages. If these projections prove accurate and labor shortages do develop, the answer to the problem would seem to be the retention of older workers—the very workers employers are currently encouraging to retire. Dennis (1986), Sheppard (1990), and Fyock (1991) all argue that an aging labor force can be a source of opportunity for employers. The smart employers, they believe, will be the ones who know how to take advantage of the opportunity.

McShulski (1997) reports the need for a "soft landing" program which eases older workers out of the labor force on a very gradual basis. Encouraging retiring employees to work a reduced number of hours and handle more limited duties for less pay, helps both the company and the employee. Future retirees can impart relevant job information to their coworkers and teach less experienced employees about specific tasks and customer needs. Thus, working for reduced hours and more limited responsibilities results in a gradual transition to retirement, which is good for the company and the employee according to McShulski.

Retirement Policies and Older Workers

Industrialized societies traditionally have low fertility rates and long life expectancy, resulting in an ever-growing number and percentage of our population that is over 65. Thus, industrialized nations very early began to shift social welfare programs from younger persons to older persons. Many economists are questioning the willingness of society to continue to support an ever-growing number of older persons through public-funded retirement incomes.

Initially, in 1935 when Social Security was passed, both management and labor were anxious to get older persons out of the labor force. Management believed that older workers were too expensive since they were high on salary schedules and had accumulated considerable fringe benefits. Labor unions believed that removing older workers would create jobs for younger workers. The public was happy since they were given economic help in support of their older family members and ultimately they looked forward to being able to retire themselves.

The post-WWII era saw major expansions in Social Security programs. Social Security was extended to cover nearly all wage earners and self-employed persons. The permissible retirement age was lowered to 62, and a national disability income program was added to Social Security. A legal interpretation of the Taft-Hartley Act resulted in private pension plans becoming legitimate items of collective bargaining. The result was that private pension plans have grown substantially from 1950 to present. As a result of these and related activities, a retirement norm has emerged in America. Most people now plan to retire and to live some part of their life out of the labor force.

Congress, with the passage of new Social Security legislation in 1983, began, for the first time, to question the desirability of removing seniors from the labor force. Concern about the financial solvency of the Social Security program led Congress and the President to increase Social Security taxes, to increase taxes on earned income of older persons, to tax Social Security benefits, and to raise the eligible age of Social Security benefits after the year 2000.

Retirement age will go up very gradually during the first quarter of the next century. Early retirement will be increased from 62 to 64 years of age. Full retirement will be increased from 65 to 67. Reduction in pension benefits for those who retire early will go up from 20% to 30% of their full retirement income. Those who stay at work after 65 will get a pension boost of 8% for each extra year of work instead of today's 3%.

The changes in Social Security benefits are clearly designed to encourage people to work longer and retire later. The question that remains, given the trend toward younger retirements, is will these changes really keep older workers in the work force longer or merely mean that more retirees will earn less and therefore more will fall below the poverty line.

Economists and labor planners have never been able to establish the fact that for every older worker who retires, a job is created for a younger worker. Changing technologies and the creation of new jobs have at different times created a greater or lesser demand for more workers. Morris (1986) states that:

> *If financial and social policy disincentives to employment could be reduced there is no prior reason to believe that the economy would be unable to expand gradually to accommodate more retired persons especially in part-time, self-employed, and service capacities (Morris 1986:291).*

TABLE 2. One-Way Analysis of Variance: Mean Perceived Health Scores for Older Workers and Retirees		
	MEAN	N=329
Work Full-Time	3.4706	51
Work Part-Time	3.2970	101
Retired/Engaged in Volunteer Activities	3.2867	143
Retired/Engaged Leisure Act.	3.2647	34

SOURCE	D.F.	SUM OF SQUARES	MEAN SQUARES	F-RATIO PROBABILITY	F
Between Groups	3	1.4682	.4891	.9956	.3951
Within Groups	325	159.6574	.4913		
TOTAL	328	161.1246			

Morris (1986) argues that half of the Social Security recipients abruptly leave the labor force and the other half engage in some short-term labor force participation after they retire.

The critical question raised by Congress in changing Social Security benefits in 1983 is can government policies change the age at which people choose to retire. If the older person is to be encouraged to remain in the labor force longer, both the individual worker and the business/industrial community must be convinced of the advantages of keeping older persons in the labor force longer. There seems to be no question that older persons can be productive members of the labor force beyond the retirement age if they have the opportunity and choose to do so.

HYPOTHESIS

1. Those working full-time or part-time will be in better health than those who have retired.
2. Those people who have retired will score higher on measures of life satisfaction than those working full or part-time.
3. Those retirees engaged in volunteer or leisure activities will score higher on measures of life satisfaction than those returning to work.
4. Those people working full-time or part-time during their later years will be more highly regarded by their peers.

METHODOLOGY

The questionnaire utilized in this study included the standard demographic variables, as well as measures of attitude toward retirement, the respondent's perceived state of health, life satisfaction, retirement adjustment, and his/her perceived status among friends.

The questionnaire was mailed to 597 members of the Older Hoosiers Federation and 200 Green Thumb workers in Indiana. The Older Hoosiers Federation is a volunteer groups of senior citizens who lobby for or against various state and federal legislation which they perceive would affect older Americans. They are primarily retired Americans over the age of 55. The Green Thumb workers are persons 55 and older who work on

various parks, roads, and community projects. They are employed by the federal government in community service projects in order to raise their income above the poverty level. A limitation of this study is that the sample was an available sample and not a random sample. It was the best available sample that the researchers could find at this time. There were 342 valid returns, which represented 42.91% of those surveyed.

FINDINGS

The first hypothesis stated that those persons working full or part-time will be in better health than those who are retired. This hypothesis was not supported by the data. As Table 2 indicates, calculating the mean score on the subjects' perceived state of health for those working full-time, those working part-time, those retired and engaged in volunteer activities, and those retired and engaged in leisure activities and then performing a one-way analysis of variance resulted in a finding of no significant difference in the means of the four groups. While past studies of when people retire have indicated that perceived health and subjects' belief that they have adequate income to retire are often identified as the critical variables in the decision of when to retire, that would not appear to be the case with this sample. There were no significant differences in the perceived state of health for those subjects who were working in comparison to those subjects who were retired (Table 2).

Hypothesis Two stated that those persons who have retired will score higher on measures of life satisfaction than those who are working full or part-time. The mean scores on life satisfaction were calculated for those working full-time, those working part-time, those retired and engaged in volunteer activity, and those retired and engaged in leisure activity. The data indicated that those retired and engaged in volunteer activities and those retired and engaged in leisure activity scored significantly higher on measures of life satisfaction than those working either full or part-time (Table 3). The hypothesis was supported by the data (Table 3).

Hypothesis Three stated that those retirees engaged in volunteer or leisure activities will score higher on measures of life

TABLE 3.
One-Way Analysis of Variance:
Mean Life Satisfaction Score for Older Workers and Retirees

	MEAN	N=318
Work Full-Time	7.6372	49
Work Part-Time	7.1875	96
Retired/Engaged in Volunteer Activities	7.9928	139
Retired/Engaged in Leisure Activities	8.0000	34

SOURCE	D.F.	SUM OF SQUARES	MEAN SQUARES	F-RATIO	F PROBABILITY
Between Groups	3	40.4064	13.4688	8.2667	.0015
Within Groups	314	803.0056	2.5573		
TOTAL	317	843.4119			

TABLE 4.
One-Way Analysis of Variance:
Mean Life Satisfaction Scores for Older Workers and Retirees

	MEAN	N=268
Returned to Work Full-Time	2.2000	5
Returned to Work Part-Time	2.0333	90
Retired/Engaged in Volunteer Activities	2.3885	139
Retired/Engaged in Leisure Activities	2.2941	34

SOURCE	D.F.	SUM OF SQUARES	MEAN SQUARES	F-RATIO	F PROBABILITY
Between Groups	3	6.9659	2.3220	5.9067	.0006
Within Groups	264	103.7804	.3931		
TOTAL	267	110.7463			

satisfaction than those who retired and then returned to work on a full-time or part-time basis. Mean life satisfaction scores were calculated for those who had retired and then returned to work full-time, those who had retired and then returned to work part-time, those who had retired and were engaged in volunteer activities, and those who had retired and were engaged in leisure activities. Those retired and engaged in volunteer or leisure activity scored significantly higher on life satisfaction than those who had retired and returned to work full or part-time. As Table 4 indicates there were only five people in this sample who had retired and returned to work full-time. Returning to work full-time was rare in this sample of people.

Hypothesis Four stated that those retirees who returned to work full or part-time will be more respected by their peers than those who have retired and engaged in volunteer or leisure activities.

In terms of their perceived respect by friends, those retired and returning to work full-time scored highest with a mean of 3.0. Those who retired and were engaged in volunteer activities scored second with a mean of 2.86. Those who retired and were engaged in leisure activities scored third with a mean of 2.76. Those who had retired and returned to work part-time perceived they were least respected by their friends with a score of 2.68.

While the analysis of variance did not find significant differences in these means at the .05 level of significance, they were significant at the .07 level of significance. Since the .05 level of significance is the normal level of acceptance of the significance of difference between groups, this hypothesis was not supported by the data (Table 5).

In order to clarify how the retirees' decision to return to work would affect their life satisfaction, an additional calculation was done. One question asked those who had returned to work was why they had done so. The choices to this question were: I needed the money, I needed to do something that makes me feel productive, and I was lonely and bored and work gave me something interesting to do. Mean scores and measures of life satisfaction were calculated for each of these three groups (Table 6). The highest mean score was for the group who returned to work in order to feel productive, and their score was 8.27. The second highest mean score was for those who had returned to work because they were lonely and bored, and their score was 7.26. The lowest mean score on life satisfaction was 6.7 for those who had been forced to return to work because they needed the money (Table 6). Thus, most of the people that returned to work did so because they needed the money, but they were the least satisfied with their lives.

TABLE 5.
One Way Analysis of Variance:
Mean Scores for Perceived Respect of Older Workers and Retirees by Their Peers

	MEAN	N=277
Returned to Work Full-Time	3.00006	4
Returned to Work Part-Time	2.6869	99
Retired/Engaged in Volunteer Activities	2.8643	140
Retired/Engaged in Leisure Activities	2.7647	34

SOURCE	D.F.	SUM OF SQUARES	MEAN SQUARES	F RATIO	F PROBABILITY
Between Groups	3	2.0236	.6745	2.4254	.0657
Within Groups	272	75.8326	.2778		
TOTAL	276	77.8556			

TABLE 6.
One Way Analysis of Variance:
Mean Scores on Life Satisfaction Based on the Reasons Individuals Returned to Work

	MEAN	N=130
Needed the money	6.7027	74
Wanted to feel productive	8.2703	37
Lonely & bored	7.2632	19

SOURCE	D.F.	SUM OF SQUARES	MEAN SQUARES	F RATIO	F PROBABILITY
Between Groups	2	60.6360	30.3180	10.7420	.0000
Within Groups	127	358.4410	2.8224		
TOTAL	129	419.0769			

CONCLUSION

The data from this study indicate that those who retire and engage in volunteer or recreational activities score higher on measures of life satisfaction than those that never retired. Of those that retired and then returned to work, those that did so because they wanted to feel productive scored highest on life satisfaction. Those that returned to work because they needed the money scored lowest on life satisfaction.

These findings would suggest that if the goal of the federal government is to keep older people in the labor force longer, some means must be found by which the older workers are kept at jobs in which they feel productive and needed. For the business community to continue, primarily for economic reasons, to encourage older workers to retire from highly skilled jobs in which they are more productive than younger workers does not seem desirable.

One possible solution to this problem might be for the federal government to give a tax incentive to businesses employing older workers so that the economic advantage business sees for retiring older workers and employing younger ones would diminish.

A major break in the cost of employing older workers in business would be for the federal government to develop a national health insurance program. One of the major costs to the employer of older workers is the amount of money they must put into health insurance for them. For the federal government to assume this cost would be a major reduction in the business cost of continuing to employ older workers.

Perhaps businesses could continue to utilize the talents of older workers by developing reduced and flexible work schedules which would pay them a lower salary but keep them involved in critical tasks for the industry, as suggested by McShulski (1997).

Since the trend of the last thirty years has been for an ever increasing number of workers to retire prior to age 65, perhaps the government's attempts to keep people in the workforce longer by increasing the age at which they can draw a Social Security check will not be successful. It is possible that through private savings, private investment programs, and pension programs financed by their employers, older workers will continue to retire prior to age 65.

On the other hand, improving technology may mean that business and industry will need fewer employees to produce the nations' good and services, and therefore they will continue to encourage their workers to retire at younger ages.

The complexity and unpredictability of the factors involved makes predicting future employment and retirement patterns for older Americans at best hazardous and at worst impossible. Observing the results of economic and political pressures placed on both business and government by an ever increasing number of the baby boom generation arriving at retirement age in the next 25 years should prove interesting.

REFERENCES

Allen, Carole and Herman Brotman. 1981. *Chartbook on Aging*. Washington, D. C.: Administration on Aging.

Beck, S. 1983. "Determinants of Returning to Work after Retirement." Final Report for Grant No. 1R23AG035:65–101, Kansas City, MO.

Berkman, Lisa F. and Lister Breslow. 1983. *Health and Ways of Living: The Alameda Country Study*. New York: Oxford University Press.

Clark, Robert. 1988. "The Future of Work and Retirement." *Research on Aging* 10:169–193.

Clifton, Bryant. 1972. *The Social Dimensions of Work*. Upper Saddle River, NJ: Prentice Hall.

Crowley, J. E. 1990. "Longitudinal Effects of Retirement on Men's Well-Being and Health." Journal *of Business and Psychology* 1:95–113.

Dennis, Helen. 1986. *Fourteen Steps to Managing an Aging Work Force*, edited by Helen Dennis, Lexington, MA: Lexington Books.

Dorfman, L. T. 1992. "Academics and the Transition to Retirement." *Educational Gerontology* 18:343–363.

Dubin, Robert. 1956. "Industrial Workers' Word: A Study of the Central Life Interests of Industrial Workers." *Social Problems* 3:131–142.

Fillenbau, G. G., L. K. George, and E. B. Palmore. 1985. "Determinants and Consequences of Retirement." *Journal of Gerontology* 39:364–371.

Fyock, Catherine. 1991. "American Work Force Is Coming of Age." *The Gerontologist* 31:422–425.

Gall, Terry, David Evans, and John Howard. May 1997. "The Retirement Adjustment Process; Changes in Well-Being of Male Retirees Across Time." *The Journal of Gerontology* 52B(3):110–117.

Gray, Robert M. and David O. Moberg. 1977. *The Church and the Older Person*, revised edition. Grand Rapids, MI: Ermanns

Hall, Richard. 1975. *Occupations and the Social Structure*. Englewood Cliffs, NJ: Prentice Hall.

Hardy, Melissa. 1991. "Employment After Retirement." *Research on Aging* 13(3):267–288.

House, James S., Karl R. Landes, and Debra Umberson. 1988. "Social Relationships and Health." *Science* 241:540–545.

Howell, Nancy Morrow. 1988. "Life Span Determinants of Work in Retirement Years." *International Journal of Aging and Human Development* 27(2):125–140.

Iams, Howard M. 1985 "New Social Security Beneficiary Women." Correlates of work paper read at the 1985 meeting of the American Sociological Association.

Markides, Kyrakos S. 1983. "Aging, Religiosity and Adjustment: A Longitudinal Analysis." *Journal of Gerontology* 38:621–625.

McShulski, Elaine. 1997. "Ease Employer and Employee Retirement Adjustment with 'Soft Landing' Program." *HR Magazine*, Alexandria: 30–32.

Mobert, David D. 1983. "Compartmentalization and Parochialism in Religion and Voluntary Action Research." *Review of Religious Research* 22(4):318–321.

Moen, Phyllis, Donna Dempster-McClain, and Robin Williams. 1992. "Successful Aging: A Life Course Perspective on Women's Multiple Roles and Health." *American Journal of Sociology* 97(6):1612–1633.

Morris, Malcolm. 1986. "Work and Retirement in an Aging Society." *Daedalus* 115:269–293.

Ortega, Suzanne T., Robert D. Crutchfield, and William A. Rusling. 1983. "Race Differences in Elderly Personal Well-Being, Friendship, Family and Church." *Research on Aging* 5(1):101–118.

Parker, Stanley. 1982. *Works and Retirement*. London: Allen & Unwin Publishers.

Quinn, Joseph and Richard Burkhauser. *1990 Handbook of Aging and the Social Sciences*, edited by Richard Beinstock and Linda K. Gorge. Academic Press.

Quinn, J. F. 1980. *Retirement Patterns of Self-Employed Workers in Retirement Policy on an Aging Society*, R. L. Clark ed., Durham, NC:. Duke University Press.

Soldo, Beth J. and Emily M. Agree. 1988. *Population Bulletin* 43(3). Population Reference Bureau.

Sammartino, Frank. 1979. "Early Retirement." in *Monographs of Aging*, No. 1, Madison: Joyce MacBeth Institute on Aging and Adult Life, University of Wisconsin.

Seccombe, K. and G. R. Lee. 1986. "Gender Differences in Retirement Satisfaction and Its Antecedents." *Research on Aging* 8:426–440.

Sheppard, Harold. 1990. *The Future of Older Workers*. International Exchange Center on Gerontology, University of South Florida, Tampa. FL.

Streib, G. F. and C. J. Schneider. 1971. *Retirement in American Society*. Cornell University Press, Ithaca, NY.

Tillenbaum, G. C. 1971. "The Working Retired." *Journal of Gerontology* 26:1:82–89. U. S. Department of Labor, Civilian Labor Force Participation Rates: Actual and Projected 1980.

Vroom, Victor. 1964. *Work & Motivation*. New York: John Wiley.

Welford, A. T. 1988. "Preventing Adverse Changes of Work with Age." *American Journal of Aging and Human Development* 4:283–291.

From *Journal of Applied Sociology*, 2001, Vol. 18, No. 1, pp. 131-149. © 2001 by Society for Applied Sociology.

UNIT 6
The Experience of Dying

Unit Selections

Key Points to Consider

- Oregon is a state that has made euthanasia (assisted suicide) legal. Why are so many of the seriously ill older persons there choosing to end their lives by refusing to eat rather than euthanasia?

- Should dying patients be told the truth about their impending death, or should the information be withheld? Defend your answer.

- Is it better for the grieving survivors if their loved one died suddenly or experienced a prolonged illness before dying?

- What were the major killers of older persons during the last two decades of the twentieth century? What were some of the changes in the causes of death among men and women?

Student Website
www.mhcls.com/online

Internet References
Further information regarding these websites may be found in this book's preface or online.

Agency for Health Care Policy and Research
http://www.ahcpr.gov

Growth House, Inc.
http://www.growthhouse.org/

Hospice Foundation of America
http://www.HospiceFoundation.org

Hospice HotLinks
http://www.hospiceweb.com/links.htm

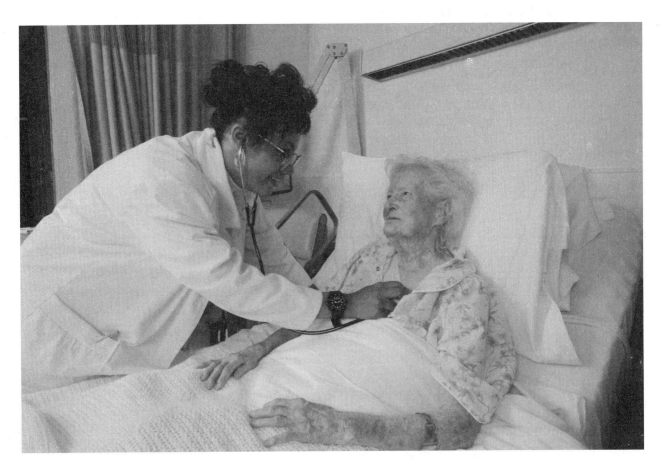

Modern science has allowed individuals to have some control over the conception of their children and has provided people with the ability to prolong life. However, life and death still defy scientific explanation or reason. The world can be divided into two categories: sacred and secular. The sacred (that which is usually embodied in the religion of a culture) is used to explain all the forces of nature and the environment that can neither be understood nor controlled. On the other hand, the secular (defined as "of or relating to the world") is used to explain all the aspects of the world that can be understood or controlled. Through scientific invention, more and more of the natural world can be controlled. It still seems highly doubtful, however, that science will ever be able to provide an acceptable explanation of the meaning of death. In this domain, religion may always prevail. Death is universally feared. Sometimes it is more bearable for those who believe in a life after death. Here, religion offers a solution to this dilemma. In the words of anthropologist Bronislaw Malinowski (1884–1942):

> Religion steps in, selecting the positive creed, the comforting view, the culturally valuable belief in immortality, in the spirit of the body, and in the continuance of life after death.

(Bronislaw Malinowski, Magic, Science and Religion and Other Essays, Glencoe, Illinois: Free Press, 1948)

The fear of death leads people to develop defense mechanisms in order to insulate themselves psychologically from the reality of their own death. The individual knows that someday he or she must die, but this event is nearly always thought to be likely to occur in the far distant future. The individual does not think of himself or herself as dying tomorrow or the next day, but rather years from now. In this way, people are able to control their anxiety about death.

Losing a close friend or relative brings people dangerously close to the reality of death. Individuals come face to face with the fact that there is always an end to life. Latent fears surface. During times of mourning, people grieve not only for the dead, but also for themselves, and for the finiteness of life.

The readings in this section address bereavement, grief, arguments for and against euthanasia, and adjustments to the stages of dying. Janet McConnaughey, in "More Hospice Patients Forgoing Sustenance," points out that in the state of Oregon, twice as many hospice patients choose to end their lives by refusing to eat as choose to die by physician-assisted suicide. The reasons for this decision were examined. The authors of "Expectancy of Spousal Death and Adjustment to Conjugal Bereavement" point out the difference in the time it takes a surviving spouse to adjust to the death of their loved one depending on whether they had or had not anticipated the death for some time before it occurred.

"Start the Conversation" explains what the dying person will experience physically and emotionally. Moreover, the inevitable caregiving choices that must be made are clearly outlined. In "Trends in Causes of Death Among the Elderly," the authors point out the major health problems that took older peoples' lives and what declines had occurred in each of these areas in the last two decades of the twentieth century.

More hospice patients forgoing sustenance

Oregon study shows more ending lives by not eating, drinking

By Janet McConnaughey

A surprising number of terminally ill hospice patients choose to speed their deaths by refusing food and drink, a study in Oregon suggests.

In fact the survey of hospice nurses found that patients pick this means of ending life–which is legal everywhere in the United States–twice as often as physician assisted suicide, which is legal only in Oregon.

The study further found that these patients are not depressed and typically die tranquilly, within two weeks.

The patients said they were ready to die, their quality of life was poor or they were afraid it would become so, and they saw no point in going on. They also wanted to die at home – where nearly all hospice care is given – and control the circumstances of their death, the nurses reported.

Nearly three-quarters of Oregon's 429 hospice nurses returned the survey. One-third of those who did said at least one of their patients had deliberately hastened death by stopping food and fluids during the previous four years.

That was only a tiny fraction of the 10,000-plus people who die under hospice care each year in Oregon. But Dr. Linda Ganzini, who directed the study, said the figure at first seemed too high to believe.

"I went back to my research assistant and said, 'Can we check this? Can we have these codes right?'" said Ganzini, who works at Oregon Health and Science University and the Portland Veterans Affairs Medical Center, and is on the board of the American Hospice Association.

After all, when she went through the medical journals, she found only three case studies about patients who had made this choice. A fourth report, from St. Christopher's Hospice in England, said that only two patients had done so in 30 years.

As striking as the numbers themselves is the fact that the nurses rated the overall quality of those deaths as "8" on a scale in which zero was "very bad" and 9 was "very good." Three-quarters of those scores were 7 or above, according to the study in Thursday's New England Journal of Medicine.

In all, 102 of the 307 nurses who answered her survey had worked with patients who ended their lives this way. At least 16 other patients stopped eating and drinking but later resumed doing so.

Over the same four years, 55 other terminally ill patients had used Oregon's assisted suicide law to get their doctors to prescribe a lethal dose of narcotics.

Other hospice professionals said that although having patients decide to refuse food and drink is far from an everyday occurrence, they found Ganzini's results completely believable. Dr. William Lamers of Malibu, Calif., medical consultant to Hospice Foundation of America, estimated that he had treated 50 such patients over 30 years of hospice practice.

"It is not an uncommon thing for people to talk about it – not uncommon for them to say, 'I'm not hungry. I don't want to eat any more, I just want to go,'" Lamers said.

EXPECTANCY OF SPOUSAL DEATH AND ADJUSTMENT TO CONJUGAL BEREAVEMENT

EDWARD F. DONNELLY

University of California, San Francisco

NIGEL P. FIELD

Pacific Graduate School of Psychology, Palo Alto, California

MARDI J. HOROWITZ

University of California, San Francisco

ABSTRACT

Previous findings on the role of expectancy of spousal death in adjustment to bereavement are inconclusive due to methodological shortcomings. This study examined the impact of subjective and objective expectancy on adjustment, while addressing the methodological problems of previous studies. At six months postbereavement, 97 midlife bereaved adults responded to interview questions regarding expectancy of their spouse's death. They also completed the Beck Depression Inventory and Texas Revised Inventory of Grief, at 6, 13, and 25 months postbereavement. Greater objective expectancy was associated with lower symptoms at all three postbereavement periods. Subjective expectancy was not related to symptoms, however. The clinical implications of objective expectancy's role on bereavement-related adjustment are addressed.

The death of a spouse is generally considered one of the most difficult experiences of life (Holmes & Rahe, 1967). Empirical studies have found that conjugally-bereaved persons experience symptoms of depression (Bornstein, Clayton, Halikas, Maurice, & Robins, 1973; Clayton, 1990; Lindemann, 1944; Lund, Caserta, & Diamond, 1986; Stroebe & Stroebe, 1992; Zisook & Shuchter, 1985; Zisook, Shuchter, Sledge, Paulus, & Judd, 1994) and grief-specific symptoms (Ball, 1977; Hill, Thompson, & Gallagher, 1988; Horowitz et al., 1984; Levy, 1991; Lindemann, 1944; Parkes & Weiss, 1983).

Although conjugal bereavement is most likely to be a difficult experience for anyone, there are individual dif-

ferences in how each widowed person responds to the loss of a loved one. An important factor that has been investigated as a contributor to these individual differences is the expectancy of spousal death (Sanders, 1988; Stroebe & Stroebe, 1987). Although there has been some support to show that expectancy plays a role in adjustment, the results have been inconclusive due to methodological shortcomings. The present study investigates the impact of expectancy on adjustment, while addressing these methodological problems.

An explanation for why expectancy may be an important factor is addressed by a contemporary cognitive schemas perspective on response to stressful life events. According to this perspective, a stressful life event is understood in terms of the extreme mismatch between the new psychological reality precipitated by the event and the person's preexisting schemas depicting life prior to the event. In the context of spousal bereavement, this can be understood in terms of the discrepancy between the bereaved person's new life situation as alone and enduring inner schemas of the prior relationship, including shared plans and hopes with the deceased.

According to schema theory (Horowitz, 1990, 1991; Janoff-Bulman, 1989, 1992), the extent of the mismatch may be larger in scope if the death is unexpected. Because the level of distress in response to the death is a direct function of the degree of mismatch, unexpected deaths are more distressing than expected deaths. In unexpected deaths, the bereaved person is more likely to experience greater distress because the schemas have had little or no opportunity to undergo revision. Furthermore, because schemas take a long time to change, the impact of expectancy on the grief-related symptomatology is likely to be evident well on after the death. On the other hand, with expected deaths the schemas of attachment have already undergone revision to incorporate the knowledge of the other's impending death; thus, the death will be less discrepant with schemas and less distressful for the bereaved person.

Even though the theoretical literature states that unexpected deaths are more distressful than expected deaths, empirical studies on the relation of expectancy to conjugal bereavement adjustment have produced mixed results. Although some support for this has been shown in a number of studies (Ball, 1977; Byrne & Raphael, 1994; Carey, 1979–1980; Hill et al., 1988; Lundin, 1984; Parkes & Weiss, 1983; Remondet, Hansson, & Winfrey, 1987; Roach & Kitson, 1989; Stroebe & Stroebe, 1992; Vachon et al., 1982; Zisook & Shuchter, 1991), little or no support has been found in other studies (Blanchard, Blanchard, & Becker, 1976; Bornstein et al., 1973; Breckenridge, Gallagher, Thompson, & Peterson, 1986; Byrne & Raphael, 1994; Carey, 1979–1980; Clayton, Halikas, Maurice, & Robins, 1973; Faletti, Gibbs, Clark, Pruchno, & Berman, 1989; Gass, 1989; Gerber, Rusalem, Hannon, Battin, & Arkin, 1975; Hill et al., 1988; Levy, 1991; Lundin, 1984; Remondet et al., 1987; Roach & Kitson, 1989; Sanders, 1982–1983; Stroebe & Stroebe, 1992; Zisook & Shuchter, 1991). Moreover, a few studies have even found an inverse relationship between expectancy and adjustment to conjugal bereavement (Clayton et al., 1973; Levy, 1991). Because most of the above studies differ in their operational definitions of expectancy and in the time in which symptoms were assessed, it is very difficult or impossible to make comparisons between studies and draw conclusions (Clayton, Parilla, & Bieri, 1980a, 1980b).

Most empirical studies on the relation of expectancy to conjugal bereavement adjustment have relied on objective expectancy measures, where objective expectancy refers to the duration of the spouse's terminal condition. A potential problem with objective expectancy involves the underlying assumption that a widowed person who had the time or opportunity to prepare for his or her spouse's death actually engaged in such preparations. Another way that expectancy has been measured, which may address this potential problem, is in terms of subjective expectancy (i.e., the extent to which a bereaved individual expected his or her loved one's death). Therefore, subjective expectancy may yield different results than objective expectancy. Thus, a comprehensive assessment of the impact of expectancy on adjustment would include both subjective and objective measures of expectancy. However, to date, only one study (Byrne & Raphael, 1994) has incorporated both measures.

Byrne & Raphael's study (1994) investigated an older aged sample (>65 years old) of 57 conjugally-bereaved men, and assessed their adjustment levels at 6 weeks and 13 months postbereavement. Subjective expectancy was measured by having the participants rate the death of their wife as either "expected," "fairly expected," "fairly unexpected," or "unexpected." They also measured objective expectancy, based on the length of the terminal interval of the wife's final illness, ranging from < *24 hours* to > *1 year*. The results showed that subjective expectancy was negatively associated with symptoms, but only at six weeks postbereavement. Objective expectancy was not related to adjustment, however.

The discrepant findings for subjective versus objective expectancy highlight the importance of employing both measures for assessing the impact of expectancy on conjugal bereavement. Although Byrne and Raphael's (1994) findings suggest that subjective expectancy is a better predictor than objective expectancy, the study has a notable limitation. In light of the fact that their sample consisted of older aged participants, the range of expectancy levels may have been more restricted compared to a younger sample. Because a restricted range decreases the likelihood of obtaining significant findings (Hinkle, Wiersma, & Jurs, 1979), this study may not have provided a fair assessment of the role of subjective expectancy in grief-related adjustment. A younger conjugally-bereaved sample should be more suitable in this regard.

The present study investigated the relationship between expectancy and adjustment to conjugal bereavement, addressing some of the aforementioned methodological shortcomings. This entailed the following methodological improvements: a) including both objective and subjective expectancy measures; b) investigating the responses of a midlife study group of conjugally-bereaved adults; c) employing both depressive and grief-specific symptom measures because grief-specific symptoms have been empirically distinguished from bereavement-related depressive symptoms as indicators of grief-related adjustment (Prigerson et al., 1996; Prigerson et al., 1995); and d) measuring adjustment to conjugal bereavement up to two years postbereavement.

This study predicted that both subjective and objective expectancy are negatively related to depressive and grief-specific symptoms in midlife conjugally-bereaved adults a 6, 13, and 25 months postbereavement.

METHOD

Participants

A midlife study group of 98 adults (33 males, 65 females) whose spouse had died within the previous three to six months were recruited by newspaper ads, posted notices, and referrals from a variety of institutions within the San Francisco Bay Area (e.g., medical centers and religious organizations).[1] The respondents ($N = 313$) were screened by structured telephone interview, which included questions addressing psychiatric and medical history. The participants were required to have been either

Table 1. Characteristics of Conjugally-Bereaved Participants

Characteristics	M	SD	Min	Max	n
Age (years)	45.92	8.21	24	61	98
Years together	15.30	10.66	0	38	96
Income	40,298	34,286	3,000	250,000	94
Beck Depression Inventory	12.36	8.50	0	37	242
Texas Revised Inventory of Grief	31.72	10.35	6	52	242

	n		%	
Sex				
Male	33		33.7	
Female	65		66.3	
Ethnicity				
Asian American	1		1.0	
African American	8		8.2	
Hispanic American	4		4.1	
Native American	3		3.1	
Caucasian	79		80.6	
Other	3		3.1	
Education				
High school	9		9.2	
Some college	42		42.9	
College degree	14		14.3	
Some graduate	16		16.3	
Master's degree	10		10.2	
Beyond Master's	2		2.0	
Doctorate	5		5.1	
Children at Home				
None	82		83.7	
Two	12		12.2	
Three	3		3.1	
Four	1		1.0	
Employment				
Not	29		29.6	
Part time	20		20.4	
Full time	48		50.0	

married to ($n = 95$) or living with their deceased partner for at least three years ($n = 3$), have no prior history of psychiatric hospitalization, and no binge eating, drug abuse, or alcohol abuse during the postbereavement time. After complete description of the study to the participants, written informed consent was obtained.

Table 1 presents the demographic characteristics of the participants.

Eleven (11.2%) participants withdrew from the study after 6 months postbereavement and 29 (30%) withdrew after 13 months postbereavement. There were no significant differences in expectancy levels in those who withdrew from those who remained in the study for subjective expectancy, $t(81) = -1.08$, ns, and objective expectancy, $t(84) = -1.92$, ns. There was no significant relationship between gender and objective expectancy, $t(96) = .60$, ns. Age, $r(98) = .20$, $p < .05$, and years together, $r(98) = .22$, $p < .05$, were associated with objective expectancy, however. Therefore, it was necessary to statistically control for age and years together in subsequent analyses.

Procedures

The respondents who met the inclusion criteria were sent a consent form and questionnaire booklet of symptom measures. Upon returning the completed questionnaires in a stamped preaddressed envelope, the participants were scheduled for a structured grief symptom interview. All questions pertaining to expectancy of spousal death were asked at the beginning of the interview. The interviews were conducted by three doctoral candidates in clinical psychology. At 13 and 25 months postbereavement, the participants were sent the same questionnaire booklet and instructions they had received at entry into the study.

Measures

Subjective Expectancy

Subjective expectancy was measured by each participant's response to the interviewer's question ("How expected was the loss of your spouse?"). Each participant used a 9-point scale, ranging from 0 (*not at all expected*), 1 (*between not at all and a little expected*), 2 (*a little expected*), 3 (*between a little and somewhat expected*), 4 (*somewhat expected*), 5 (*between somewhat and quite expected*), 6 (*quite expected*), 7 (*between quite and highly expected*), to 8 (*highly expected*), to indicate the subjective expectancy of his or her spouse's death. Although no reliability and validity information is available on this specific measure, and for that matter any other subjective expectancy measure, the scores were well distributed across the scale ($M = 3.67$, $SD = 3.38$).

Objective Expectancy

Objective expectancy was measured by the length of each participant's forewarning of spousal death, defined as participants' reports of the interval between receiving the first news of the spouse's terminal condition and the spouse's death. A 9-point scale, ranging from 0 (*less than 24 hours forewarning*), 1 (*greater than 24 hours to 1 week forewarning*), 2 (*greater than 1 week to 2 weeks forewarning*), 3 (*greater than 2 weeks to 1 month forewarning*), 4 (*greater than 1 month to 6 months forewarning*), 5 (*greater than 6 months to 1 year forewarning*), 6 (*greater than 1 year to 2 years forewarning*), 7 (*greater than 2 years to 3 years forewarning*), 8 (*more than 3 years forewarning*), was used to identify each participant's objective expectancy of his or her spouse's death. Although no reliability and validity information is available on this specific measure, and for that matter any other objective expectancy measure, the scores were well distributed across the scale ($M = 4.40$, $SD = 2.81$).

Grief-Specific Symptoms

The Texas Revised Inventory of Grief (TRIG; Faschingbauer, 1981; Faschingbauer, Zisook, & DeVaul, 1987) is a well-established measure of grief-specific symptoms. It consists of 13 items that measure the respondent's present thoughts, feelings, memories, opinions, and attitudes, in relation to the deceased.

Depressive Symptoms

The Beck Depression Inventory (BDI; Beck, Steer, & Garbin, 1988; Beck, Ward, Mendelson, Mock, & Erbaugh, 1961) is a widely-used 21-item measure of depression.

RESULTS

The overall group means and standard deviations for the BDI and TRIG are shown in Table 1. Correlations between the expectancy measures and symptom measures indicated that objective expectancy was predictive of depressive symptoms at 6 months postbereavement, $r(97) = -.29$, $p < .01$, 13 months postbereavement, $r(87) = -.34$, $p < .001$, and 25 months bereavement, $r(58) = -.51$, $p < .001$. Objective expectancy was also predictive of grief-specific symptoms at 6 months postbereavement, $r(97) = -.36$, $p < .001$, 13 months postbereavement, $r(87) = -.33$, $p < .01$, and 25 months postbereavement, $r(58) = -.33$, $p < .01$. Subjective expectancy showed no relationship to depressive and grief-specific symptoms, however it did exhibit a significant relationship with objective expectancy, $r(98) = .35$, $p < .001$. Because of the nonsignificant findings for subjective expectancy, only objective expectancy was considered in subsequent analyses.

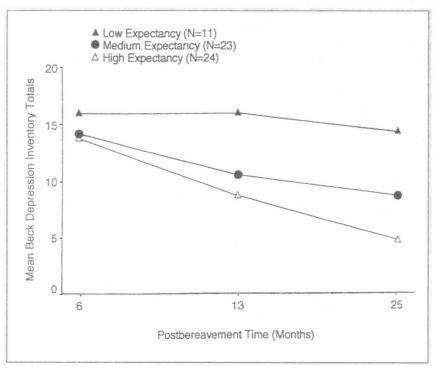

Figure 1. Mean Beck Depression Inventory totals for low objective expectancy, medium objective expectancy, and high objective expectancy groups at 6, 13, and 25 months postbereavement. (Low expectancy = forewarning 2 weeks or less; medium expectancy = forewarning over 2 weeks to 1 year; high expectancy = over 1 year forewarning.)

Predictors of Adjustment at 6, 13, and 25 Months Postbereavement

A hierarchical regression analysis was performed to determine if objective expectancy remained predictive of symptoms when controlling for age and years together as potential confounds. Age and years together were entered in step 1 and objective expectancy in step 2 of each of the regression analyses.

The results showed that objective expectancy remained predictive of depressive symptoms at 6 months postbereavement, β (3, 94) = -.24, $p < .05$, 13 months postbereavement $\beta(3,81)$ = -.31, $p < .01$, and 25 months postbereavement, $\beta(3,53)$ = -.46, $p < .001$. Objective expectancy also remained predictive of grief-specific symptoms, at 6 months postbereavement, $\beta(3,91)$ = -.30, $p < .01$, 13 months postbereavement, $\beta(3,81)$ = -.26, $p < .05$, and 25 months postbereavement, $\beta(3,53)$ = -.30, $p < .05$.

Repeated Measures Analysis

A repeated measures analysis of variance (ANOVA) was conducted to investigate if objective expectancy's relationship to symptoms was stable over time. This entailed trichotomizing the objective expectancy scores into three groups, such that scores between 6 and 8 were designated as *high expectancy* ($n = 38$), while scores between 3 and 5 were designated as *medium expectancy* ($n = 36$), and those between 0 and 2 were *low expectancy* ($n = 24$). Based on the correlational analyses, one would expect to find a significant main effect for expectancy over time.

For depressive symptoms, consistent with initial correlations analyses, the main effect for objective expectancy was significant, $F(2,55)$= 4.9, $p < .01$. There was also a significant main effect for postbereavement time, $F(2,110)$ = 16.49, $p < .001$, and a significant interaction between objective expectancy and postbereavement time, $F(4,110)$ = 2.58, $p < .05$. For grief-specific symptoms, also consistent with initial correlational analyses, the main effect for objective expectancy was significant, $F(2,55)$ = 5.9, $p < .01$.[2] There was also a significant main effect for postbereavement time, $F(2,110)$ = 39.07, $p < .001$, however, the interaction between objective expectancy and postbereavement time was not significant, $F(4,110)$ = 1.98, *ns*. As shown in Figures 1 and 2, the differences among the objective expectancy groups endured up to 2 years postbereavement for depressive symptoms and beyond 13 months for grief-specific symptoms. Although the interaction between objective expectancy and postbereavement time was significant for depressive symptoms, the pattern of findings were similar to those found for grief-specific symptoms.

Finally, post hoc tests (Scheffé's Test with an alpha level of .05) were utilized to determine how each expectancy group and postbereavement time contributed to the significant ANOVA findings. The results showed that the low expectancy group had significantly greater depressive symptoms than the medium and high expectancy

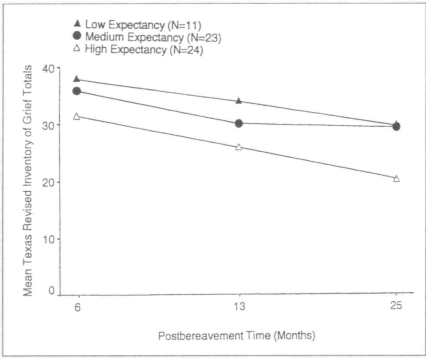

Figure 2. Mean Texas Revised Inventory of Grief totals for low objective expectancy, medium objective expectancy, and high objective expectancy groups at 6, 13, and 25 months postbereavement. (Low expectancy = forewarning 2 weeks or less; medium expectancy = forewarning over 2 weeks to 1 year; high expectancy = over 1 year forewarning.)

groups, and significantly greater grief-specific symptoms than the high expectancy group. In addition, the medium expectancy group had significantly greater grief-specific symptoms than the high expectancy group. Regarding postbereavement time, depressive and grief-specific symptoms were significantly greater at 6 months postbereavement than at both 13 and 25 months postbereavement. No other differences were significant.

DISCUSSION

Objective expectancy was a significant predictor of both depressive and grief-specific symptoms in midlife conjugally-bereaved adults at 6, 13, and 25 months postbereavement. However, subjective expectancy showed no relationship to symptoms.

The consistently significant findings for objective expectancy indicate that it is an important factor in predicting depressive and grief-specific symptoms in conjugally-bereaved adults. In fact, the findings for objective expectancy were upheld even when controlling for age and years together as potential confounds. Furthermore, the predictive power of objective expectancy seems to endure over time, lasting up to two years.

One of the main limitations of this study was the way in which participants were recruited. Because the most distressed were likely to have participated in this research (Bornstein et al., 1973; Clayton, Halikas, & Maurice, 1972; Stroebe & Stroebe, 1989), the findings may exaggerate the impact of the loss. Employing a random sample would help answer this question, and needs to be done in future studies.

There are a number of reasons that might explain why subjective expectancy was not related to symptoms. In terms of measurement, it was difficult to obtain a valid and reliable assessment of subjective expectancy because, unlike objective expectancy, there is no general consensus on how to measure subjective expectancy. It was also difficult to know whether the subjective expectancy ratings were accurate, in light of the fact that they were derived from participants' recollection of their experience six months ago and were therefore possibly confounded by such factors as denial.

There are several reasons that may explain why objective expectancy predicted adjustment. In terms of measurement, it seems that objective expectancy was easier to measure than subjective expectancy. The general consensus in conjugal bereavement research is that objective expectancy refers to the length of time of the deceased spouse's terminal condition. On the whole, bereaved individuals are probably more aware of the duration between the spouse's terminal condition and death than how they experienced or processed that information. Therefore, their response to the objective expectancy question was probably more accurate than their response to the subjective expectancy question. In fact, in contrast to the subjective expectancy question, none of the participants reported any difficulties with understanding the objective expectancy question.

Although a previous study measured both subjective and objective expectancy (Byrne & Raphael, 1994), the present study was the first to demonstrate that, contrary to the theoretical literature which advocates that subjective expectancy is more important than objective expectancy (Breckenridge et al., 1986; Byrne & Raphael, 1994; Faletti et al., 1989; Fulton & Gottesman, 1980; Levy, 1991; Rando, 1986, 1987), objective expectancy is a better predictor of adjustment than subjective expectancy. However, because this study did not utilize a random sample, the findings are limited in terms of their generalizability to all bereaved populations. Nonetheless, given the predominant characteristics of the sample, the findings are most applicable to middle-class, well-educated, Caucasian Americans.

CONCLUSIONS

Longer terminal illnesses, which allow for a period of expecting the death in spousal survivors, may buffer husbands and wives from the more intense mourning which follows the loss. In contrast, acute illnesses and accidents may lead to conjugal losses without advance mental activities that might enable adaptation. In such instances, extended distress for at least two years may be more likely, and additional supportive or therapeutic services are then indicated.

ACKNOWLEDGMENTS

The data for this research was obtained from the John D. and Catherine T. MacArthur Foundation, Program on Conscious and Unconscious Mental Processes, directed by Mardi J. Horowitz. This paper originated from the first author's doctoral dissertation in clinical psychology at the California School of Professional Psychology at Alameda. The authors wish to thank Samuel Gerson, Carole Huffine, and Ciril Wyatt-Donnelly for assistance with manuscript preparation.

NOTES

1. This study is part of a larger John D. and Catherine T. MacArthur Foundation research program on midlife conjugal bereavement. It involved a longitudinal design in which research participants were administered a diverse set of measures including questionnaires, structured and semi-structured interviews, cognitive tasks, and physiological measures. This research program encompassed a series of independent studies (Bonanno, Keltner, Holen, & Horowitz, 1995; Horowitz et al., 1997), all sharing a set of standardized symptom outcome measures.
2. Because Mauchly's sphericity test was significant for grief-specific symptoms, $W = .88, p < .05$, the Greenhouse-Geisser corrected F, df, and p values were utilized. Consistent with the results for depressive symptoms, a significant main effect was shown for objective expectancy with grief-specific symptoms, $F(1.79,49) = 2.58, p < .01$.

REFERENCES

Ball, J. F. (1977). Widow's grief: The impact of age and mode of death. *Omega, 7,* 307–333.

Beck, A. T., Steer, R. A., & Garbin, M. G. (1988). Psychometric properties of the Beck Depression Inventory: Twenty-five years of evaluation. *Clinical Psychology Review, 8,* 77–100.

Beck, A. T., Ward, C. H., Mendelson, M., Mock, J., & Erbaugh, J. (1961). An inventory for measuring depression. *Archives of General Psychiatry, 4,* 561–571.

Blanchard, C. G., Blanchard, E. B., & Becker, J. V. (1976). The young widow: Depressive symptomatology throughout the grief process. *Psychiatry, 39,* 394–399.

Bonanno, G. A., Keltner, D., Holen, A., & Horowitz, M. J. (1995). When avoiding unpleasant emotions might not be such a bad thing. *Journal of Personality and Social Psychology, 69,* 975–990.

Bornstein, P. E., Clayton, P. J., Halikas, J. A., Maurice, W. L., & Robins, E. (1973). The depression of widowhood after thirteen months. *British Journal of Psychiatry, 122,* 561–566.

Breckenridge, J. N., Gallagher, D., Thompson, L. W., & Peterson, J. (1986). Characteristic depressive symptoms of bereaved elders. *Journal of Gerontology, 41,* 163–168.

Byrne, G. J. A., & Raphael, B. (1994). A longitudinal study of bereavement phenomena in recently widowed elderly men. *Psychological Medicine, 24,* 411–421.

Carey, R. G. (1979–1980). Weathering widowhood: Problems and adjustment of the widowed during the first year. *Omega, 10,* 163–174.

Clayton, P. J. (1990). Bereavement and depression. *Journal of Clinical Psychiatry, 51,* 34–58.

Clayton, P. J., Halikas, J. A., & Maurice, W. L. (1972). The depression of widowhood. *British Journal of Psychiatry, 120,* 71–77.

Clayton, P. J., Halikas, J. A., Maurice, W. L., & Robins, E. (1973). Anticipatory grief and widowhood. *British Journal of Psychiatry, 122,* 47–51.

Clayton, P. J., Parilla, R. H., Jr., & Bieri, M. D. (1980a). Methodological problems in assessing the relationship between acuteness of death and the bereavement outcome. In J. Reiffel, R. DeBellis, L. C. Mark, A. H. Kutscher, P. R. Patterson, & B. Schoenberg (Eds.), *Psychosocial aspects of cardiovascular disease: The life-threatened patient, the family, and the staff* (pp. 267–275). New York: Columbia University Press.

Clayton, P. J., Parilla, R. H., Jr., & Bieri, M. D. (1980b). Survivors of cardiovascular and cancer deaths. In J. Reiffel, R. DeBellis, L. C. Mark, A. H. Kutscher, P. R. Patterson, & B. Schoenberg (Eds.), *Psychosocial aspects of cardiovascular disease: The life-threatened patient, the family, and the staff* (pp. 277–293). New York: Columbia University Press.

Faletti, M. V., Gibbs, J. M., Clark, M. C., Pruchno, R. A., & Berman, E. A. (1989). Longitudinal course of bereavement in older adults. In D. A. Lund (Ed.), *Older bereaved spouses: Research with practical implications* (pp. 37–51). New York: Hemisphere.

Faschingbauer, T. R. (1981). *Texas Revised Inventory of Grief Manual.* Houston: Honeycomb Publishing.

Faschingbauer, T. R., Zisook, S., & DeVaul, R. (1987). The Texas Revised Inventory of Grief. In S. Zisook (Ed.), *Biopsychosocial aspects of bereavement* (pp. 109–124). Washington, D.C.: American Psychiatric Press.

Fulton, R., & Gottesman, D. J. (1980). Anticipatory grief: A psychosocial concept reconsidered. *British Journal of Psychiatry, 137,* 45–54.

Gass, K. A. (1989). Health of older widowers: Role of appraisal, coping, resources, and type of spouse's death. In D. A. Lund (Ed.), *Older bereaved spouses: Research with practical implications* (pp. 95–110). New York: Hemisphere.

Gerber, I., Rusalem, R., Hannon, N., Battin, D., & Arkin, A. (1975). Anticipatory grief and aged widows and widowers. *Journal of Gerontology, 30*, 225–229.

Hill, C. D., Thompson, L. W., & Gallagher, D. (1988). The role of anticipatory bereavement in older women's adjustment to widowhood. *The Gerontologiest, 28*, 792–796.

Hinkle, D. E., Wiersma, W., & Jurs, S. G. (1979). *Applied statistics for the behavioral sciences.* Boston, MA.: Houghton Mifflin Company.

Holmes, T. H., & Rahe, R. H. (1967). The social readjustment rating scale. *Journal of Psychosomatic Research, 11*, 213–218.

Horowitz, M. J. (1990). A model of mourning: Change in schemas of self and other. *Journal of the American Psychoanalytic Association, 38*, 297–324.

Horowitz, M. J. (1991). Person schemas. In M. J. Horowitz (Ed.), *Person schemas and maladaptive interpersonal patterns* (pp. 13–31). Chicago: The University of Chicago Press.

Horowitz, M. J., Milbrath, C., Bonanno, G. M., Field, N. P., Stinson, C., & Holen, A. (1997). Predictors of complicated grief. *American Journal of Psychiatry, 154*, 904–910.

Horowitz, M. J., Weiss, D., Kaltreider, N., Krupnick, J., Wilner, N., Marmar, C., & DeWitt, K. (1984). Reactions to the death of a parent: Results from patients to field subjects. *Journal of Nervous and Mental Diseases, 172*, 383–392.

Janoff-Bulman, R. (1989). Assumptive worlds and the stress of traumatic events: Applications of the schema construct. *Social Cognition, 7*, 113–136.

Janoff-Bulman, R. (1992). *Shattered assumptions: Towards a new psychology of trauma.* New York: Free Press.

Levy, L. H. (1991). Anticipatory grief: Its measurement and proposed reconceptualization. *The Hospice Journal, 7*, 1–28.

Lindemann, E. (1944). Symptomatology and management of acute grief. *American Journal of Psychiatry, 101*, 141–148.

Lund, D., Caserta, M., & Diamond, M. (1986). Testing for gender differences through two years of bereavement among the elderly. *The Gerontologist, 26*, 314–320.

Lundin, T. (1984). Morbidity following sudden and unexpected bereavement. *British Journal of Psychiatry, 144*, 84–88.

Parkes, C. M., & Weiss, R. S. (1983). *Recovery from bereavement.* New York: Basic Books.

Prigerson, H. G., Bierhals, A. J., Kasl, S. V., Reynolds, C. F., III, Shear, M. K., Newsom, J. T., & Jacobs, S. (1996). Complicated grief as a disorder distinct from bereavement-related depression and anxiety: A replication study. *American Journal of Psychiatry, 153*, 1484–1486.

Prigerson, H. G., Frank, E., Kasl, S. V., Reynolds, C. F., III, Anderson, B., Zubenko, G. S., Houck, P. R., George, C. J., & Kupfer, D. J. (1995). Complicated grief and bereavement-related depression as distinct disorders: Preliminary empirical validation in elderly bereaved spouses. *American Journal of Psychiatry, 152*, 22–30.

Rando, T. A. (Eds.). (1986). *Loss and anticipatory grief.* Lexington, MA: Lexington Books.

Rando, T. A. (1987). The unrecognized impact of sudden death in terminal illness and in positively progressing convalescence. *Israel Journal of Psychiatry and Related Sciences, 24*, 125–135.

Remondet, J. H., Hansson, B. R., & Winfrey, G. (1987). Rehearsal for widowhood. *Journal of Social and Clinical Psychology, 5*, 285–297.

Roach, M. J., & Kitson, G. C. (1989). Impact of forewarning on adjustment to widowhood and divorce. In D. A. Lund (Ed.), *Older bereaved spouses: Research with practical implications* (pp. 185–200). New York: Hemisphere.

Sanders, C. M. (1982–1983). Effects of sudden vs. chronic illness death on bereavement outcome. *Omega, 13*, 227–241.

Sanders, C. M. (1988). Risk factors in bereavement outcome. *Journal of Social Issues, 44*, 97–111.

Stroebe, M. S., & Stroebe, W. (1989). Who participates in bereavement research? A review and empirical study. *Omega, 20*, 1–29.

Stroebe, W., & Stroebe, M. S. (1987). *Bereavement and health.* New York: Cambridge University Press.

Stroebe, W., & Stroebe, M. S. (1992). Bereavement and health: Processes of adjusting to the loss of a partner. In L. Montada, S. H. Filipp, & M. J. Lerner (Eds.), *Life crises and experiences of loss in adulthood* (pp. 3–22). Hillsdale, NJ: Lawrence Erlbaum Associates.

Vachon, M. L. S., Rogers, J., Lyall, W. A., Lancee, W. J., Sheldon, A. R., & Freeman, S. J. J. (1982). Predictors and correlates of adaptation to conjugal bereavement. *American Journal of Psychiatry, 139*, 998–1002.

Zisook, S., & Shuchter, S. R. (1985). Time course of spousal bereavement. *General Hospital Psychiatry, 7*, 95–100.

Zisook, S., & Shuchter, S. R. (1991). Early psychological reaction to the stress of widowhood. *Psychiatry, 54*, 320–333.

Zisook, S., Shuchter, S. R., Sledge, P. A., Paulus, M., & Judd, L. L. (1994). The spectrum of depressive phenomena after spousal bereavement. *Journal of Clinical Psychiatry, 55*, 29–36.

From *Omega*, Vol. 42, No. 3, 2000-2001, pp. 195-208 by Edward F. Donnelly, Nigel P. Field, and Mardi J. Horowitz. © 2001 by Baywood Publishing Company, Inc. Reprinted by permission.

Start the Conversation

The MODERN MATURITY guide to end-of-life care

The Body Speaks

Physically, dying means that "the body's various physiological systems, such as the circulatory, respiratory, and digestive systems, are no longer able to support the demands required to stay alive," says Barney Spivack, M.D., director of Geriatric Medicine for the Stamford (Connecticut) Health System. "When there is no meaningful chance for recovery, the physician should discuss realistic goals of care with the patient and family, which may include letting nature take its course. Lacking that direction," he says, "physicians differ in their perception of when enough is enough. We use our best judgment, taking into account the situation, the information available at the time, consultation with another doctor, or guidance from an ethics committee."

Without instructions from the patient or family, a doctor's obligation to a terminally ill person is to provide life-sustaining treatment. When a decision to "let nature take its course" has been made, the doctor will remove the treatment, based on the patient's needs. Early on, the patient or surrogate may choose to stop interventions such as antibiotics, dialysis, resuscitation, and defibrillation. Caregivers may want to offer food and fluids, but those can cause choking and the pooling of dangerous fluids in the lungs. A dying patient does not desire or need nourishment; without it he or she goes into a deep sleep and dies in days to weeks. A breathing machine would be the last support: It is uncomfortable for the patient, and may be disconnected when the patient or family finds that it is merely prolonging the dying process.

The Best Defense Against Pain

Pain-management activists are fervently trying to reeducate physicians about the importance and safety of making patients comfortable. "In medical school 30 years ago, we worried a lot about creating addicts," says Philadelphia internist Nicholas Scharff. "Now we know that addiction is not a problem: People who are in pain take

pain medication as long as they need it, and then they stop." Spivack says, "We have new formulations and delivery systems, so a dying patient should never have unmet pain needs."

In Search of a Good Death

If we think about death at all, we say that we want to go quickly, in our sleep, or, perhaps, while fly-fishing. But in fact only 10 percent of us die suddenly. The more common process is a slow decline with episodes of organ or system failure. Most of us want to die at home; most of us won't. All of us hope to die without pain; many of us will be kept alive, in pain, beyond a time when we would choose to call a halt. Yet very few of us take steps ahead of time to spell out what kind of physical and emotional care we will want at the end.

The new movement to improve the end of life is pioneering ways to make available to each of us a good death—as we each define it. One goal of the movement is to bring death through the cultural process that childbirth has achieved; from an unconscious, solitary act in a cold hospital room to a situation in which one is buffered by pillows, pictures, music, loved ones, and the solaces of home. But as in the childbirth movement, the real goal is choice—here, to have the death you want. Much of death's sting can be averted by planning in advance, knowing the facts, and knowing what options we all have. Here, we have gathered new and relevant information to help us all make a difference for the people we are taking care of, and ultimately, for ourselves.

In 1999, the Joint Commission on Accreditation of Healthcare Organizations issued stern new guidelines about easing pain in both terminal and nonterminal patients. The movement intends to take pain seriously:

to measure and treat it as the fifth vital sign in hospitals, along with blood pressure, pulse, temperature, and respiration.

The best defense against pain, says Spivack, is a combination of education and assertiveness. "Don't be afraid to speak up," he says. "If your doctor isn't listening, talk to the nurses. They see more and usually have a good sense of what's happening." Hospice workers, too, are experts on physical comfort, and a good doctor will respond to a hospice worker's recommendations. "The best situation for pain management," says Scharff, "is at home with a family caregiver being guided by a hospice program."

The downsides to pain medication are, first, that narcotics given to a fragile body may have a double effect: The drug may ease the pain, but it may cause respiratory depression and possibly death. Second, pain medication may induce grogginess or unconsciousness when a patient wants to be alert. "Most people seem to be much more willing to tolerate pain than mental confusion," says senior research scientist M. Powell Lawton, Ph.D., of the Philadelphia Geriatric Center. Dying patients may choose to be alert one day for visitors, and asleep the next to cope with pain. Studies show that when patients control their own pain medication, they use less.

Final Symptoms

Depression This condition is not an inevitable part of dying but can and should be treated. In fact, untreated depression can prevent pain medications from working effectively, and antidepressant medication can help relieve pain. A dying patient should be kept in the best possible emotional state for the final stage of life. A combination of medications and psychotherapy works best to treat depression.

Anorexia In the last few days of life, anorexia—an unwillingness or inability to eat—often sets in. "It has a protective effect, releasing endorphins in the system and contributing to a greater feeling of well-being," says Spivack. "Force-feeding a dying patient could make him uncomfortable and cause choking."

Dehydration Most people want to drink little or nothing in their last days. Again, this is a protective mechanism, triggering a release of helpful endorphins.

Drowsiness and Unarousable Sleep In spite of a coma-like state, says Spivack, "presume that the patient hears everything that is being said in the room."

Agitation and Restlessness, Moaning and Groaning The features of "terminal delirium" occur when the patient's level of consciousness is markedly decreased; there is no significant likelihood that any pain sensation can reach consciousness. Family members and other caregivers may interpret what they see as "the patient is in pain" but as these signs arise at a point very close to death, terminal delirium should be suspected.

Hospice: The Comfort Team

Hospice is really a bundle of services. It organizes a team of people to help patients and their families, most often in the patient's home but also in hospice residences, nursing homes, and hospitals:

• Registered nurses who check medication and the patient's condition, communicate with the patient's doctor, and educate caregivers.
• Medical services by the patient's physician and a hospice's medical director, limited to pain medication and other comfort care.
• Medical supplies and equipment.
• Drugs for pain relief and symptom control.
• Home-care aides for personal care, homemakers for light housekeeping.
• Continuous care in the home as needed on a short-term basis.
• Trained volunteers for support services.
• Physical, occupational, and speech therapists to help patients adapt to new disabilities.
• Temporary hospitalization during a crisis.
• Counselors and social workers who provide emotional and spiritual support to the patient and family.
• Respite care—brief noncrisis hospitalization to provide relief for family caregivers for up to five days.
• Bereavement support for the family, including counseling, referral to support groups, and periodic check-ins during the first year after the death.

Hospice Residences Still rare, but a growing phenomenon. They provide all these services on-site. They're for patients without family caregivers; with frail, elderly spouses; and for families who cannot provide at-home care because of other commitments. At the moment, Medicare covers only hospice services; the patient must pay for room and board. In many states Medicaid also covers hospice services (see How Much Will It Cost?). Keep in mind that not all residences are certified, bonded, or licensed; and not all are covered by Medicare.

Getting In A physician can recommend hospice for a patient who is terminally ill and probably has less than six months to live. The aim of hospice is to help people cope with an illness, not to cure it. All patients entering hospice waive their rights to curative treatments, though only for conditions relating to their terminal illness. "If you break a leg, of course you'll be treated for that," says Karen Woods, executive director of the Hospice Association of America. No one is forced to accept a hospice referral, and patients may leave and opt for curative care at any time. Hospice programs are listed in the Yellow Pages. For more information, see Resources.

The Ultimate Emotional Challenge

A dying person is grieving the loss of control over life, of body image, of normal physical functions, mobility and strength, freedom and independence, security, and the illusion of immortality. He is also grieving the loss of an earthly future, and reorienting himself to an unknowable destiny.

At the same time, an emotionally healthy dying person will be trying to satisfy his survival drive by adapting to this new phase, making the most of life at the moment, calling in loved ones, examining and appreciating his own joys and accomplishments. Not all dying people are depressed; many embrace death easily.

Facing the Fact

Doctors are usually the ones to inform a patient that he or she is dying, and the end-of-life movement is training physicians to bring empathy to that conversation in place of medspeak and time estimates. The more sensitive doctor will first ask how the patient feels things are going. "The patient may say, 'Well, I don't think I'm getting better,' and I would say, 'I think you're right,' " says internist Nicholas Scharff.

At this point, a doctor might ask if the patient wants to hear more now or later, in broad strokes or in detail. Some people will need to first process the emotional blow with tears and anger before learning about the course of their disease in the future.

"Accept and understand whatever reaction the patient has," says Roni Lang, director of the Geriatric Assessment Program for the Stamford (Connecticut) Health System, and a social worker who is a longtime veteran of such conversations. "Don't be too quick with the tissue. That sends a message that it's not okay to be upset. It's okay for the patient to be however she is."

Getting to Acceptance

Some patients keep hoping that they will get better. Denial is one of the mind's miracles, a way to ward off painful realities until consciousness can deal with them. Denial may not be a problem for the dying person, but it can create difficulties for the family. The dying person could be leaving a lot of tough decisions, stress, and confusion behind. The classic stages of grief outlined by Elisabeth Kübler-Ross—denial, anger, bargaining, depression, and acceptance—are often used to describe post-death grieving, but were in fact delineated for the process of accepting impending loss. We now know that these states may not progress in order. "Most people oscillate between anger and sadness, embracing the prospect of death and unrealistic episodes of optimism," says Lang. Still, she says, "don't place demands on them

Survival Kit for Caregivers

A study published in the March 21, 2000, issue of **Annals of Internal Medicine** shows that caregivers of the dying are twice as likely to have depressive symptoms as the dying themselves.

No wonder. Caring for a dying parent, says social worker Roni Lang, "brings a fierce tangle of emotions. That part of us that is a child must grow up." Parallel struggles occur when caring for a spouse, a child, another relative, or a friend. Caregivers may also experience sibling rivalry, income loss, isolation, fatigue, burnout, and resentment.

To deal with these difficult stresses, Lang suggests that caregivers:

• Set limits in advance. How far am I willing to go? What level of care is needed? Who can I get to help? Resist the temptation to let the illness always take center stage, or to be drawn into guilt-inducing conversations with people who think you should be doing more.
• Join a caregiver support group, either disease-related like the Alzheimer's Association or Gilda's Club, or a more general support group like The Well Spouse Foundation. Ask the social services department at your hospital for advice. Telephone support and online chat rooms also exist (see Resources).
• Acknowledge anger and express it constructively by keeping a journal or talking to an understanding friend or family member. Anger is a normal reaction to powerlessness.
• When people offer to help, give them a specific assignment. And then, take time to do what energizes you and make a point of rewarding yourself.
• Remember that people who are critically ill are self-absorbed. If your empathy fails you and you lose patience, make amends and forgive yourself.

to accept their death. This is not a time to proselytize." It is enough for the family to accept the coming loss, and if necessary, introduce the idea of an advance directive and health-care proxy, approaching it as a "just in case" idea. When one member of the family cannot accept death, and insists that doctors do more, says Lang, "that's the worst nightmare. I would call a meeting, hear all views without interrupting, and get the conversation around to what the patient would want. You may need another person to come in, perhaps the doctor, to help 'hear' the voice of the patient."

What Are You Afraid Of?

The most important question for doctors and caregivers to ask a dying person is, What are you afraid of? "Fear aggravates pain," says Lang, "and pain aggravates fear." Fear of pain, says Spivack, is one of the most common problems, and can be dealt with rationally. Many people do not know, for example, that pain in dying is not inevitable. Other typical fears are of being separated from loved ones, from home, from work; fear of being a burden, losing control, being dependent, and leaving things undone. Voicing fear helps lessen it, and pinpointing fear helps a caregiver know how to respond.

How to Be With a Dying Person

Our usual instinct is to avoid everything about death, including the people moving most rapidly toward it. But, Spivack says, "In all my years of working with dying people, I've never heard one say 'I want to die alone.' " Dying people are greatly comforted by company; the benefit far outweighs the awkwardness of the visit. Lang offers these suggestions for visitors:

• Be close. Sit at eye level, and don't be afraid to touch. Let the dying person set the pace for the conversation. Allow for silence. Your presence alone is valuable.

• Don't contradict a patient who says he's going to die. Acceptance is okay. Allow for anger, guilt, and fear, without trying to "fix" it. Just listen and empathize.

• Give the patient as much decision-making power as possible, as long as possible. Allow for talk about unfinished business. Ask: "Who can I contact for you?"

• Encourage happy reminiscences. It's okay to laugh.

• Never pass up the chance to express love or say goodbye. But if you don't get the chance, remember that not everything is worked through. Do the best you can.

Taking Control Now

Sixty years ago, before the invention of dialysis, defibrillators, and ventilators, the failure of vital organs automatically meant death. There were few choices to be made to end suffering, and when there were—the fatal dose of morphine, for example—these decisions were made privately by family and doctors who knew each other well. Since the 1950s, medical technology has been capable of extending lives, but also of prolonging dying. In 1967, an organization called Choice in Dying (now the Partnership for Caring: America's Voices for the Dying; see Resources) designed the first advance directive—a document that allows you to designate under what conditions you would want life-sustaining treatment to be continued or terminated. But the idea did not gain popular understanding until 1976, when the parents of Karen Ann Quinlan won a long legal battle to disconnect her from respiratory support as she lay for months in a vegetative state. Some 75 percent of Americans are in favor of advance directives, although only 30–35 percent actually write them.

Designing the Care You Want

There are two kinds of advance directives, and you may use one or both. A Living Will details what kind of life-sustaining treatment you want or don't want, in the event of an illness when death is imminent. A durable power of attorney for health care appoints someone to be your decision-maker if you can't speak for yourself. This person is also called a surrogate, attorney-in-fact, or health-care proxy. An advance directive such as Five Wishes covers both.

Most experts agree that a Living Will alone is not sufficient. "You don't need to write specific instructions about different kinds of life support, as you don't yet know any of the facts of your situation, and they may change," says Charles Sabatino, assistant director of the American Bar Association's Commission on Legal Problems of the Elderly.

The proxy, Sabatino says, is far more important. "It means someone you trust will find out all the options and make a decision consistent with what you would want." In most states, you may write your own advance directive, though some states require a specific form, available at hospital admitting offices or at the state department of health.

When Should You Draw Up a Directive?

Without an advance directive, a hospital staff is legally bound to do everything to keep you alive as long as possible, until you or a family member decides otherwise. So advance directives are best written before emergency status or a terminal diagnosis. Some people write them at the same time they make a will. The process begins with discussions between you and your family and doctor. If anybody is reluctant to discuss the subject, Sabatino suggests starting the conversation with a story. "Remember what happened to Bob Jones and what his family went through? I want us to be different...." You can use existing tools—a booklet or questionnaire (see Resources)—to keep the conversation moving. Get your doctor's commitment to support your wishes. "If you're asking for something that is against your doctor's conscience" (such as prescribing a lethal dose of pain medication or removing life support at a time he considers premature), Sabatino says, "he may have an obligation to transfer you to another doctor." And make sure the person you name as surrogate agrees to act for you and understands your wishes.

Filing, Storing, Safekeeping...

An estimated 35 percent of advance directives cannot be found when needed.

• Give a copy to your surrogate, your doctor, your hospital, and other family members. Tell them where to find the original in the house—not in a safe deposit box where it might not be found until after death.

Five Wishes

Five Wishes is a questionnaire that guides people in making essential decisions about the care they want at the end of their life. About a million people have filled out the eight-page form in the past two years. This advance directive is legally valid in 34 states and the District of Columbia. (The other 16 require a specific state-mandated form.)

The document was designed by lawyer Jim Towey, founder of Aging With Dignity, a nonprofit organization that advocates for the needs of elders and their caregivers. Towey, who was legal counsel to Mother Teresa, visited her Home for the Dying in Calcutta in the 1980s. He was struck that in that haven in the Third World, "the dying people's hands were held, their pain was managed, and they weren't alone. In the First World, you see a lot of medical technology, but people die in pain, and alone." Towey talked to MODERN MATURITY about his directive and what it means.

What are the five wishes? Who do I want to make care decisions for me when I can't? What kind of medical treatment do I want toward the end? What would help me feel comfortable while I am dying? How do I want people to treat me? What do I want my loved ones to know about me and my feelings after I'm gone?

Why is it so vital to make advance decisions now? Medical technology has extended longevity, which is good, but it can prolong the dying process in ways that are almost cruel. Medical schools are still concentrating on curing, not caring for the dying. We can have a dignified season in our life, or die alone in pain with futile interventions. Most people only discover they have options when checking into the hospital, and often they no longer have the capacity to choose. This leaves the family members with a guessing game and, frequently, guilt.

What's the ideal way to use this document? First you do a little soul searching about what you want. Then discuss it with people you trust, in the livingroom instead of the waiting room—before a crisis. Just say, "I want a choice about how I spend my last days," talk about your choices, and pick someone to be your health-care surrogate.

What makes the Five Wishes directive unique? It's easy to use and understand, not written in the language of doctors or lawyers. It also allows people to discuss comfort dignity, and forgiveness, not just medical concerns. When my father filled it out, he said he wanted his favorite afghan blanket in his bed. It made a huge difference to me that, as he was dying, he had his wishes fulfilled.

For a copy of Five Wishes in English or Spanish, send a $5 check or money order to Aging With Dignity, PO Box 1661, Tallahassee, FL 32302. For more information, visit www.agingwithdignity. org.

• Some people carry a copy in their wallet or glove compartment of their car.
• Be aware that if you have more than one home and you split your time in several regions of the country, you should be registering your wishes with a hospital in each region, and consider naming more than one proxy.
• You may register your Living Will and health-care proxy online at uslivingwillregistry.com (or call 800-548-9455). The free, privately funded confidential service will instantly fax a copy to a hospital when the hospital requests one. It will also remind you to update it: You may want to choose a new surrogate, accommodate medical advances, or change your idea of when "enough is enough." M. Powell Lawton, who is doing a study on how people anticipate the terminal life stages, has discovered that "people adapt relatively well to states of poor health. The idea that life is still worth living continues to readjust itself."

Assisted Suicide: The Reality

While advance directives allow for the termination of life-sustaining treatment, assisted suicide means supplying the patient with a prescription for life-ending medication. A doctor writes the prescription for the medication; the patient takes the fatal dose him- or herself. Physician-assisted suicide is legal only in Oregon (and under consideration in Maine) but only with rigorous preconditions. Of the approximately 30,000 people who died in Oregon in 1999, only 33 received permission to have a lethal dose of medication and only 26 of those actually died of the medication. Surrogates may request an end to life support, but to assist in a suicide puts one at risk for charges of homicide.

Good Care: Can You Afford It?

The ordinary person is only one serious illness away from poverty," says Joanne Lynn, M.D., director of the Arlington, Virginia, Center to Improve Care of the Dying. An ethicist, hospice physician, and health-services researcher, she is one of the founding members of the end-of-life-care movement. "On the whole, hospitalization and the cost of suppressing symptoms is very easy to afford," says Lynn. Medicare and Medicaid will help cover that kind of acute medical care. But what is harder to afford is at-home medication, monitoring, daily help with eating and walking, and all the care that will go on for the rest of the patient's life.

"When people are dying," Lynn says, "an increasing proportion of their overall care does not need to be done by doctors. But when policymakers say the care is nonmedical, then it's second class, it's not important, and nobody will pay for it."

Bottom line, Medicare pays for about 57 percent of the cost of medical care for Medicare beneficiaries.

Another 11 percent is paid by Medicaid, 20 percent by the patient, 10 percent from private insurance, and the rest from other sources, such as charitable organizations.

Medi-what?

This public-plus-private network of funding sources for end-of-life care is complex, and who pays for how much of what is determined by diagnosis, age, site of care, and income. Besides the private health insurance that many of us have from our employers, other sources of funding may enter the picture when patients are terminally ill.

•**Medicare** A federal insurance program that covers health-care services for people 65 and over, some disabled people, and those with end-stage kidney disease. Medicare Part A covers inpatient care in hospitals, nursing homes, hospice, and some home health care. For most people, the Part A premium is free. Part B covers doctor fees, tests, and other outpatient medical services. Although Part B is optional, most people choose to enroll through their local Social Security office and pay the monthly premium ($45.50). Medicare beneficiaries share in the cost of care through deductibles and co-insurance. What Medicare does not cover at all is outpatient medication, long-term nonacute care, and support services.

•**Medicaid** A state and federally funded program that covers health-care services for people with income or assets below certain levels, which vary from state to state.

•**Medigap** Private insurance policies covering the gaps in Medicare, such as deductibles and co-payments, and in some cases additional health-care services, medical supplies, and outpatient prescription drugs.

Many of the services not paid for by Medicare can be covered by private long-term-care insurance. About 50 percent of us over the age of 65 will need long-term care at home or in a nursing home, and this insurance is an extra bit of protection for people with major assets to protect. It pays for skilled nursing care as well as non-health services, such as help with dressing, eating, and bathing. You select a dollar amount of coverage per day (for example, $100 in a nursing home, or $50 for at-home care), and a coverage period (for example, three years—the average nursing-home stay is 2.7 years). Depending on your age and the benefits you choose, the insurance can cost anywhere from around $500 to more than $8,000 a year. People with pre-existing conditions such as Alzheimer's or MS are usually not eligible.

How Much Will It Cost?

Where you get end-of-life care will affect the cost and who pays for it.

•**Hospital** Dying in a hospital costs about $1,000 a day. After a $766 deductible (per benefit period), Medicare reimburses the hospital a fixed rate per day, which varies by region and diagnosis. After the first 60 days in a hospital, a patient will pay a daily deductible ($194) that goes up (to $388) after 90 days. The patient is responsible for all costs for each day beyond 150 days. Medicaid and some private insurance, either through an employer or a Medigap plan, often help cover these costs.

•**Nursing home** About $1,000 a week. Medicare covers up to 100 days of skilled nursing care after a three-day hospitalization, and most medication costs during that time. For days 21–100, your daily co-insurance of $97 is usually covered by private insurance—if you have it. For nursing-home care not covered by Medicare, you must use your private assets, or Medicaid if your assets run out, which happens to approximately one-third of nursing-home residents. Long-term-care insurance may also cover some of the costs.

•**Hospice care** About $100 a day for in-home care. Medicare covers hospice care to patients who have a life expectancy of less than six months. (See Hospice: The Comfort Team.) Such care may be provided at home, in a hospice facility, a hospital, or a nursing-home. Patients may be asked to pay up to $5 for each prescription and a 5 percent co-pay for in-patient respite care, which is a short hospital stay to relieve caregivers. Medicaid covers hospice care in all but six states, even for those without Medicare.

About 60 percent of full-time employees of medium and large firms also have coverage for hospice services, but the benefits vary widely.

•**Home care without hospice services** Medicare Part A pays the full cost of medical home health care for up to 100 visits following a hospital stay of at least three days. Medicare Part B covers home health-care visits beyond those 100 visits or without a hospital stay. To qualify, the patient must be homebound, require skilled nursing care or physical or speech therapy, be under a physician's care, and use services from a Medicare-participating home-health agency. Note that this coverage is for medical care only; hired help for personal nonmedical services, such as that often required by Alzheimer's patients, is not covered by Medicare. It is covered by Medicaid in some states.

A major financial disadvantage of dying at home without hospice is that Medicare does not cover out-patient prescription drugs, even those for pain. Medicaid does cover these drugs, but often with restrictions on their price and quantity. Private insurance can fill the gap to some extent. Long-term-care insurance may cover payments to family caregivers who have to stop work to care for a dying patient, but this type of coverage is very rare.

Resources

MEDICAL CARE

For information about pain relief and symptom management:
Supportive Care of the Dying (503-215-5053; careofdying.org).

For a comprehensive guide to living with the medical, emotional, and spiritual aspects of dying:
Handbook for Mortals by Joanne Lynn and Joan Harrold, Oxford University Press.

For a 24-hour hotline offering counseling, pain management, downloadable advance directives, and more:
The Partnership for Caring (800-989-9455; www.partnershipforcaring.org).

EMOTIONAL CARE

To find mental-health counselors with an emphasis on lifespan human development and spiritual discussion:
American Counseling Association (800-347-6647; counseling.org).

For disease-related support groups and general resources for caregivers:
Caregiver Survival Resources (caregiver911.com).

For AARP's online caregiver support chatroom, access **America Online** every Wednesday night, 8:30–9:30 EST (keyword: AARP).

Education and advocacy for family caregivers:
National Family Caregivers Association (800-896-3650; nfcacares.org).

For the booklet,
Understanding the Grief Process (D16832, EEO143C), e-mail order with title and numbers to member@aarp.org or send postcard to AARP Fulfillment, 601 E St NW, Washington DC 20049. Please allow two to four weeks for delivery.

To find a volunteer to help with supportive services to the frail and their caregivers:
National Federation of Interfaith Volunteer Caregivers (816-931-5442; nfivc.org).

For information on support to partners of the chronically ill and/or the disabled:
The Well Spouse Foundation (800-838-0879; www.wellspouse.org).

LEGAL HELP

AARP members are entitled to a free half-hour of legal advice with a lawyer from **AARP's Legal Services Network**. (800-424-3410; www.aarp.org/lsn).
For **Planning for Incapacity**, *a guide to advance directives in your state*, send $5 to Legal Counsel for the Elderly, Inc., PO Box 96474, Washington DC 20090-6474. Make out check to LCE Inc.
For a **Caring Conversations** *booklet on advance-directive discussion:*

Midwest Bioethics Center (816-221-1100; midbio.org).

For information on care at the end of life, online discussion groups, conferences:
Last Acts Campaign (800-844-7616; lastacts.org).

HOSPICE

To learn about end-of-life care options and grief issues through videotapes, books, newsletters, and brochures:
Hospice Foundation of America (800-854-3402; hospice-foundation.org).

For information on hospice programs, FAQs, and general facts about hospice:
National Hospice and Palliative Care Organization (800-658-8898; nhpco.org).

For **All About Hospice: A Consumer's Guide** (202-546-4759; www.hospice-america.org).

FINANCIAL HELP

For **Organizing Your Future**, *a simple guide to end-of-life financial decisions*, send $5 to Legal Counsel for the Elderly, Inc., PO Box 96474, Washington DC 20090-6474. Make out check to LCE Inc.

For **Medicare and You 2000** *and a* **2000 Guide to Health Insurance for People With Medicare** (800-MEDICARE [633-4227]; medicare.gov).

To find your State Agency on Aging: **Administration on Aging, U.S. Department of Health and Human Services** (800-677-1116; aoa.dhhs.gov).

GENERAL

For information on end-of-life planning and bereavement: (www.aarp.org/endoflife/).

For health professionals and others who want to start conversations on end-of-life issues in their community:

Discussion Guide: On Our Own Terms: Moyers on Dying, based on the PBS series, airing September 10–13. The guide provides essays, instructions, and contacts. From PBS, www.pbs.org/onourownterms Or send a postcard request to On Our Own Terms Discussion Guide, Thirteen/WNET New York, PO Box 245, Little Falls, NJ 07424-9766.

Funded with a grant from The Robert Wood Johnson Foundation, Princeton, N.J. *Editor* Amy Gross; *Writer* Louise Lague; *Designer* David Herbick

---

"Start the Conversation" by Louise Lague reprinted from *AARP Modern Maturity,* September/October 2000. © 2000 by Louise Lague and American Association for Retired Persons (AARP). Reprinted with permission of the author and AARP.

Trends in Causes of Death Among the Elderly

By Nadine R. Sahyoun, Ph.D., RD
Harold Lentzner, Ph.D.
Donna Hoyert, Ph.D.
Kristen N. Robinson, Ph.D.

Highlights

The leading causes of death among the elderly are chronic diseases, notably cardiovascular disease and cancer. Other major causes of death include:

- Chronic respiratory diseases such as emphysema and chronic bronchitis
- Diseases common among the elderly such as Alzheimer's and renal diseases
- Infectious diseases and injuries

Significant trends in mortality among the elderly have emerged:

- Death from heart disease and atherosclerosis has declined dramatically for all groups.
- Death from cancer decreased for men in the 1990's after increasing in the previous 2 decades.
- Hypertension declined among older white men, but drastically increased among older black men.
- Biomedical advances, public health initiatives, and social changes may reduce mortality and increase longevity.

Overview

Since 1900, life expectancy in the United States has dramatically increased, and the principal causes of death have changed. At the beginning of the 20th century, many Americans died young. Most did not live past the age of 65, their lives often abruptly ended by one of a variety of deadly infectious diseases. But over time, death rates dropped at all ages, most dramatically for the young. By the dawn of the 21st century, the vast majority of children born in any given year could expect to live through childhood and into their eighth decade or beyond.

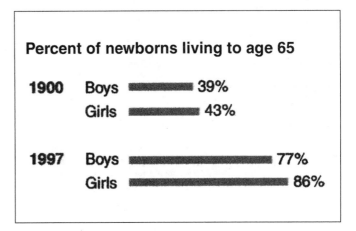

Percent of newborns living to age 65

1900	Boys	39%
	Girls	43%
1997	Boys	77%
	Girls	86%

Life expectancy has increased, but will the expansion continue?

For those born in the second half of the 20th century, chronic diseases replaced acute infections as the major causes of death. Today, death in the United States is largely reserved for the elderly. Roughly three-fourths of all deaths are at ages 65 and older.

Will we see major advances in life expectancies in the 21st century? Experts disagree. Some say we cannot continue to reduce mortality at the oldest ages without making dramatic and unforeseen medical advances against such major killers as cardiovascular disease and cancer.[1-3] But others counter that it is not only possible—other societies like Japan have already achieved significantly higher life expectancies—but likely as we reap the benefits of a more robust, better educated population taking better care of themselves and using modern medical technologies and therapies.[4-7]

Top 3 leading causes of death in the United States

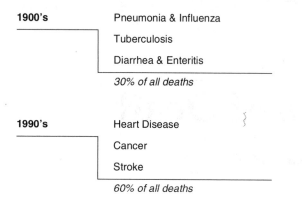

1900's
- Pneumonia & Influenza
- Tuberculosis
- Diarrhea & Enteritis

30% of all deaths

1990's
- Heart Disease
- Cancer
- Stroke

60% of all deaths

Countries with highest life expectancy, 1995

Men		Women	
Japan	76.4 yrs.	Japan	82.9 yrs.
Sweden	76.2	France	82.6
Israel	75.3	Switzerland	81.9
Canada	75.2	Sweden	81.6
Switzerland	75.1	Spain	81.5
Greece	75.1	Canada	81.2
Australia	75.0	Australia	80.9
Norway	74.9	Italy	80.8
Netherlands	74.6	Norway	80.7
Italy	74.4	Netherlands	80.4

Life expectancy in the U.S. was 72.5 yrs. for men and 78.9 yrs. for women.

Quality of life is an important concern

Perhaps a more pressing question is this: If we succeed in extending life expectancy, what will these added years bring? Will they be spent in active, productive, fulfilling endeavors, or will they be overshadowed by declining health, loss of memory, and lingering illness? How valuable is a longer life if we simply increase the time we spend functionally limited by such debilitating ailments as heart disease, osteoporosis, or Alzheimer's disease?

As we face the challenge of extending and improving life, we must be aware of trends in important measures of health, so that we identify the most effective ways to use resources to achieve these goals. Specifically, we should be familiar with trends in:

- Elderly mortality and the leading causes of death
- Quality of life including measures of illness and disability
- Factors associated with healthy aging

- The cost of illness

This new series of reports features information to help monitor the health of our aging population

Older Americans can expect to live longer than ever before. Under existing conditions, women who live to age 65 can expect to live about 19 years longer, men about 16 years longer. Whether the added years at the end of the life cycle are healthy, enjoyable, and productive depends, in part, upon preventing and controlling a number of chronic diseases and conditions.

This report is one of a series undertaken by the National Center for Health Statistics, with support from the National Institute on Aging, to help meet the challenge of extending and improving life. By monitoring the health of the elderly, using information compiled from a variety of sources, we hope to help focus research on the most effective ways to use resources and craft health policy.

What are the leading causes of death?

Chronic diseases are the leading causes of death

Heart disease and cancer have been the two leading causes of death among persons 65 years of age and older for the past 2 decades, accounting for nearly a million deaths (995,187) in 1997. Over one-third (35 percent) of all deaths are due to heart disease, including heart attacks and chronic ischemic heart disease. Cancer accounted for about one fifth (22 percent) of all deaths.

Other important chronic diseases among persons 65 years of age and older include stroke (cerebrovascular disease), chronic obstructive pulmonary diseases, diabetes, and pneumonia and influenza.

The leading causes of death are the same for different age-race-sex groups, but their ranking order varies. Heart disease remains the leading cause of death for most of the groups. Cancer is as common as heart disease within the youngest age group, 65–74 years of age, but decreases in importance with age, ranking third among women 85 years of age and older.

The third leading cause of death is most often stroke. However, among white men and women 65–74 years old, the third leading cause is chronic obstructive pulmonary diseases and allied conditions (COPD), which includes chronic bronchitis, emphysema, asthma, and other chronic respiratory diseases. Deaths from COPD are believed to be caused primarily by cigarette smoking. COPD ranks as the fourth or fifth cause of death for almost all other age-race-sex groups. The remaining leading causes vary in rank among different age, race, and sex groups.

Elderly decedents frequently suffer from more than one life-threatening condition at the time of death. It is sometimes difficult for the attending physician or other official charged with filling out the death certificate to

Leading causes of deaths for persons 65 years of age and older

White	Black	American Indian	Asian or Pacific Islander	Hispanic
1. Heart Disease	Heart Disease	Heart Disease	Heart Disease	Heart Disease
2. Cancer	Cancer	Cancer	Cancer	Cancer
3. Stroke	Stroke	Diabetes	Stroke	Stroke
4. COPD	Diabetes	Stroke	Pneu/Influenza	COPD
5. Pneu/Influenza	Pneu/Influenza	COPD	COPD	Pneu/Influenza

identify the initiating cause among several grave conditions. While a single cause, known as the underlying cause of death, is used in nearly all statistical reporting systems, the death certificate also allows for the listing of other causes in addition to a single underlying cause—up to 20 diseases and conditions.

Other major causes of death among the elderly include Alzheimer's disease and renal diseases

Alzheimer's disease and several important renal diseases (including nephritis, nephrotic syndrome, and nephrosis) have gained importance as causes of death among the elderly over the past 2 decades. Alzheimer's disease is now among the 10 leading causes of death for older white persons, but not for other racial groups. This cause of death increased significantly from 1979 to 1988, stabilized for a few years, and gradually increased after 1992.[8] The increase may be due to improvements in diagnosis and reporting of Alzheimer's disease, wider knowledge of the condition within the medical community, and other unidentifiable factors. This disease became a ranked condition in 1994.

Nephritis, nephrotic syndrome, and nephrosis ranks between sixth and tenth as a cause of death. It is a relatively more common cause of death among black than among white persons.

Older adults are vulnerable to common infectious diseases

Although infectious diseases are no longer the most common causes of death, pneumonia, influenza, and septicemia remain among the top causes of death. They were responsible for 5.5 percent or 95,640 deaths of people 65 years of age and older in 1997. However, the role infectious diseases play in declining health and mortality is not fully apparent. This is because several other medical conditions caused by infectious diseases, such as endocarditis and rheumatic heart disease, are classified as diseases of the heart despite their infectious origins. A study of deaths attributed to diseases known to be caused by infectious organisms showed a 25 percent increase in mortality between 1980 and 1992 for persons 65 years of age and older.[9]

The combined death rate from pneumonia and influenza has increased in recent years for all age-race-sex groups. This increase may be partly due to the higher tendency by medical certifiers to record pneumonia as the underlying cause of death with advancing age. But it also may reflect an increase in the severity of pneumonia, attributed to changes in the population at risk of contracting pneumonia or other respiratory pathogens, the increasing occurrence of drug-resistant microorganisms, and the detection of new respiratory infections.[10]

Pneumonia is now one of the most serious infections in elderly persons, especially among women and the oldest old. In a study of nursing home-acquired pneumonia patients, pneumonia resulted in death among 40 percent of individuals who required hospitalization.[11]

Septicemia ranks as the sixth leading cause of death for black women 85 years of age and older, but is less important for other demographic groups. This disease is nonspecific and often occurs as a consequence of other bacterial infections of the urinary tract, skin, or respiratory system.

Injuries remain a major cause of death well into old age

Death from injury is the leading cause of death among children and young adults. And although its relative importance decreases among the elderly, it remains a frequent cause of death among people 65 years of age and older (2 percent, or 31,400 deaths in 1997). Injuries from motor vehicle crashes, firearms, suffocation, and falls account for most deaths.

What are the significant trends?

Important changes in mortality have occurred over 2 decades

Between 1979–81 and 1995–97, the death rate from all causes decreased among persons 65–74 years of age (by 6 percent for women and 19 percent for men) and those 75–84 years of age (by 8 percent for women and 16 percent for men). The death rate increased slightly for women 85 years of age and older, but declined by about 3 percent for men of the same age. Among all three age groups, the decrease has been much greater for men.

Circulatory diseases have declined

A primary reason for the overall decline in mortality is the decrease in the death rate for heart disease and stroke. Heart disease declined by 30–40 percent for both women and men ages 65–74 and 75–84; stroke declined by about 35–40 percent for men and women in the same two age groups. Declines at the oldest age group for heart disease and stroke were more modest, but still significant (heart disease, 14 percent for women and 19 percent for men; stroke, 27 percent for women and 29 percent for men).

For the two racial groups examined, diseases of the heart decreased at a slower rate for black than for white persons (20 vs 37 percent for ages 65–74; 16 vs 32 percent for ages 75–84; and 8 vs 18 percent for ages 85+). The decline in stroke followed a similar pattern with the reduction more modest among the black population.

The decrease in mortality from atherosclerosis is striking

Death from atherosclerosis, which includes arteriosclerosis or "hardening of the arteries," has dropped over 2 decades for all age, sex, and racial groups. In 1979, atherosclerosis ranked as one of the top five causes of death, especially within the oldest age group. As an underlying cause, this disease declined over the years so that today it does not even rank among the top 10 leading causes of death for most age groups.

Such a drastic decline in atherosclerosis may reflect both a decrease in incidence over time and a change in reporting practice. Atherosclerosis is now frequently regarded as a preclinical process or a risk factor so the condition may have been recorded less frequently over time as physicians choose a more specific cause of death.[12]

Cancer rates among men decreased in the 1990's

Since 1990, there has been an overall downward trend among white men 65–74 (3 percent decline) and 75–84 years of age (6 percent) and among black men 65–74 (9 percent) and 75–84 years of age (2 percent), although the trend varies greatly by type of cancer. This decrease does not hold among women or the oldest old. For example, respiratory and intrathoracic cancer (largely lung cancer) increased until 1990 and then decreased among white men 65–84 years of age. But it continued to increase among black men, the oldest old, and all women. Breast cancer increased until 1990 and then stabilized among white women 65–84 years old; it continued to increase among the oldest group of white women and among black women over 75 years of age.

Chronic bronchitis, emphysema, and other COPD conditions increased as causes of death, especially among women

Nonspecific or undifferentiated chronic lung disease is the largest contributor to the increase in COPD; emphysema has also increased among women. The increase is more pronounced among older age groups, particularly women, and among black persons. Although research points to a true increase in COPD over time, a portion of this increase may be artificial and could be the result of changes in reporting practices.

Deaths from motor vehicle injuries and suicide

Deaths from motor vehicle injuries decreased over time for white men except the oldest old, but there was no common trend among older black men. Motor vehicle deaths increased for older white women, but remained the same for black women. The number of deaths from suicide and homicide has remained relatively small, although suicides increased by about 25 percent from 4,500 in 1981 to 5,700 in 1997. The rate of suicide is higher for elderly white men than for any other age group, including teenagers.

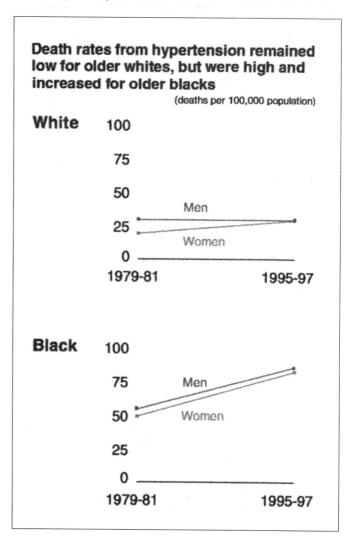

Death rates from hypertension remained low for older whites, but were high and increased for older blacks

(deaths per 100,000 population)

Hypertension mortality declined among white men, but drastically increased among older black men of all ages

When we examine the data by race and age, the differences are striking. Between 1979–81 and 1995–97, mortality from hypertension decreased among older white men (75–84 and 85+ years particularly), but dramatically increased among older black men. Similarly, although mortality from hypertension increased among older white women, the increase was much greater among older black women.

What are the possibilities for future progress?

Biomedical breakthroughs, technological advances, public health initiatives, and social changes may reduce mortality and increase the length of life

While most advances in life expectancy are the measured consequence of advances in social and economic well-being, biomedical science, and public health, scientific and medical breakthroughs have, at times, brought impressive gains over a short period. For example, in the late 19th and early 20th centuries, death from infectious diseases plummeted after the discovery of the germ theory of disease and the broad public health initiatives that followed. Could we be entering such a breakthrough period today? Could emerging medical technologies drawn from new scientific discoveries dramatically reduce or postpone deaths at older ages from such major killers as heart disease, cancer, and respiratory diseases and thus increase life expectancy? Or will the move toward a longer life expectancy be more deliberate?

Since mortality from any one cause of death may fluctuate from year to year, we averaged the death rate over 3 years and compared rates for 1979–81 to those for 1995–97 to obtain the percent change.

For heart disease, advances in prevention and treatment offer the hope that death rates will continue to decline. Adopting healthy lifestyles (such as reasonable physical activity, a balanced diet, and stable lean body weight) that are known to reduce risk factors for heart disease may not be magic bullets, but should reduce the onset of circulatory problems, particularly if all segments of the population accept them. Developments in treating heart disease, including aspirin therapies, antibiotics, and more effective emergency and surgical procedures, may well reduce or delay deaths from heart disease.

For cancer, a better understanding of the genetics of cancer (the goal of the Cancer Genome Anatomy Project) may lead eventually to new prevention strategies, targeted screening, or better treatment regimes.[13] Recently approved hormonal treatments for breast cancer may reduce or delay mortality,[14] and gene therapies offer hope that prostate cancer can be effectively treated.[15]

In general, we may expect real changes to continue to come through broader and slower avenues. As knowledge of disease etiology and medical technology progresses at a rapid pace, the multi-pronged approach of public health education, screening, and early intervention and treatment of disease could yield positive results. Because chronic diseases are the result of a long process, it takes time to reap the benefits of efforts made now.

But unbroken progress toward lengthening our life span is not inevitable. Elderly persons, like children, are particularly vulnerable to epidemics. A major epidemic such as influenza or disease-resistant strains of gastrointestinal infections could produce a sharp increase in mortality among the frail elderly and at least temporarily halt the progress in life expectancy. Public health surveillance of known and emerging infections is critical to the long-term health of our aging population.

Moreover, meaningful reductions in mortality, even at the older ages, require reductions in the racial, class, and rural/urban disparities that influence health and well-being.

Improved quality of life?

There is concern that extending life will merely increase the number of years in declining health. Many wonder, for example, whether an improvement in treating potentially fatal heart attacks or strokes will simply lengthen the survival of persons who are physically incapacitated, cognitively impaired, or emotionally distraught. This unhappy scenario, coupled with an unparalleled growth in the population of older persons (projected to reach 70 million by the year 2030), would place severe demands on our health care system as more people spend more years of life chronically disabled.

However, recent findings on levels of disability obtained from several large national surveys suggest that in addition to living longer lives, our noninstutionalized elderly may now be stronger, healthier, and better able to care for themselves.[16,17]

More about the multiple-cause-of-death system

Good public health policies depend on complete information. By considering not just the single underlying cause of death listed on the death certificate, but also the other accompanying health problems listed on the certificate—the comorbid conditions—we arrive at a much more complete picture of the true cause of death. These comorbid conditions may play as important a role in contributing to death as the underlying cause, especially among the elderly. Understanding their role is necessary if additional advances if life expectancy are to be made.

What happens when we switch to this approach? A number of diseases are more likely to be identified as comorbid conditions present at the time of death rather than as the underlying cause. Of these, the most important are:

Diabetes: In 1996 the multiple-cause death rate for diabetes was about 3.3 times higher than the underlying cause rate for older decedents. This means that while approximately 153,000 decedents had diabetes on their death certificate, only about 46,400 had the disease listed as the underlying cause. Many adults develop noninsulin-dependent diabetes mellitus (NIDDM) as they age; the disease can cause weight loss, vision deficits, increased susceptibility to infections, and coma leading to death if the diabetes is not controlled. According to death certificates, roughly 70 percent of all elderly diabetics who died also had heart disease, and in about half of those deaths, heart disease was listed as the underlying cause of death.

COPD: The conditions categorized as COPD (chronic obstructive pulmonary diseases) are more likely to be listed as contributing conditions than as the underlying cause of death; the multiple cause of death rate is over twice the underlying cause rate. In 1996, approximately 203,300 elderly decedents had a chronic respiratory disease listed on the death certificate. Nearly 40 percent of these decedents had heart disease or malignant neoplasms listed as the underlying cause of death.

Atherosclerosis: Atherosclerosis is now rarely mentioned as the underlying cause of death, although the disease is a precursor of circulatory diseases that are the major causes of death. Over 71,000 elderly persons had atherosclerosis listed as a cause of death, more than 4.5 times the number who had the disease listed as the underlying cause.

About the data

Information on mortality comes from death certificates collected by the States and forwarded to NCHS for processing and publishing. Geographic coverage has been complete since 1933, and the high quality and availability of the data (and variety of social, economic, and health factors) have made death rates the best barometer of the health and well-being of a population. However, all data collection systems have limitations, and some of these limitations must be considered when using information to estimate levels and trends of cause-specific mortality in older persons. Here are three examples.

First, changes in coding conventions, in the death certification format or in the training of those who fill out the death certificates may lead to discontinuities in trends in cause of death. For example, when attending physicians, coroners, and funeral home directors began using the new international coding conventions (ICD-9) in 1979,

the number of deaths attributed to septicemia jumped abruptly. The level eventually stabilized after these certifiers received instructions to record more specific causes of death as the underlying cause. As another example, in 1989, after the format was changed to include more space to encourage certifiers to provide more complete information, a study found that the mortality trend for some causes of death changed significantly.[18] Similarly, diabetes as a cause of death rapidly increased after instructions on the death certification included diabetes as an example. This may have reminded certifiers to include this disease on the death certificate.

Second, death certificates for the elderly are often incomplete. The completeness of the death certificate depends on the thoroughness of the certifier and of the amount of information available. Studies show that the quality of the decedent's medical history and thus the physicians' report of underlying cause of death diminishes with the age of the deceased. This may be because medical conditions of younger decedents are more acute and directly associated with death. The incompleteness for the elderly decedents may be a particular problem for those dying in long-term care institutions where medical certification is handled with less precision, less is known about the decedents' medical histories, and less diagnostic information is available from laboratory tests and autopsy results.[19]

Third, the age on the death certificate is often incorrect for older persons. Misreporting the age of decedents has been documented (both under- and over-reporting), particularly among black decedents, and reported that the errors were greater for women than for men.[20] This results in rates that are either too high or too low.

These factors need to be considered when using mortality data, which remain the most reliable and favored indicator of public health researchers.

Notes

1. Fries JF. Aging, natural death and the compression of morbidity. New Engl. J Med. 303: 130–5, 1980.
2. Fries JF. Strategies for reduction of morbidity. Am J Clin Nutr. 55: 1257S–62S, 1992.
3. McCormick J, Skrabanek P. Coronary heart disease is not preventable by population interventions. Lancet. ii: 839–41, 1988.
4. Rothenberg R, Lentzner HR, Parker RA. Population aging patterns: the expansion of mortality. J Gerontol. 46 (2): S66–70, 1991.
5. Manton KG, Stallard E, Corder L. Changes in morbidity and chronic disability in the U.S. elderly population: evidence from the 1982, 1984, and 1989 National Long Term Care Surveys. J Gerontol. 50B (4): S194–S204, 1995.
6. Manton KG, Vaupel JW. Survival after the age of 80 in the United States, Sweden, France, England and Japan. New Engl J Med. 333 (18): 1232–5, 1995.
7. Schneider EL, Brody JA. Aging, natural death and the compression of morbidity: another view. New Engl J Med. 309 (14): 854–6, 1983.
8. Hoyert DL. Mortality trends for Alzheimer's disease, 1979–91. National Center for Health Statistics. Vital Health. 20 (28), 1996.
9. Pinner RW, Teutsch SM, Simonsen L, Klug LA, Graber JM, Clarke MJ, Berkelman RL. Trends in infectious diseases mortality in the United States. J Am Med Assoc. 275 (3): 189–93, 1996.

10. CDC. Pneumonia and influenza death rates, United States, 1979–1994. MMWR Morb Mortal Wkly Rep. 44 (28): 535–7, July 21, 1995.

11. Marrie TJ. Pneumonia. Clin Geriatr Med. 8: 721–34, 1992.

12. Hoyert DL, Rosenberg H, MacDorman MF. Effect of changes in death certificate format on cause-specific mortality trends, United States, 1979–92. Office for National Statistics. Studies on Medical and Population Subjects. 64: 47–58, 2000.

13. Sandhu JS, Keating A, Hozumi N. Human gene therapy. Crit Rev Biotechnol. 17 (4): 307–326, 1997.

14. Thurlimann B. Hormonal treatment of breast cancer: new developments. Oncology. 55 (6): 501–507, 1998.

15. Brinkmann U, Vasmatzis G, Lee B, Yerushalmi N, Essand M, Pastan I. PAGE-1 and X chromosome-linked GAGE-like gene that is expressed in normal and neoplastic prostate, testis, and uterus. Proc Natl Acad Sci USA. 95 (18): 10757–62, 1998.

16. Manton KG, Corder L, Stallard E. Chronic disability trends in elderly United States populations: 1982–1994. Proc Natl Acad Sci. 94: 2593–2598, 1997.

17. Freedman VA, Martin LG. Understanding trends in functional limitations among older Americans. Am J Public Health, 88: 1457–1462, 1998.

18. Hoyert DL, Rosenberg H, MacDorman MF. Effect of changes in death certificate format on cause-specific mortality trends. United States, 1979–82. Office for National Statistics. Studies on Medical and Population Subjects. 64: 47–58, 2000.

19. Feinlieb MF, ed. Proceedings of 1988 International Symposium on data on aging. National Center for Health Statistics. Vital Health Stat. 5 (6), 1991.

20. Elo IT, Preston SH. Estimating African-American mortality from inaccurate data. Demography. 31: 427–58, 1994.

From *Aging Trends*, No.1, March 2001, pp. 1-9. Published by the Centers for Disease Control and Prevention.

UNIT 7

Living Environment in Later Life

Unit Selections

Key Points to Consider

- How does Bill Thomas propose changing the nursing home so that people don't think of it as just a place where people go to die?

- What are the advantages to old persons that move into continuing care communities?

- What are the things family members should investigate and consider before placing a loved one in an assisted living facility?

- In the city of Laguna Woods, how did the older people unite to protect their interests?

Student Website

www.mhcls.com/online

Internet References

Further information regarding these websites may be found in this book's preface or online.

American Association of Homes and Services for the Aging
http://www.aahsa.org

Center for Demographic Studies
http://cds.duke.edu

Guide to Retirement Living Online
http://www.retirement-living.com

The United States Department of Housing and Urban Development
http://www.hud.gov

Unit 4 noted that old age is often a period of shrinking life space. This concept is crucial to an understanding of the living environments of older Americans. When older people retire, they may find that they travel less frequently and over shorter distances because they no longer work and most neighborhoods have stores, gas stations, and churches in close proximity. As the retirement years roll by, older people may feel less in control of their environments due to a decline in their hearing and vision as well as other health problems. As the aging process continues, the elderly are likely to restrict their mobility to the areas where they feel most secure. This usually means that an increasing amount of time is spent at home. Estimates show that individuals age 65 and over spend 80 to 90 percent of their lives in their home environments. Of all the other age groups, only small children are as house- and neighborhood-bound.

The house, neighborhood, and community environments are, therefore, more crucial to the elderly than to any other adult age group. The interaction with others that they experience within their homes and neighborhoods can be either stimulating or foreboding, pleasant or threatening. Across the country, older Americans find themselves living in a variety of circumstances, ranging from desirable to undesirable.

Approximately 70 percent of the elderly live in a family setting, usually a husband-wife household; 20 percent live alone or with nonrelatives; and the remaining number live in institutions such as nursing homes. Although only about 5 percent of the elderly will be living in nursing homes at any one time, 25 percent of people 65 and over will spend some time in a nursing home setting. The longer one lives, the more likely he or she is to end up in a total-care institution. Because most older Americans would prefer to live independently in their own homes for as long as possible, their relocation—to other houses, apartments, or nursing homes—is often accompanied by a considerable amount of trauma and unrest. Because the aged tend to be less mobile and more neighborhood-bound than any other age group makes their living environment most crucial to their sense of well-being.

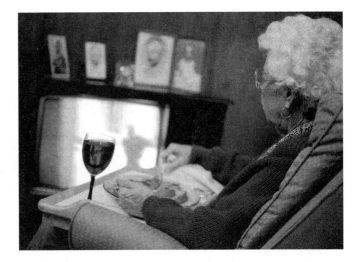

Articles in this section focus on some of the alternatives available to the aged: from family care to assisted living to nursing homes.

In "(Not) the Same Old Story," Chuck Salter reviews recommendations from gerontologist Bill Thomas for changing nursing homes to make them livable and enjoyable to the residents. In "A Home for the Rest of Your Life," Jane Bennett Clark describes continuing care communities where you may initially move into your own apartment, later move into an assisted living area, and, if necessary, ultimately move into a nursing home. Consumer Reports in the article "Assisted Living: How much assistance can you really count on?" points out many of the past problems people have encountered living in assisted living facilities and makes suggestions on how to choose the best facility for yourself or your loved ones.

In "The City of Laguna Woods: A Case of Senior Power in Local Politics," the authors describe how the incorporation of the senior living facilities in Orange County, California, allowed the residents to block the building of a nearby airport.

THE BIG **FIX**

(not)
the same old story

Eden Alternative is a change-minded organization determined to save a critically ill patient: long-term care for the elderly. The nursing-home industry should be about living, argues founder Bill Thomas, not about dying. Here's his prescription—and lessons for changing any industry.

By Chuck Salter

In 1999, after writing a book about improving long-term care for the elderly, Bill Thomas did what authors do: He hit the road for a promotional tour. He appeared on radio and television. He also met with public officials, offering his perspective as a gerontologist—a doctor who specializes in treating the elderly—on what was wrong with nursing homes: They were utterly devoid of hope, love, humor, meaning—the very stuff of life. He gave lectures on the changes he had in mind, which included adding pets, plants, and children to nursing-home life. But at each stop, he also demonstrated why this is no ordinary book and this was no ordinary tour—and why he is certainly no ordinary doctor.

> "Does anyone **want** to leave his home and go live in a nursing home? That's why we're turning the industry upside down."

Thomas, now 42, didn't write a prosaic account of the principles behind Eden Alternative, the nonprofit organization that he and his wife, Jude, operate out of their farm in Sherburne, New York. Instead, he told a story, a fantastic tale interweaving fact and fiction. *Learning from Hannah: Secrets for a Life Worth Living* (VanderWyk & Burnham, 1999) is a novel that doesn't call itself a novel. It begins with Thomas and his wife completing a book about the medical aspects of aging and then taking a much-needed vacation. While sailing south from San Juan toward the island of Montserrat, they get caught in a storm that leaves them shipwrecked. For nearly a year, they live in a mysterious place called Kallimos, where they learn the ways of a society in which the elderly play a vibrant role in the community. Instead of living apart from younger generations, the oldest inhabitants are embraced by them. The wisdom and experience of the elderly are valued as a resource. When Thomas and wife eventually return home, the lessons from Hannah, the old woman who mentored them, become the inspiration and foundation for Eden Alternative.

It wasn't enough for Thomas to communicate his vision for better long-term care through an imaginative book. He also developed a one-man show based on the tale. In the summer of 1999, the Harvard-educated doctor turned novelist turned actor launched the Eden Across America Tour, traveling by private bus to 27 cities in 31 days with his wife, their five children, and his parents. It's not hard to imagine Thomas on stage; he's alternately funny, exuberant, and sincere, offering glimpses of a natural theatricality. After a performance at a medical school in the Midwest, he wrote in his online journal, "I had the strange sense that the ghosts of medical professors past were looking on us and clucking their tongues. I didn't care."

For Thomas, the Eden Across America Tour never ended. It can't. Not if he's going to fix long-term care in this country. For all practical purposes, he says, the industry is broken. "Does anyone want to leave his home and go live in a nursing home?" he asks. "Does anyone want to put a parent, spouse, or loved one there? That's why we're turning the industry upside down."

It's an audacious mission and a truly big fix—one that requires more than just fresh ideas. It demands an unorthodox approach to mobilizing and motivating a wide range of forces, many of which have little incentive to change. "You need to have people go a little nuts about what you want to do," Thomas says. On its own, the industry isn't going to do an about-face and overhaul its core ideas. And individual nursing homes are often too overwhelmed by the day-to-day demands of caring for residents in a heavily regulated field to try anything new. Hoping to prod people into going a little nuts about radical reform, Thomas appeals to their imaginations and their hearts. Hence the book, the tour, and the play. "A lot of innovators don't focus enough on the story that they're telling," he says. "But the story is the only thing that ever gets people to change. It captures your passion and conviction and inspires others to feel the same way."

"Some homes think that **Eden** and the operation of the facility are two separate things. But Eden is all over. It affects everything you do."

It's no accident that Eden Alternative evokes another story: that of the Garden of Eden. A garden is the central metaphor behind Thomas's vision. "Human beings aren't meant to live in institutions," he says, "but that's what most nursing homes are: big, impersonal, cold institutions that don't treat people the way they want to be treated. People are meant to live in a garden, a place where they can grow and thrive as human beings."

So far, about 300 nursing homes in the United States (as well as a handful in Europe and Australia) have been "Edenized." Which is to say that these institutions have been deinstitutionalized and turned into warm, nurturing human habitats. The results have proven not only good for residents but also good for business. Impressed by the improved quality of care, residents' health, and staff retention, several states have begun offering Eden grants—using the fines that more backward-looking facilities pay for violating regulations.

Typically, an Eden nursing home is divided into neighborhoods, with a staff that knows the residents personally—their background and interests as well as their medications. There's all sorts of activity: children playing, dogs and cats visiting rooms, birds chirping. The institution becomes a close-knit community teeming with life.

The transformation, however, is often arduous. Creating an Eden home involves major organizational and cultural change, because the facility has to think differently about care, priorities, and old habits. For instance, the residents have more input into how the facility operates, as do the staff members who work closest with them—a shift that often proves difficult for traditional-minded administrators.

"Caring for the elderly is not simply about health care or medicine or technology… It's about creating the right environment and **caring** relationships that sustain an older adult in his last years." says Bill Thomas

"Out of all the people we've talked to about creating Eden homes, no one says, 'This is a horrible idea,'" says Jude Thomas, who conducts Eden workshops with her husband. "But some people think that all they have to do is bring in a dog, and everything will be better. It won't be. This is an entirely different philosophy. It's a total change."

Voices in the Garden (Part I) *Jane Lough, administrator, Toomsboro Nursing Center, Toomsboro, Georgia: "This one lady, Mrs. Miller, dressed nicely every day and got her hair done once a week for the first year and a half she was here. Then she went into the hospital for pneumonia, and when she came back, she wouldn't get out of bed. She gave up. So I got her a blue parakeet named Mercy, and we put the cage on an IV pole next to her bed. She would feed it crackers and sing to it. After three or four months, she got up, got her hair done, and started going everywhere with Mercy. She'd tell people she loved that bird."*

MISSION: OVERCOMING THE THREE PLAGUES

After graduating from Harvard Medical School, Bill Thomas had his heart set on the emergency room. He liked the action and the adrenaline rush. But in 1991, after completing his residency in family medicine at the University of Rochester, he tried something different: becoming the physician at Chase Memorial Nursing Home in New Berlin, New York. He discovered that he enjoyed working with the elderly, getting to know them, hearing their stories. He also discovered that nursing homes were seriously flawed—even the best-performing facilities. At Chase, the equipment was up-to-date, the staff was dedicated, and the inspection record was spotless. Yet the residents were

how does your garden grow?

Through Eden Alternative, Bill Thomas is making a difference in long-term care for the elderly. He's turning institutions into places where residents actually enjoy living. Here's how he's fixing things.

Have a good story to tell. Stories help people understand your ideas. Through your passion, stories inspire others to get on board and make your vision a reality. "You need a mythic, heroic story that people will respond to," Thomas says. "Ours is about creating gardens for our elders where they can thrive. That's something that people want for their mothers and fathers."

Watch your language. Eden has a vocabulary all its own, most of which grew (pun intended) out of its defining metaphor of cultivating gardens. Eden practitioners know what they mean by "warming the soil" and "experiencing a frost." It may sound goofy, but it's a way of changing the conversation within an organization.

Don't mistake tokens for real change. The most visible component of Eden is the animals that reside in nursing homes. But "fur and feathers," says Thomas, aren't a shortcut to transformation. Unless you change the culture and philosophy, the facility won't be different. It will still be an institution—but with pets. Big deal.

Make innovation a group activity. Thomas doesn't claim to have all the answers for improving nursing homes. The Eden program gives a framework and some ideas, but individual facilities decide which changes are best to make. Administrators share ideas through Eden's Web site and at get-togethers. Thomas has the same "open source" philosophy about the Greenhouse Project, which involves building homes for small groups of elders. He's sharing his ideas online and letting others build on them. "You can't do it alone," he says.

Expect setbacks. Failure is an inevitable part of the change process. So you'd better be prepared for it, or you won't be able to bounce back. Understand that people are going to get scared and revert back to doing things the old way. Forgive them and move forward—and expect it to happen again. "Frost always comes," says Thomas. "We've never been wrong on that one."

miserable. "What appalled me was how lonely and bored they were," Thomas says. "It was painfully obvious to me that they were dying in front of my eyes."

He concluded that nursing-home residents suffer from three plagues: loneliness, helplessness, and boredom. They feel lonely because they've been uprooted from their family, friends, and even their pets. They feel helpless because they've lost control of their lives; for the most part, they eat, sleep, get dressed, and bathe according to the institution's schedule. Finally, they feel bored because the few activities that are available to them, such as watching television, aren't meaningful or fulfilling. "Care for the elderly is not simply about health care or medicine or technology," Thomas says. "It's about creating the right environment and caring relationships that sustain an older adult in his last years."

While working at Chase, Thomas received a $200,000 grant to improve life for the facility's residents. The experiment gave rise to Eden Alternative. Bringing animals into nursing homes was not a new idea, but in the past, they were usually brought in for visits. They didn't live on the premises, as Thomas prefers. That way, the animals become companions, and the residents grow attached to them. As one of the 10 Eden principles says, "Loving companionship is the antidote to loneliness."

If the elders—Thomas finds the term more dignified—are able, they lend a hand in grooming or feeding the animals, watering plants, or reading with children. These activities not only allow residents to engage in everyday physical therapy, but they also satisfy another fundamental human need, one that often gets neglected: giving care, as opposed to only receiving it.

At Eden facilities, residents and staff are partners. Whenever possible, the two groups work together, voting on what type of pet to add or what type of decorations to put up. Staff members understand that what they call the workplace is a far more intimate and personal place to residents: It's home. And that understanding shapes decisions. Eden removes hierarchical or autocratic management. Like the residents, the certified nurse assistants, who make up the bulk of the staff, have more control over their schedules and help make decisions about how to divvy up work. "What you find is that as the managers do to the staff, the staff does to the elders," says Thomas. "So if you treat the staff well, the elders will benefit."

That's the case in the Toomsboro Nursing Center, a 62-bed facility in rural Georgia. Since adopting the Eden model, the staff has become more responsive and more unified, and the care has become more compassionate and individualized, says Jane Lough, an administrator at the center. Instead of giving orders, Lough tells the certified nurse assistants, "You know this resident. Tell me what you think she needs." By working in teams—the Conquerers, Earth Angels, Outrageous Girlfriends, and Untouchables—employees began seeing beyond their roles as cook, laundry aide, nurse, and housekeeper. They realized that every staff member provides care in one way or another. As the stickers that they wear declare, "I'm a world-maker." "That's one of Dr. Thomas's terms," says Lough. "In a nursing home, very little of the outside world comes in, except for the staff. They are the residents' world, and they have the opportunity to make it a special place."

Eden does not reverse the aging process, of course, but studies, including one done by the Texas Long Term Care Institute in San Marcos, Texas, indicate that the residents' overall health does improve: They had fewer infections and required less medication. Meanwhile, the staff absenteeism went down and retention went up—a significant improvement in an industry that is notorious for high turnover.

"Relationships are the foundation of good health care," Thomas says. "This is nothing new. But it's not something that the industry has made a priority." In fact, some institutions actively discourage relationships between staff and residents. "When I started out, I was told, 'You don't share yourself with residents, because it hurts too much when they die,'" says Lough. "That's definitely not the attitude here."

Voices in the Garden (Part II) *Kathleen Perra, director of nursing, St. Luke's Home, New Hartford, New York: "Every day last summer, we had school-age day care here. There were kids screaming down the hall, cats jumping on tables. It was bedlam, but it was great. You want those unpredictable things happening for the residents. Of course, health-care workers favor predictability. We work around schedules. I'd say the biggest change with the Eden program is for the staff."*

METHOD: WARMTH, SUCTION, FROST

Nursing homes that are designed like gardens provide an apt metaphor for Bill Thomas's program, because, like a garden, Eden Alternative doesn't occur naturally. It requires preparation, hard work, and continuous scrutiny as it evolves. Otherwise, if the changes are taken for granted or neglected, Eden eventually shrivels up and dies.

Since founding their organization, Bill and Jude Thomas have become change experts out of necessity. Merely tweaking facilities wasn't effective. Creating an Eden involves a complete transformation. "Some homes think that Eden and the operation of the facility are two separate things," he says. "But Eden is all over. It affects everything you do."

> Says director of nursing Kathleen Perra: "Every day last summer, we had school-age day care here. There were kids screaming down the hall, cats jumping on tables. It was **bedlam**, but it was great"

The duration and success of the change process depends on what Bill Thomas calls the "warmth" of the organization. A warm culture is open to change, because employees have trust and generosity for one another, whereas a cold culture is characterized by pessimism and cynicism. After conducting a survey to determine an organization's temperature, the Thomases or one of 5,000 Eden associates nationwide begin "warming the soil." In some cases, managers hold a potluck dinner at someone's house, where they can't discuss work. Employees also perform good deeds, or mitzvahs, for their colleagues and the residents without expecting anything in return. "You open people's minds by opening their hearts," Thomas says.

Before virtually every step—before adding pets, before switching to self-scheduling—the staff votes. If the outcome isn't unanimous, the group continues the education process. "You can't force change on anybody," says Thomas. "Consensus is the only way. You have to get the entire staff to see the

advantages for themselves and become excited about what you're going to do. We call it creating 'suction.'"

Thomas also expects setbacks, or "frost," as he puts it. It's a natural part of change. "I tell the leaders to expect that what they're changing will be smashed to bits, and when that happens, they have to be ready to pick up the pieces and move forward," says Thomas. "People are going to get scared. They're going to make mistakes." Every year, about 5% of Eden homes drop the program. But Thomas doesn't give up hope for them. He prefers to think that they're experiencing a long frost.

Voices in the Garden (Part III) *Ron Rothstein, president and COO, Levindale Hebrew Geriatric Center and Hospital, Baltimore, Maryland: "You don't cure the three plagues overnight. Some of our residents have been here a while, and they've become depressed. It takes time to bring out the best in them. I'm a type A personality—a 'gotta get it done today' type. But culture change is slow. And subtle. You don't necessarily see the relationships between people every day."*

MOMENTUM: PROGRESSIVES VS. STALWARTS

Eden Alternative's headquarters isn't located in an actual garden. But almost. It's on a lush farm in the rolling hills of upstate New York, 60 miles southeast of Syracuse. On 220 acres that had been abandoned for 50 years, Bill and Jude Thomas brought Summer Hill Farm to life, building a house, barn, retreat center, and 14-room lodge. It's here that you fully appreciate how much of a Renaissance man Thomas is. In the fields behind his house, he uses draft horses to pull the machinery that cuts and rakes the hay. Come wintertime, he takes the family on a horse-drawn-carriage ride into the snowy woods to tap maple sap in order to produce Summer Hill Syrup.

In a very real sense, Summer Hill is the Thomases' personal Eden, a home with dogs and children and individuals who need long-term medical care. Hannah and Haleigh Thomas, 5 and 7, suffer from a rare neurological disorder that prevents them from being able to see, speak, and walk. During a break in the Eden training, Jude checks on them and their nurse and dotes on the dark-haired girls in the double stroller. "When people ask if the Eden program can make a difference in someone who's in a nursing home, I tell them that it can, because I see how Hannah and Haleigh respond to loving care," says Jude. "I honestly believe they're alive because of Eden."

When her husband isn't at Summer Hill, he's spreading the word to nursing-home administrators, regulators, insurance companies, policy makers, and industry associations. He gives about 40 talks a year. Thomas is an optimist—"It can be different," his business card says—but he's also a realist. He knows that he can't fix the country's nursing homes on his own. He relies on Eden associates to promote the program, share success stories, and conduct training sessions in their communities.

Part of changing an industry is about choosing wisely where to focus your energy. In long-term care, as in any field, the stalwarts vastly outnumber the progressives. In general, Thomas says, the progressives have ideas and enthusiasm but lack real authority or management skills, and the stalwarts have authority and experience but resist changes in the status quo. Thomas doesn't turn down invitations to address the latter, but he doesn't court them either. "The reason I'm not racing to Edenize 17,000 nursing homes across the country is because I know that I'll never win over the stalwarts," he says. "I'm focusing on the progressives, because they're interested in changing things."

Ultimately, Eden Alternative is a repair for a broken industry. The replacement, says Thomas, is his Greenhouse Project. It involves houses that are built for small groups of elders and that have a dedicated staff. They are actual homes, instead of an institution that calls itself a home. St. Luke's Home, where Thomas used to be the medical director, expects to break ground on the first greenhouses within the next couple of years.

After that, he says, the next logical stage is an Eden Village, where the greenhouses and the elders are part of a larger community.

But why stop there? he wonders. Why not apply these principles to other institutions, such as schools and prisons? Thomas jokes about starting a group called "Institutions Anonymous." Maybe he's only half joking. "Don't get me started," he says.

Chuck Salter (csalter@fastcompany.com) is a FAST COMPANY senior writer based in Baltimore. Learn more about **Eden Alternative** on the Web (www.edenalt.com), or contact **Bill Thomas** by email (thomaswh@edenalt.com).

A **HOME**
for the rest of your life

Continuing-care communities promise independence now and all the help you need later on.

Jane Bennett Clark

FOUR DAYS. That's how long Lucy and Dick Thomson had to make the decision of a lifetime: Stay in Saginaw, Mich., where they had met before World War II, or pull up stakes and move to a cottage that they had never seen in a new development that was swimming in mud. The couple had placed a small deposit on a cottage at the unfinished site in Lake Forest, Ill., at the urging of their son, who lives nearby. But they were taken aback when the call came that the cottage was available. The message: Grab it now or lose your place in line. That was six years ago.

Today, the Thomsons smile at the memory as they show off their two-bedroom cottage, a sunny space decorated in pale green, yellow and cream. The couple, both 84, enjoy good health and a full calendar at Lake Forest Place, a continuing-care retirement community run by the Presbyterian Homes, in Evanston, Ill. Should their health fail, they are assured of getting help, either in their home or elsewhere on campus. Says Lucy, "it was the best decision we've made in our whole life."

Lake Forest Place is one of 2,100 continuing-care communities across the country that offer independent living, in either cottages or apartments, along with various levels of care. Unlike assisted-living facilities, which can ask you to leave when your money runs out or you need skilled nursing, these communities promise to keep you for life, usually in exchange for an upfront six-figure deposit and monthly fees. Most offer amenities such as fitness clubs, restaurant-style meals and a busy social schedule. Says Linda Fodrini-Johnson, a geriatric-care manager with an office in San Francisco, "It's a nice choice for the healthy senior who wants to be socially engaged."

Continuing-care communities also present a conundrum: To qualify, you must be reasonably healthy—healthy enough that you could still stay in your own home. In fact, most retirees remain in their homes or go directly to assisted living at about age 80 or older. Those who do enter a life-care community typically wait until they are at least 75.

But moving to the right place at the right time can prolong your vitality, says Karen Love, founder of the Consumer Consortium on Assisted Living. The communities are "wonderful environments because they're supportive," she says. "Typically, the food is excellent. There's transportation. If I want a buddy to go shopping with, there are tons of people to pick from." You could actually live longer and healthier in such settings, says Larry Minnix, president of the American Association of Homes and Services for the Aging. "They give the services that people need when they need them, in a place they can call home," Minnix says.

The Thomsons had no immediate plans to leave Saginaw six years ago, but they did have compelling reasons to move someday. All four of their parents had ended their days in grim nursing homes, and the couple's four children had already moved away. "We were wondering what our parents were going to do," says Richard Jr., known as Tom. When Lake Forest Place sprang up near his home outside of Chicago, the family saw an opening. Says Dick, a pilot who parachuted out of his aircraft after it was hit over Hungary during World War II, "It was time to hit the silk."

GO IN WITH YOUR EYES OPEN

IT'S EASY TO SEE why the Thomsons are pleased with their decision. The sea of mud is long gone, and their cottage, which backs to a beautifully landscaped area, boasts a full kitchen, a laundry room and a garage. In the Town Center, the community's main building across the road, the paneling, arched windows and overstuffed chairs easily compete with the ambiance of any country club. Residents can work out in the fitness club or take a dip in one of the community's several pools.

But Dick steers clear of the parts of the complex that offer nursing care or help with eating and dressing. "When it comes to assisted living, I'm in denial," he admits. And he's not alone, says Laurie Duncan, a CPA who owns Choices for Aging, a geriatric-care management company in Arlington, Va. "People like to look at the apartments, the dining facilities—but when you suggest a visit to the health facilities, they say, 'No thanks.'"

As understandable as the ostrich approach might be, anyone looking to secure a comfortable future should "make sure they tour every bit of a community, including the assisted-living and nursing-home areas," says Nicole Muller of Brecht Associates, a firm that specializes in senior housing. Odors, poor housekeeping or residents who look parked are obvious red flags. "The atmosphere should feel comfortable to the person looking at it, not scary."

Lake Forest Place can rightly boast of its caregiving: It's accredited by the Commission on Accreditation of Rehabilitation Facilities. (To find out if a facility has earned the commission's okay, go to www.carf.org.) State inspection reports, required for assisted-living and nursing-home units, provide another glimpse into quality control—if you can decipher them. Geriatric-care managers offer insight into such reports, as well as the skinny on local retirement communities. To find one in your area, call the National Association of Professional Geriatric Care Managers, at 520-881-8008, or go to www.caremanager.org.

Whatever the measuring stick, facilities that come up short, says Duncan, usually share the same problem: poor staffing. "You can have a beautiful lobby, but if you don't have the staff, you're not going to give good care," she says. "If you're paying minimum wage and don't have good training—that's where the rubber meets the road."

The bottom line is that good caregiving requires plenty of willing arms, Duncan says. "In the nursing units, if you have one aide for every nine residents, each resident is getting much less than one hour of one-on-one care during a shift. If one aide is out, then are residents going to get showered or moved? On the assisted-living end, people who need help getting in and out of bed or a chair won't get help if there's only one aide for 15 residents."

Assuming the care and staff are top-notch, you'll need to explore how much help can be brought into your apartment before the community moves you from one level to another, especially when dementia is involved. Grouping cognitively impaired residents isn't necessarily bad, says Gail Kohn, of Linking Partners, a long-term-care consulting firm. But be sure to ask whether and how it is done.

Some states dictate the circumstances in which you will be moved from an assisted-living to a nursing unit; in others, the managers of the community—preferably with the input of family members—make the call. Either way, ask how many nursing beds have been set aside for residents, says Chris Cooper, a registered financial adviser in Toledo who specializes in geriatrics. In a large community, "if there are only 12 beds, they could be full when you need them."

The path between independent living and the nursing unit doesn't have to be one-way. At Lake Forest Place, for instance, stroke victims and surgery patients can practice getting in and out of a full-scale car or climb stairs in the rehab center, giving them a leg up on recovery. The Erickson Retirement Communities, based in Baltimore, go a step further: They have doctors and other health-care providers on their campuses. "That's a big innovation," Minnix says.

A NEW BEGINNING

JUST HOW DO two people trade the house where they have lived for 45 years—and the town where they met, married and raised four kids—for a community of total strangers? Piece of cake, says Lucy Thomson. "We've met tons of people. We invite them over for a drink, then go to the town center for dinner. When you go, you have to mingle and it's boy-girl-boy-girl. Everyone has been reading something different. You exchange ideas."

Her son Tom, who heads the microbiology laboratory at Evanston Northwestern Health Care, happily concurs. "We thought it would be hard for our parents to pull up roots from the town where our family had been for generations, but it just worked," he says. "In Saginaw, they knew everyone and had done everything. This has been a social rebirth."

The Thomsons connected in their new setting in part because the residents of life-care communities tend to be likeminded, says Fodrini-Johnson. "These are bright people who are used to doing the research and finding the answers to complex problems." Dick, who spent his career manufacturing automotive parts, agrees with that assessment. "The whole campus is composed of top professionals."

Still, each community has its own flavor. For instance, the Kendal Communities—most of whose small campuses are located near liberal-arts colleges—attract residents who want to take classes or participate in campus functions. The Erickson communities draw members who like a wide range of activities. Religion, politics and socioeconomic status each play a role in the matchmaking process, says Kohn.

But little things like dining-room seating arrangements can be an important indication of how thoughtfully a community brings you into the mix. At the Erickson communities, for instance, residents are led to tables by a hostess rather than left to hunt for a seat. "You never sit alone," says Trudy Couch, who lives in Riderwood Village, in Silver Spring, Md. Couch spent several nights in the guest suites at Riderwood to get a feel for the place before moving in. "I noticed how friendly the staff members were."

Although the Thomsons first visited Lake Forest Place as a mudhole, any uncertainty about their move has vanished. Lucy attends yoga class or walks the trail beyond her house in the morning. Dick has taken a spot on the finance committee. They meet friends for dinner in the dining room three or four times a week. Says Lucy, "We've never been happier."

Assisted living

How much assistance can you really count on?

Since they started to dot the U.S. landscape in the early 1980s, assisted-living facilities have become the best hope of America's seniors for avoiding confinement in a nursing home. Instead of a hospital environment, assisted living promised private apartments and communal dining in hotel-like settings, and some help with daily needs such as dressing and bathing.

In CR's three-month investigation, we found that assisted living now presents quite a different picture. Settings vary dramatically. Among the dozen facilities we visited, there are high-rise apartment buildings, down-at-the-heels mansions, and single-family houses. They are run by large public companies, states, families, small businesses, and nonprofits.

Each one has a different notion of how much or what kind of assistance assisted living should provide. Some facilities offer an apartment, meals, and some activities. Others provide several levels of help, each at a higher price. Some facilities require residents to be ambulatory; others have units for people with Alzheimer's disease.

Seniors and their families, anxious to avoid nursing homes, have come to look upon assisted living as the preferred placed to go when health starts failing. Assisted-living operators, out of compassion or a need to fill beds, accept and keep residents even if their condition has worsened.

As a result, many of the nearly 1 million people now in assisted-living facilities are more likely to be frail and sick

CR Quick Take

In our three-month investigation of assisted living, we visited a dozen sites and talked to experts as well as residents and their families. We found that picking an appropriate assisted-living facility can be extremely difficult because:

- Most facilities are operated by small private companies that don't provide information—including data on their financial strength—needed to make a decision.
- Neither size, décor, nor amenities necessarily determines the quality of care or assistance available at a facility.
- There is no standard for care that should be provided and no clear guideline to indicate who belongs in assisted living and who doesn't.
- The nearly 1 million people who now live in assisted-living residences have become frailer, raising concerns about their safety and care.
- States regulate assisted living but provide little oversight or protection for residents.

than independent. And that has created a troubling mismatch between the care a resident needs and the care a facility and its staff can give.

The result can be neglect or poor care for residents. Example: A draft report of a 2004 national survey conducted by the

National Academy for State Health Policy found that 28 states reported that problems with medication occurred frequently or very often.

More critically, no one seems to be watching very closely. While the federal government protects nursing-home residents—albeit not always effectively—with rigid regulations and state-run inspections about once a year, states monitor assisted living with a hodgepodge of licensing, inspection, and staff-training standards of varying strictness.

Finding a good, safe, and affordable facility has thus become problematic for seniors and their families. There's a lot to consider: the setting, the cost, the array of services, the condition of the other residents, the solvency of the company, not to mention the rights of residents to stay, or the necessity for them to go, if their condition deteriorates.

Getting information to make your choice can be difficult. Posing as adult children from out of state whose parent was considering assisted living, we contacted at least three locations for each of the 10 largest assisted-living chains in the country. We asked each to send us all the information we'd need to decide on the facility, including the services it provides, pricing structures for different levels of care, and its contract. None gave us everything we requested. Mostly we received glossy brochures showing happy, peppy seniors. (See Big 10 providers.)

THE PLAYERS

Assisted living is based on a Scandinavian model of "social" care, where residents live in private units within a larger community, much different from nursing homes whose patients need constant medical care. In the late 1980s, social-care facilities in the U.S. began referring to themselves as assisted living.

Marriott and Hyatt jumped into the business in the late 80s, seeing assisted living as a natural extension of their lodging business. Marriott built more than a hundred 70- to 90-unit facilities, but "they couldn't fill them up," says Steve Monroe, editor of The SeniorCare Investor, which tracks the mergers, acquisitions and financing of senior-care companies. Marriott sold most of its interest to Sunrise Senior Living in 2003. Hyatt currently runs 17 luxury assisted-living residences and has 3 more under development.

In the U.S. there are two large publicly traded chains: Sunrise, with 364 facilities for 43,000 seniors in the U.S., the U.K., Canada, and Germany; and Emeritus Assisted Living, which can house 18,400 residents at 182 locations in 34 states. Most other providers, including the next three largest—Alterra Healthcare, Atria Senior Living, and Merrill Gardens—are private companies. Smaller companies tend to be regional chains.

The assisted-living business boomed in the mid-1990s, and some 15 companies went public. But by 2000, the intense overbuilding caught many providers short on capital. Several declared bankruptcy. The industry has since settled down, with mergers more common than bankruptcies. But independent facilities do go bust, and residents stand to lose any deposits or prepayments. At the very least, they have to find a new place to live.

Assessing the financial strength of an assisted-living company is anything but easy, however. Information on Sunrise and Emeritus, as well as Assisted Living Concepts and Manor Care, all public companies, is available to consumers on company Web sites. But most residents live in units operated by small private companies that are not likely to release financial data.

THE SETTINGS

Assisted living now offers a wide choice of settings and price levels. Typical of full-service facilities is Crosby Commons in Shelton, Conn., a 67-unit brick facility run by United Methodist Homes. It provides an on-site beauty shop, a gift and toiletry store, a fitness center, and a gourmet menu, which recently featured herb-rubbed leg of lamb and fish Florentine. (Studios and one-bedrooms range from $2,780 to $3,570.)

Other facilities are not as elaborate. Avalon in Falls Church, Va., houses a maximum of 8 people, all with dementia, in individual rooms ($105 a day) and has live-in attendants. The Washington Elms in Bennington, Vt., a towering gray Victorian, houses 24, most of whom share dormitory-like bedrooms with 2 or 3 roommates for $80 a day. Some of the floors, walls, and porches were dilapidated, though Melissa Greason, the owner, says, "We are doing major repair work."

Neither the size, décor, nor amenities determines the quality of care. We found residents at the Avalon, which has no pool or other amenities, happily playing poker in the living room. But at the glossy Renaissance Gardens in Springfield, Va., which has pleasant grounds, a fitness center, and a swimming pool, we saw two residents in wheelchairs complaining about long waits to get a caregiver's attention, and a staff member who ignored a resident who repeatedly asked to enter an enclosed flower garden.

Mel Tansill, senior director of public affairs for Erickson Health, the company that owns Renaissance Gardens, told us in an e-mail that "residents deemed safe are not required to be accompanied while enjoying the courtyard." Moreover, he added, one of the residents in a wheelchair was waiting for a rehabilitation appointment that had been rescheduled from the morning. He said that past surveys show that residents never wait more than 10 minutes. At Washington Elms in Vermont, most of the residents sat slumped in darkened rooms or in front of a television set. Greason, the owner, says that the facility has no activities director, but "we have bingo, church groups come in, and we do crafts around the holidays."

MORE HELP FOR MORE MONEY

Just because the facility calls itself assisted living doesn't mean that residents get as much help as they want—at least not without paying for it. Most facilities offer a basic service plan. Although that plan varies from one facility to another, it typically provides a 24-hour staff, weekly light housekeeping and laundry services, two to three meals a day, social activities such as bingo and movies, and help with some of the activities of daily living (ADLs), for example, bathing, dressing, and going to the bathroom. A MetLife survey showed that the average monthly basic rate ranged from $1,340 a month in Miami to $4,327 in Stamford, Conn., in 2003.

how to choose

TWELVE STEPS TO FINDING THE RIGHT PLACE

Many consumers start the difficult search for an assisted-living facility in the midst of a crisis—when a spouse or parent has been injured in a fall, for example. You should start learning about assisted living and other services when you notice a senior showing some signs of decline, recommends Karen Love, founder and chairwoman of the Consumer Consortium for Assisted Living, an advocacy group in Falls Church, Va. Deciding early can be crucial because better residences often have long waiting lists. According to assisted-care experts, regulators, and residents' children, here are the steps you should take.

1. Create a list of possibles. To find facilities, contact the local Area Agency on Aging office. The national Eldercare Locator can lead you to yours (800-677-1116, or www.eldercare.gov). Try for a list of seven to eight facilities of varying size.

2. Call your state's long-term-care ombudsman. Ask whether there have been complaints about facilities on your list and how to obtain inspection reports, if there are any.

3. Meet with a geriatric-care manager. These pros are social workers, nurses, or gerontologists who can tell you about the facilities you've selected and how well they match your relative's needs. For an initial assessment, expect to pay $300 to $800; subsequent hour-long sessions cost $100 to $150. Names are available on the Web site of the National Association of Professional Geriatric Care Managers (www.caremanager.org).

4. Tour the top four or five choices. Don't get carried away by the "chandelier effect"—the appeal of expensive-looking furnishings. Look instead for senior-friendly furniture: armchairs that are sturdy yet light enough to be maneuvered, with wheels on front legs for mobility. Check for grab bars in bathrooms and along hallways and nonskid flooring in baths. And view occupied rooms—you'll be able to tell how thoroughly the staff cleans.

5. Request the documents you need to help you make a decision. See Big 10 providers.

6. Talk to the residents. Ask how they like the food, the staff, and the activities, what they like and don't like, and whether they are satisfied with the handling of complaints. Ask visiting relatives the same questions.

7. Observe what people are doing. Are they up and about or passively watching TV?

8. Ask to meet with the administrator. The person in charge should care about those in his or her charge and also have the ability to run the facility efficiently.

9. Study the staff. Ask how many employees are in the building during the day and in the evening. Find out about their training to see whether it corresponds to the needs of the prospective resident. Ask any residents who are sitting unattended whether they are waiting for help. Note the degree to which attendants talk to or spend time with residents.

10. Visit unannounced. Stop by the facility two or three more times when the staff is not expecting you so that you can speak with residents without someone looking over your shoulder. Plan each stop at different times of day on different days of the week to see how many staff members are on duty.

11. If you are shopping for a relative, bring him or her on your visits. Stay for a meal and an activity and taste the food. Consider having your relative stay overnight as a tryout.

12. Monitor the care. After a relative moves into assisted living, visit often to make sure there are no problems. Your family member's health may deteriorate, so you have to be honest with yourself and with him or her when it's time to move to a nursing home. A geriatric-care manager can help with the decision.

Some facilities charge a flat rate, while others offer a choice of service levels or complicated à la carte pricing. Atria, the nation's fourth-largest chain, has 18 different fees based on the required level of care (there are six) and which apartment style you select (three are available) at its Stratford, Conn., location. Prices range from $3,400 a month for a studio (which includes the room, meals, utilities, activities, daily housekeeping, weekly laundering of bed linens, and some transportation, but no assistance with ADLs) to a $6,400 two-bedroom option for residents with dementia. Most facilities also require an up-front fee, which may range from the equivalent of one month's charges to tens of thousands of dollars; it may or may not be partially refundable if a resident leaves.

Most assisted-living residences provide some health care. Small staffs run by a nurse may be in the building or on call around the clock. At some locations, there's no nurse at all. Generally, residents consult their own doctors; but personal physicians do not necessarily communicate with staff at the facility. Medication administration may also be offered at an additional charge.

The question of what and how much care residents should receive can pit seniors—and their families—against the facility. Marty Margeson, for example, has battled to make the Pioneer, a state-run assisted-living facility in Anchorage, Alaska, reinstate care for her 91-year-old father, William, who is in the later stages of dementia. Though he has been at Pioneer since 1997, in the fall of 2004, the facility cut his baths from twice to once a week and now checks his vital signs once a month instead of once a week.

"The standard of care here is one bath a week and checking vitals once a month," says David Frain, the Anchorage Pioneer's administrator. The facility had previously offered William Margeson a higher level of care because, says Frain, "We try to bend over backwards for someone who is struggling, but at some point you have to say, it's time to place your loved one in a nursing home."

The difference between Pioneer and a nursing home isn't that clear, however. The chain's Web site states, "Many residents receive a level of service that would otherwise be delivered in a nursing home." In any case, Frain recently sent Marty Margeson a letter saying that her father would have to leave because she had not signed the required plan of care or service contract. She says she has not signed because of the reduction in care. Moreover, she doesn't want to take her dad to a nursing home because she fears the move would be fatal.

PAYING FOR IT

Most people in assisted living pay for it out of their own (or a relative's) pocket or with proceeds from long-term-care insurance, if the policy allows. If money runs out, a resident usually has to move out to a nursing home where he or she may qualify for Medicaid or to a relative's home. A few providers pledge to keep residents even if they deplete their funds. Some nonprofits can tap charitable donations to reduce a needy resident's fees.

Unlike nursing-home care, assisted living doesn't generally qualify for payment by Medicaid. However, 42 states have a Medicaid waiver program that allows some funds to pay for skilled nursing care in assisted living. The resident must generally meet certain low-income requirements: generally owning no more than $2,000 in liquid assets and with income of no more than $1,600 to $1,700 a month. Worse, states limit the number who may qualify to 300 to 400 people at any one time.

Assisted-living meals, lodging, and medical care may be tax deductible as medical expenses. However, you may only deduct medical and dental expenses that exceed 7.5 percent of your adjusted gross income.

THE PATIENTS: FRAILER AND SICKER

"When assisted living started, people who developed Alzheimer's had to move to nursing homes," says Karen Love, founder and chairwoman of the Consumer Consortium on Assisted Living, a consumer advocacy and education group in Falls Church, Va. "Now chains like

Sunrise build special floors for Alzheimer's patients." Indeed, a study published in October 2004 of 2,078 residents in 193 assisted-living homes in four states, funded by the National Institute on Aging, found that more than half the residents suffer from dementia.

"As our residents have grown older, many want to stay in assisted living and avoid nursing homes, so our providers try to accommodate them," says Richard Grimes, president of the Assisted Living Federation of America, a trade group. "Our hallmark is flexibility."

Yet, a 2002 National Academy for State Health Policy survey of providers in all 50 states and the District of Columbia concluded that increased state flexibility in assisted living has raised concerns about the adequacy of care and the inappropriate retention or discharge of residents.

If potentially violent or troublesome residents are retained, they can harm others. Herb Boyle, 82, was such a victim, contends his daughter, Ingrid Shaginoff. On the afternoon of April 1, 2005, he said he was assaulted by his next-door neighbor, a 77-year-old man with dementia. Boyle, who had Parkinson's disease, had moved into Palmer Pioneers' Home, a state-run facility in Palmer, Alaska, nine days earlier because his family feared he might fall and injure himself. Doctors told the family that Boyle's vertebrae and ribs were broken. Subsequently, he contracted pneumonia and died. "I am just outraged this happened when we put him there to be safe," Shaginoff says. "When I went in to pack my dad's stuff, that man was still living next door, free to roam around." Lynda Garcia, the home's administrator, says that Boyle's injuries resulted from "an unwitnessed two-person fall." She adds, "Our internal investigation revealed that nothing inappropriate happened." The police are investigating, and the autopsy report had not been released at press time.

OVERSIGHT: LITTLE TO NOT MUCH

Finding out about such incidents isn't easy. "Every state has a long-term-care ombudsman who looks into complaints consumers have," says Carol Scott, the Missouri long-term-care ombudsman. She adds that consumers would probably

FIGURE OUT WHERE PARENTS BELONG

WHO Marty Margeson and her father, William, Anchorage Alaska.
SITUATION Margeson says that her 91-year-old dad, who is in the later stages of dementia, saw his care cut back to one bath a week by Pioneer Home, his assisted-living facility. And attendants now take his vital signs only once a month, instead of once a week. Pioneer says that this is its standard of care for all residents and that Mr. Margeson now belongs elsewhere. Says his daughter, "I'm afraid the change would kill him."

not think to call the state department of health, which would track cases of assault or abuse.

Inspections, usually conducted by a state's department of health, should ideally track everything from staff-training certificates to kitchen-refrigeration temperatures. Yet, Massachusetts and Oregon inspect every other year; Colorado inspects for health one year and safety the next; and California, with more assisted-living facilities than any other state, inspects only once every five years.

Staffing and training requirements also vary. Georgia requires 1 person on duty for every 15 residents during the day; 1 for every 25 at night. But Alabama and Oregon require only "sufficient staff." Also Oregon does not specify who may administer medication as long as the procedure is approved by a pharmacist, registered nurse, or physician. It's no wonder that medication problems have been cited by many states in two National Academy for State Health Policy surveys of providers. Ethel Mitty, a nurse and project adviser at the Hartford Institute for Geriatric Nursing at New York University, points out, "You do not have the same controls on medication administration in assisted living that you have in nursing homes."

Consumers considering a facility aren't likely to know whether it is properly staffed until a problem occurs. When police responded to a 911 call from a Sunrise assisted-living facility in Alexandria, Va., at 3 a.m. on July 31, 2004, they could not get staff to respond to the after-hours call button, phone

closeup
Do the Big 10 providers give you the information you need?

In a word, no. According to an April 2004 U.S. Government Accountability Office study, assisted-living facilities do not routinely provide information about involuntary-discharge criteria or staff training and qualifications. That information, the contract, medication policies, costs, and details about different levels of care is vital to compare assisted-living alternatives. In late March 2005, we made one call each to at least three locations for each of the 10 largest assisted-living providers and said we were shopping for a facility for a relative who lives nearby. We asked for all the information in the categories listed below. Although many facilities sent us glossy brochures and monthly menus and activity lists, none sent us everything we requested. Chains are listed in alphabetical order.

PROVIDER	NO. OF FACILITIES CONTACTED	NO. THAT SENT INFORMATION ON:					
		Contracts	Discharge information	Detailed cost data	Staff training	Staffing levels	Who administers medications
Alterra Healthcare	3	0	0	0	0	0	0
American Lifestyles	3	0	1	3	0	0	0
Assisted Living Concepts	3	0	1	3	1	0	0
Atria Senior Living Group	3	0	0	1	0	0	0
Emeritus	5	0	1	4	0	0	1
HCR ManorCare	3*	0	1	2	1	0	0
Hearthstone Assisted Living	3	0	0	3	0	0	0
Leisure Care	3	1	1	2	0	0	0
Merrill Gardens	3	0	2	3	1	1	1
Sunrise Senior Living	7	0	2	4	1	1	2

* Only 2 facilities sent us information.

calls, or their cruiser sirens, according to a court document. Officers gained entry through an unlocked rear door and found Harold Podall, a 79-year-old paraplegic. He had called 911 after trying to summon Elizabeth Thorpe-Saffa, a care manager on duty, for more than an hour for help with his catheter.

On that same call, officers found an 87-year-old on the floor of his room, unable to get up. When police located Thorpe-Saffa, 54, who was in charge of the overnight care of residents on two floors, she admitted she had been sleeping. In November 2004 she pleaded guilty to one charge of neglect and was given a 45-day jail sentence, which was served at home with electronic monitoring. Sunrise was fined $500. Sarah Evers, a spokeswoman for Sunrise, says, "We had policies in place that required team members to be awake at all times while on their shifts. Thorpe-Saffa willingly violated this

KNOW WHAT TO EXPECT

WHO Susan Olshan and her mother, Sally, 75, at Crane's Mill, West Caldwell, N.J.

SITUATION When her mom had a stroke eight years ago, Olshan chose Sunrise at West Essex in Fairfield, N.J. The experience didn't live up to the sales pitch, she says, adding, "I expected them to do more than just cook meals. It's called assisted living, but you have to pay extra for any real assistance." Olshan paid for laundry, but her mom's clothes turned blue after they were tossed in the washing machine without being sorted. Olshan moved her mom two years ago. Sunrise says it made its services and prices clear at the outset.

policy and was terminated. We assisted police in her prosecution."

The Virginia incident shows that assisted living has serious shortcomings. Whether federal regulation can correct them isn't clear. At the very least, states should put standards in place that will—as they do not now—assure the safety and well-being of residents.

Until that happens, consumers have to be ultra-cautious in choosing an assisted-living facility that can provide the care they need. And the facilities themselves need to be forthright at the beginning about the services they can render.

The City of Laguna Woods: A Case of Senior Power in Local Politics

This study examined an example of the potential for senior power in local politics. On March 2, 1999, a gated retirement community in Orange County, California, known as Leisure World, incorporated with three adjacent senior-living facilities and several businesses to form the first city in the nation—Laguna Woods—almost exclusively populated by seniors. An immediate threat to the community's lifestyle—the building of a nearby airport—set off city incorporation and allowed the residents to fight the airport more effectively. City-generated revenues are mostly dedicated to satisfy the needs of senior residents and finance age-relevant services such as building golf cart trails for nondrivers. This case suggests that, when crisis arises, "able seniors" may become influential political activists. Although the senior power model may not be robust on the federal or state levels, it may become more so on the local level.

ROSS ANDEL
PHOEBE S. LIEBIG
University of Southern California

During the twentieth century, the American population underwent major demographic changes, particularly, a steady increase in the aging population. According to the U. S. Senate Committee on Aging (1991), in 1900, 1 in 25 American citizens was over the age of 65. In 1997, the proportion had changed to 1 in 8. Prospectively, 1 in 5 Americans will be at least 65 years of age by the year 2030. Although the American population has already been aging rapidly over the past decades, an even more dramatic increase in the number of older Americans can be expected as the baby boom generation approaches the later stages of life. Projections indicate that a baby boomer will turn 50 every seven seconds for the next two decades (Price 1997: 112).

With this demographic shift, some important questions arise. Among the most intriguing questions is whether these changing conditions will result in more senior power. The purpose of this case study is to describe the circumstances that preceded and accompanied city incorporation of a large retirement community—Leisure World in Laguna Hills, CA—into the city of Laguna Woods. We also elaborate on what this successful political action by seniors may represent for the politics of aging in the twenty-first century.

SENIOR ACTIVISM: PARTICIPATION, POWER, OR PERIL?

Rosenbaum and Button (1989) explored the level and outcomes of senior political activism in several Florida counties and municipalities. They summarized their findings in three hypotheses that address national concerns about the prospect of increasing political power among the aged: gray participation, gray power, and gray peril.

GRAY PARTICIPATION

The "gray participation" hypothesis refers to a gradual rise in political activism among the aged that may occur within the next several decades, as aging cohorts continue to show gains in education and socioeconomic status compared to the current older cohort. Findings of cross-sectional studies examining voter turnout during national elections consistently indicate that the aged show disproportionately higher voter participation than any other age group (Binstock 1997, 2000; Strate et al. 1989; Van Doorn 1992). For example, in 1992, 70.1 percent of registered voters 65 years of age or older cast their votes during presidential elections, while only 53.2 percent of registered voters between 25 and 34 years of age did so (Van Doorn 1992). Compared to younger cohorts, a relatively high percentage of older Americans also register to vote (Hey 1988).

McManus (1996) and Dobson (1983) suggest that older people are better informed about politics than members of younger cohorts. In their examination of the theory of life span development, Strate et al. (1989) conclude that interest and political knowledge—both components of civic competence—increase with age and decline only slightly in advanced old age, while showing minimal dependence on education. Because current trends suggest growing senior participation, the first Rosenbaum and Button's (1989) hypothesis seems relevant.

GRAY POWER

In their second hypothesis, Rosenbaum and Button (1989) present the anticipation of "gray power." They predict that a growing consciousness of shared political attitudes and interests will result in the aged being a major determinant of elections and policy outcomes. Some policy analysts are convinced that political power of the aged expressed through uniform political activism and advocacy, growing political participation, and bloc voting will increase the ability of the aged to influence local, state, and national politics (e.g., Cutler 1977; Cutler, Pierce, and Steckenrider 1984; Hudson 1988). Others suggest that the aged are likely to continue to gain political clout through the growing impact of aging interest groups (Binstock and Day 1995; Day 1990, 1998) and through their increasingly effective lobbying efforts (Pratt 1976, 1997). Finally, older people may benefit from a relatively high representation of older cohorts in political offices (Binstock and Day 1995; Blondel 1980; Hudson and Strate 1985).

Seniors, in spite of consistently showing high voter turnouts, have failed to capitalize on their political participation in terms of policy outcomes in national (Binstock 1997, 2000; Jennings and Markus 1988; Strate et al. 1989; Liebig 1992, Wallace et al. 1991) and state and local politics (Jirovec and Enrich 1992; Rosenbaum and Button 1989). For example, in the 1984 and 1988 presidential elections, older people voted for presidential candidates regardless of the likely impacts of their stance on aging policies such as Social Security, Medicare, and senior housing (Wallace et al. 1991). Older Americans do not seem to vote as a bloc (Barrow 1989; Binstock 1997, 2000; Liebig 1992), and other factors, such as social class and party affiliation, seem to be a better predictor of voting behavior than age (Binstock and Day 1995; Campbell and Strate 1981; Wallace et al. 1991). As a result, senior political participation, although extensive, may lack the political substance and direction commonly generated by shared goals, interests, and attitudes.

Binstock (2000) concludes that the aged have largely benefited from "electoral bluff," or the perception that seniors are a politically powerful group because of their relatively high voting turnout. Although the potential clout of seniors may scare politicians, it soon dissipates in the face of differences in ethnicity, race, social class, religion, partisanship, and other im-

portant political variables (Binstock 1997, 2000; Binstock and Day 1995; Hudson and Strate 1985; Rhodebeck 1993; Street 1999).

Frequency of voting behavior may be a misleading indicator of political power because it requires little effort and can be performed without a political purpose. Studies have found a relatively high and steady involvement among older adults in voting, but a marked decline in the more demanding modes of political activity such as campaigning and political meeting participation (Binstock 1972; Jennings and Markus, 1988; Jirovec and Erich 1992; Miller, Gurin, and Gurin 1980; Strate et al. 1989). This observed decline in nonvoting political participation can be explained by the concept of differential disengagement outlined by Streib and Schneider (1971). According to Streib and Schneider, aging individuals tend to discontinue political activities that have high-energy demands but continue low-energy activities at the same or even increased levels.

High senior voter turnouts may also reflect only habitual rather than purposive behavior, often with no underlying objective besides a desire for continued social involvement. Voting allows aging individuals to affirm their civic virtue during the life period when some may develop a sense of political powerlessness (Angello 1973).

GRAY PERIL

Rosenbaum and Button's (1989) third hypothesis refers to seniors as the "gray peril" of the American politics. This hypothesis predicts that the size and political vigor of the aged will ultimately thwart any efforts to implement policies that may disadvantage the aged. However, given the heterogeneity of attitudes and opinions among the aged (Binstock 2000; Jennings and Markus 1988; Rosenbaum and Button 1992), this hypothesis may be less viable.

POLITICAL ACTIVISM IN RETIREMENT COMMUNITIES

Retirement communities are still a fairly recent phenomenon in the United States. They represent unique entities with interesting consequences for policy making. Streib, Folts, and LaGreca (1985) and Anderson and Anderson (1978) conducted studies using retirement community samples. In both studies, senior political activism seemed relatively dormant except for high voting turnouts. However, when a critical event or a circumstance occurred with potential adverse effects for the community's well-being, residents demonstrated an exceptional ability to mobilize and confront the political threat.

Smelser's (1963) theory of collective behavior offers a theoretical explanation for this selective mobilization of retirement community seniors. Smelser suggests that people can be mobilized in large numbers for purposes that bridge their narrow self-interests and are associated with some greater sense of social need. Such collective action may be value oriented, norm oriented, or a result of a hostile outburst in response to an undesirable state of affairs. It may be that collective political action of community-dwelling seniors can only be triggered by an undesirable state of affairs, while their political participation remains passive in the absence of a significant mobilizing event.

Most studies examining senior political activity have used national samples during presidential elections (Binstock 1972, 1997, 2000; Jennings and Markus 1988; Strate et al. 1989). Two important consequential issues that stem from such research should be given some attention. First, the diversity of issues in presidential elections, combined with diversity among the elderly, precludes researchers from obtaining a coherent picture of voting preferences among seniors. It is important to recognize that the same aging issue may have unequal impacts on seniors of different socioeconomic background, gender, race, or religion.

Second, seniors are much less likely to agree on complex national issues than on immediate and specific local issues. Therefore, they may mobilize more readily in response to local issues, while showing little unity nationally. National surveys can hardly capture this distinction in senior political activity. Although aging interest groups have shown the ability to block unfavorable policy proposals on the national level (Binstock and Day 1995; Liebig 1992; Street 1999), effective political actions by seniors may be more likely to occur in local and state politics where mobilization around a single issue seems more feasible.

THE "ABLE ELDERLY"—A SLEEPING GIANT OF AMERICAN POLITICS

The elderly are a heterogenous group, not only in terms of political views but also in terms of their ability to remain active. According to Hudson (1988), the "able elderly"—those who are mentally and physically healthy, economically independent, and educated—manifest attributes that are correlated with political activity and involvement. The "able elderly" are becoming a distinct subgroup of the aged, with the potential for turning into an influential political entity. Although the relatively healthy and wealthy elderly tend to identify with general aging issues less than the more frail elderly (Miller et al. 1980), a clear threat to their collective well-being may still make them a powerful, cohesive bloc of seniors (Hudson 1988: Rose 1965).

Another plausible reason for collective coherence and mobilization of political activity among the able elderly can be a common need and desire to realize productive capacities (Hudson 1988) and replace social roles that are taken away by an age-graded society. A perceived need to be involved in the society even in older age (Atchley 1989; Cutler 1977; Cutler et al. 1984) may compel the able old to continue (or begin) to participate in politics. Atchley (1989), in his continuity theory, suggests that life-span development occurs on a continuum of retaining similar but developing attitudes and interests in related activities. A relatively high involvement of older people in voluntary organizational activities (Cutler 1977; Glenn and Grimes 1968) and the high turnout of elderly voters (e.g., Bin-

stock 2000) may reflect a continued need for self-expression and involvement in society, supporting Atchley's proposition.

Method

This case study analyzes developments related to incorporation of a large retirement community in Leisure World, Laguna Hills, California, into the City of Laguna Woods. Leisure World is the main part of the city, encompassing about 3.3 square miles of the 4-square-mile city. About 18,000 people reside in Leisure World, and about 500 Laguna Woods residents live outside the gates of Leisure World.

The average age in the new city is about 77 years. At least one member of each household in Leisure World must be 55 years of age or older. A spouse or a caregiver of an older resident may reside in Leisure World if they are at least 45 years old. Although no age limit exists in the city outside of Leisure World, only about 20 people who are younger than 55 years live in the remaining city area, according to city manager Leslie Keane (personal communication, May 18, 2001).

MEASURES

To capture the sequence and relative importance of events, we analyzed the content of newspaper articles that we considered relevant to the incorporation of Leisure World. First, we searched electronic archives of the two major newspapers in Orange County—the *Los Angeles Times, Orange County Edition*, and the *Orange County Register*—for information pertaining to either Leisure World or Laguna Woods. Then, we used the Leisure World Historical Society archives to obtain an account of articles from local and national newspapers that referred to the events surrounding the city incorporation. This search allowed us to extend our article database to articles from the community newsletter *Leisure World News* and relevant articles form the *New York Times* and the *Chicago Tribune*. The articles were organized chronologically and according to their relevance to the outcome of this study—senior mobilization in Leisure World, the subsequent city incorporation, and the operation of the city.

In addition to these analyses, we conducted interviews with key players involved in the pro- and anti-city movements and with members of the city council. We used the unstructured or conversational interviewing technique (Hendricks 1995) to capture personal accounts by those who were involved in the process that led to city incorporation. The advantage of conversational interviewing is that it allows the interviewer to establish a more emphatetic relationship with the interviewee. By permitting a greater degree of self-expression, it provides for an examination more sensitive to the differences in individual interpretations of the events and is less contaminated by generic outcomes of more rigid survey research. We believe that the combination of newspaper article analysis and conversational interviewing enabled us to explore and understand the interactions of circumstances and events that eventually led to the incorporation of Leisure World into the City of Laguna Woods.

The City of Laguna Woods

On March 2, 1999, an unprecedented event happened in Southern California's Orange County. An age-restricted gated community, Leisure World, joined with three adjacent senior assisted living facilities and several businesses to become an incorporated city—the City of Laguna Woods. Laguna Woods is the first municipality in the United States that consists almost entirely of senior citizens.[1]

HISTORY OF FAILED ANNEXATION ATTEMPTS

Leisure World residents had earlier opted against city annexation twice in the 36-year history of the retirement community. The first attempt came in 1982 when the annexation to the city of Irvine was proposed. However, this attempt failed even before it went to a vote, as almost half of Leisure World residents signed a petition against it, largely due to concerns about changes to the residential community's established rules.

The second attempt occurred in 1989. A nearby, unincorporated community, Laguna Hills, offered to incorporate with Leisure World to form the city of Laguna Hills. This appeal initially received a more favorable answer from the Leisure World residents. In part, an increased willingness to consider incorporation came as a result of an Orange County announcement that services such as police and trash collection would be limited in unincorporated areas like Laguna Hills or Leisure World. Nevertheless, concerns about lifestyle changes, including the lifting of move-in restrictions that were presumed to be part of the incorporation, led Leisure World residents to oppose incorporation by a large margin of nearly two to one. Laguna Hills subsequently became a city by itself in 1991. This earlier resistance to annexation may well support opinions that older people resist change. The former Laguna Woods Mayor, Bert Hack, and the president of Leisure World Residents for Cityhood, Betty Hohwiesner, perceive this as more than a truism (personal communication, October 26, 1999).

NEW DEVELOPMENTS FAVOR INCORPORATION

The 1999 successful attempt at city incorporation took place under vastly different conditions from those that accompanied the previous two annexation attempt. First, over the past two decades, Orange County has become more reluctant to provide services such as security, maintenance, and health care to unincorporated areas such as Leisure World. Limiting or even taking away these services could have had severely negative effects on the community. Second, Leisure World residents were forced to travel over 50 miles to county offices in Santa Ana to complete legal transactions.

Finally and most important, recent developments in local politics seemed to have directly led to a greater penchant of Leisure World residents for a greater political clout associated with a city status. In 1992, politicians in Orange and adjacent countries began to consider various reuse projects for closure of the El Toro Marine Corps Air Base scheduled for 1999. An interna-

tional commercial airport emerged as the most popular proposition. The El Toro Base is located only a few miles east of Leisure World. Not surprisingly, building a commercial airport so close by alarmed Leisure World residents, and warnings about the expected impact of the airport on the overall quality of life in the community and health and life expectancy of the residents started to spread.

The new attempt at city incorporation possessed yet another strength. Since the incorporation involved Leisure World as the main and central part of the proposed city, concerns about maintaining the community's autonomy and avoiding changes to regulations by an outside entity were essentially eliminated. As current Laguna Woods Mayor Brenda Ross indicated, she had never met a senior who would not want to be independent (personal communication, October 19, 1999). A threat to the political independence and autonomy of the community by annexation with another large community could have impeded the process of city incorporation, as it had in the previous attempts.

CITY INCORPORATION

It is our contention that the willingness and ability of the able old to participate actively in politics, and circumstances that mobilized and united a senior community, accompanied the creation of the first major "City of Seniors"—Laguna Woods. Although not all residents of Leisure World are retired, the community, has acquired an image of a secluded recreational entity. While Leisure World seniors have shown interest in current events and political issues, most internal and external observers, characterized the involvement of Leisure World residents in societal issues as observation rather than active participation (personal communication, October 26, 1999). Therefore, mobilization of the residents around the issue of city incorporation and the subsequent creation of Laguna Woods may have come as a surprise to many.

THE PROCESS OF POLICY-MAKING

In spite of a seemingly better outlook for cityhood, this attempt was initially met with rather gloomy prospects. A survey conducted in October 1998 of a random sample of Leisure World residents found that 42 percent were undecided (Blodgett 1999). So how did this attempt become successful? The first and most important factor was the existence of a clear and present threatening issue—the proposed commercial airport. A pronounced shift in public mood (Kingdon 1995) toward incorporation occurred when Leisure World residents began to recognize their ability to oppose the airport was impeded by the community's status as an unincorporated community. The airport, by presenting an immediate threat to community well-being, seemed to instigate a sense of cohesiveness and an explicit reason for political mobilization. The inability to act was most apparent to Leisure World residents in 1998 when they could not stop Orange County policymakers from using their taxes to support the pro-airport campaign.

An important part of political softening up (see Kingdon 1995) by pro-city activists was an increasing awareness of Leisure World residents about the potential adverse health effects of living in close proximity to an airport. In his letter to the editor of the *Los Angeles Times*, Hack (1999) reported on a 1993 study by Meecham and Shaw conducted near the Los Angeles International Airport. The results indicated that living near that airport was related to a two-year loss in life expectancy among seniors 74 years of age and older. The negative factors that contributed to a decline in life expectancy were excessive noise levels and air pollution. As worries of the Leisure World residents concerning the noise and pollution associated with the airport grew, so did the success of pro-city activists.

The fact that pro-city activists were able to clarify their goals, values, and objectives in their campaign was also an important factor that may have eventually affected the outcome of the election. The MuniFinancial Group from Temecula, California, hired by the pro-city activists, performed a fiscal analysis. The city proposal was submitted to the Local Agency Formation Commission (LAFCO) for evaluation. LAFCO, along with the Orange County Board of Supervisors, examined the proposal for the financial and organizational consequences of cityhood. LAFCO finally approved a city election and set the election day for March 2, 1999 (Haldane 1998).

Pro-city activists worked hard to communicate their ideas to Leisure World residents. The president of Leisure World Residents for Cityhood, Better Hohwiesner, recalled that cityhood supporters distributed flyers and conducted numerous official and unofficial discussions about incorporation-related issues (personal communication, October 26, 1999). Four two-hour leadership development seminars titled "How a City Operates" were organized by the Leisure World Community Association and moderated by an experienced city management expert, Len Wood. Recordings of the seminars were made available to the residents on a local TV cable channel and on tapes.

Anti-city activists worked hard as well, stating concerns about the proposed city's long-term financial health as serious enough to negate incorporation. Helen Ensweiler, the president of Leisure World Residents against Cityhood, said that in spite of assurances from LAFCO urban developers, "many Leisure World residents still feared that the new city would not have enough funds to operate" (personal communication, December 3, 1999). In her opinion, annexation to a neighboring city would have been a better option. That would have enabled Leisure World residents to fight against the airport and provided better financial resources than the new city could ever provide for itself.

The pro-city activists countered with three main arguments. First, as suggested by city management experts, property taxes and surrounding businesses would provide enough tax money to keep the city solvent. Second, the new city would have no authority over any policies within the gated community. And third, the city could become a major player in the anti-airport campaign.

As the election outcome reveals, pro-city activists succeeded in conveying the advantages of a new municipality, although the results were far from overwhelming. A relatively high 68.6 percent of all voters registered their opinion at the polls on March 2, 1999 (Tessler and Gottlieb 1999). In spite of the publicity and the significance of city incorporation for effective opposition to the airport, Laguna Woods was approved only by a slight majority of 51.7 percent (or 342 votes) of more than 10,000 Leisure World residents who voted.

The relatively close outcome of the election and the fact that nearly one-third of registered voters did not participate suggest that seniors may be hesitant to take on a major change, even when their welfare maybe threatened. This inference seems to undermine the validity of the senior power model. It may be that other relevant issues besides fighting the airport and the innate resistance to change among seniors prevented Leisure World seniors from gaining a stronger impetus toward incorporation.

LAGUNA WOODS: SENIOR POWER OF ABLE OLD IN LOCAL POLITICS

The city began to function officially on March 24, 1999, only three and a half weeks after the election. "Most cities take three to six months to organize and become active," said Mayor Pro Tem and former Mayor Bert Hack (personal communication, October 26, 1999). One of the first issues addressed by the newly elected city council was participation in the anti-airport campaign. In its first meeting, the council agreed to use its new power by joining the El Toro Reuse Planning Authority in the fight against the proposed airport, thereby clearly demonstrating the importance of the airport issue in the new city's policies.

In another action, the council approved and encouraged support of the Safe and Healthy Communities Act, also known as Measure F. Volunteers from the new city gathered signatures to get this measure on the March 2000 ballot. This required the county to get a two-thirds vote before building a new jail, passenger airport, or noxious waste dump. Laguna Woods led the county in voter turnout with 68 percent of registered votes (Willon and Reyes 2000). Laguna Woods votes were second only to El Toro with 93 percent voting in favor of Measure F. Although the initiative received an overwhelming majority, it was eventually deemed unconstitutional by the Orange County judge (Pasco and James 2000).

In addition to the airport issue, an important agenda item early in the existence of Laguna Woods was the contract with the county for maintenance, security, and health services. Although the responsibility for maintenance, security, and health services was transferred from the county to the city on incorporation, the city council unanimously decided that the county should continue to provide those services via contracts. The decision to become a "contract city" is typical of newly formed cities in California.

Not all issues in Laguna Woods were dealt with as smoothly and unanimously as the anti-airport project and community services issues. During the council meeting on July 21, 1999, Mayor Jim Thorpe abruptly decided to resign his seat (Glazer and Willon 1999; Walker 1999). His resignation appeared to be a result of a critical letter sent to other council members by one member, Ann Snider, criticizing the length and ineffectiveness of city meetings. The mayor attributed his decision to step down to the lack of experience and competence among the members of the City Council and sluggishness of the meetings. Council member Bert Hack, as mayor pro tem, replaced Thorpe and became the second mayor of Laguna Woods. Hack acknowledged that political operations tend to be more difficult among senior council members in Laguna Woods because of a natural tendency of older people to become more diverse in their attitudes and opinions (personal communication, October 26, 1999).

In April 2000, a new council was selected, which then selected a third mayor—Brenda Ross—in the second year of the city's existence. Despite its changing leadership, the city has managed to be financially sound. "The city doubled its projected budget surplus of $900,000 for the fiscal year 1999," said city manager Leslie Keane (personal communication, November 30, 2000). Most revenues came from motor vehicle licensing, state funds for new cities, and sales taxes (Pasco 1999). Plans were approved for increasing city revenues through a shopping mall, additional businesses, and a hotel on city property. The main expenses for the first year included contracting with the county for law enforcement services and road maintenance, and salaries (Pasco 1999).

The gated community within Laguna Woods creates an interesting situation from a financial standpoint. First, all property within the gates of Leisure World is private, which precludes the city from spending its revenues on maintenance and development of this major part of the city. Any facilities or housing financed by public funds within the gated community must be available to the general public—a situation Leisure World residents want to avoid. Using city land adjacent to the gated community is the only way to utilize city funds. Second, although the city is obliged to yield a part of property taxes to pay for state and local school bonds, no schools exist on the city land, precluding any additional expenditures for school maintenance or expansion.

As a result of these unique factors, more funds are available for other projects that can be devoted specifically to the needs of senior residents. For example, the council recently approved funds to build golf cart trails and overpasses to improve mobility and safety of nondrivers. These new roadways will connect the gated community with neighboring stores and businesses, enabling the city residents to maintain their independence without having to drive or worry about traffic. The council has also agreed to build a dog park on city property. The passage of this proposal was supported when council members cited psychosocial benefits for seniors of owning and interacting with a pet (e.g., Raina et al. 1999).

Discussion and Conclusions

WHAT CAN WAKE THE SLEEPING GIANT?

This case study indicates that the senior power model (Cutler 1977; Pratt 1997; Rosenbaum and Button 1989; Street 1999) may be a reality in today's aging politics. Its demonstration

may, however, be contingent on several factors. First, a major critical issue has to be at stake for seniors to exhibit their political potential. While seniors tend to engage in passive forms of political participation such as voting and withdraw from more energy-demanding activities such as campaigning and contacting politicians (Jennings and Markus 1988; Streib and Schneider 1971), they may show high levels of active political activism when their welfare is threatened (Anderson and Anderson 1978; Streib et al. 1985).

Second, a political issue is more likely to provoke effective senior activism if it affects a homogeneous senior group rather than American seniors in general. Even major national political events such as presidential elections (Binstock 1997, 2000; Strate et al. 1989) or important issues such as Social Security and Medicare (Street 1999) may not support the senior power model. However, a specific local issue threatening to affect a well-defined group of seniors may give rise to an effective local response as it did in the case of Laguna Woods.

Finally, the "able old" (Hudson 1988) may be especially likely to demonstrate senior political power. A relatively high income, education, and high levels of activity assert that Laguna Woods residents fit Hudson's definition of the able elderly. Leisure World requires that residents have an annual income of more than $30,000 and more than $50,000 in assets. Although data on residents' education are not available, higher income is generally correlated with higher levels of education (e.g., Osberg et al. 1987). Leisure World includes more than 250 clubs and organizations that promote high levels of activity, such as tennis, arts and computer clubs, horseback riding, and an orchestra. These Leisure World entities enjoy large memberships and plenty of volunteer activity.

Hudson (1988) predicted that a collective sense of being discriminated against and a struggle for group autonomy could lead to effective political mobilization. Streib et al. (1985) found self-government and control over one's future important for retirement community residents. Political activism in Laguna Woods corroborates that the able old may represent a group that can effectively respond to unfavorable political developments.

The relatively narrow margin of victory in the 1999 city election and less than 70 percent voting turnout suggest that not all seniors become politically involved when their welfare is directly contested by political circumstances. Nevertheless, the support for opposing the proposed El Toro airport among Leisure World residents demonstrates that seniors can unite and mobilize against threats to their health, lifestyle, and well-being.

IS DIRECTED POLITICAL ACTIVISM AGE SPECIFIC?

The incorporation of Laguna Woods was a concerted political action of a functionally competent, active group of adults who felt their health and lifestyle would be threatened if an airport were built nearby. Although the airport issue may not appear "senior-specific," some of the consequences of living near an airport may seem more threatening to an older person. The adverse health effects and increased mortality occasioned by living near an airport (e.g., Meecham and Shaw 1993; Pope et al. 1995) were among the pivotal arguments that drove pro-city activism. By contrast, while younger persons may also have health concerns about being located near an airport, they may consider the economic and transportation benefits of such a facility as more important. In addition, seniors may be more determined to maintain the status quo in terms of living conditions than younger cohorts (Campbell and Strate 1981; Streib et al. 1985). Therefore, a greater magnitude of political mobilization can be expected from seniors than other age groups on issues that disrupt continuation of preexisting conditions.

While the initial effort to create a city in Leisure World was inspired by airport opposition, the new city's existence has enabled Laguna Woods residents to get involved in actions that could result in unprecedented benefits for seniors. Since the city is almost exclusively occupied by seniors, senior-related services such as the proposed golf cart paths for nondrivers are always among the main items on the city's agenda. This unique opportunity to focus on aging issues could make this California city an appealing model for other senior communities. Laguna Woods appears to represent a case of gray power (Rosenbaum and Button 1989) in local politics, with special circumstances playing a major role in senior mobilization. Whether it will remain the only "senior city" or whether other senior communities will respond to political crises in a similar way remains to be seen.

NOTE

1. A small community, now composed mostly of seniors, became a municipality in Ocean Breeze Park, Florida, in 1960. However, the age distribution was more diverse when city incorporation took place (personal communication, April 19, 2001).

REFERENCES

Agnello, Thomas J., Jr. 1973. "Aging and the Sense of Political Powerlessness." *Public Opinion Quarterly* 37:251–59.

Anderson, William A. and Norma D. Anderson, 1978. "The Politics of Age Exclusion: Adults Only Movement in Arizona." *The Gerontologist* 18:6–12.

Atchley, Robert C. 1989. "A Continuity Theory of Normal Aging." *The Gerontologist* 29:183–90.

Barrow, Georgia M. 1989. *Aging, the Individual, and Society.* St. Paul, MN: West Publishing.

Binstock, Richard H. 1972. "Interest Group Liberalism and the Politics of Aging." *The Gerontologist* Autumn Part I:265–80.

____. 1997. "The 1996 Election: Older Voters and Implications for Policies on Aging." *The Gerontologist* 37:15–19.

____. 2000. "Older People and Voting Participation: Past and Future." *The Gerontologist* 40:18–31.

Binstock, Richard H. and Christine L. Day. 1995. "Aging and Politics." Pp. 362–87 in *Handbook of Aging and Social Science*, edited by R. H. Binstock and L. K. George. San Diego, CA: Harcourt Brace.

Blodgett, Dave. 1999. "'Twas April Fools Day." *Leisure World News*, April 8, p. 3.

Blondel, Jean. 1980. *World Leaders: Heads of Government in the Postwar Period.* Beverly Hills, CA: Sage.

Campbell, John. C. and John M. Strate. 1981. "Are Old People Conservative?" *The Gerontologist* 21:580–91.

Cutler, Neal E. 1977. "Demographic, Social-Psychological, and Political Factors in the Politics of Aging: A Foundation for Research in 'Political Gerontology.'" *The American Political Science Review* 71:1011–25.

Cutler, Neal E., Robert C. Pierce, and Janie S. Steckenrider. 1984. "How Golden Is the Future?" *Generations* 9:38–43.

Day, Christine L. 1990. *What Older Americans Think.* New Jersey: Princeton University Press.

____. 1998. "Old Age Interest Groups in the 1990s: Coalitions, Competition, and Strategy." Pp. 131–50 in *New Perspectives on Old Age Policies*, edited by J. Steckenrider and T. Parrott. Albany: State University of New York Press.

Dobson, Douglas. 1983. "The Elderly as a Political Force." Pp. 123–44 in *Aging and Public Policy: The Politics of Growing Old in America*, edited by W. P. Browne and L. K. Olson. Westport, CT: Greenwood.

Glazer, Andrew and Phil Willon. 1999. "Laguna Woods Mayor Quits in Indignation." *The Los Angeles Times, Orange County Edition*, July 22, p. B1.

Glenn, Norval D. and Michael Grimes. 1968. "Aging, Voting, and Political Interest." *American Sociological Review* 33:563–75.

Hack, Bert. 1999. "In Laguna Woods, Those Who Recall the Past Look to the Future." *The Los Angeles Times, Orange County Edition*, April 18, p. B11.

Haldane, David. 1998. "Leisure World Vote on Cityhood Approved." *The Los Angeles Times, Orange County Edition*, September 16, p. B1.

Hendricks, Jon. 1995. "Qualitative Research: Contributions and Advances." Pp. 52–72 in *Handbook of Aging and the Social Sciences*, edited by R. H. Binstock and L. K. George. San Diego, CA: Academic Press.

Hey, R. R. 1988. "Elderly Voters Are Organizing and Candidates Are Paying Attention." *Christian Science Monitor*, January 25, p. 1.

Hudson, Robert B. 1988. "Politics and the New Old." Pp. 59–72 in *Retirement Reconsidered*, edited by R. Morris and S. A. Bass. New York: Springer.

Hudson, Robert B. and John M. Strate. 1985. "Aging and Political Systems." Pp. 554–85 in *Handbook of Aging and the Social Sciences*, edited by R. H. Binstock and E. Shanas. New York: Van Nostrand Reinhold.

Jennings, M. Kent and Gregory B. Markus. 1988. "Political Involvement in the Later Years: A Longitudinal Survey." *American Journal of Political Science* 32:302–16.

Jirovec, Ronald L. and John A. Erich. 1992. "The Dynamics of Political Participation Among the Urban Elderly." *Journal of Applied Gerontology* 11:216–27.

Kingdon, John W. 1995. *Agendas, Alternatives, and Public Policies.* New York: HarperCollins.

Liebig, Phoebe S. 1992. "Federalism and Aging Policy in the 1980s: Implications for Changing Interest Group Roles in the 1990s." *Journal of Aging and Social Policy* 4:17–33.

McManus, Susan A. 1996. *Young vs. Old: Generational Combat in the 21st Century.* Boulder, CO: Westview.

Meecham, William C. and Neil A. Shaw. 1993. *"Increase in Mortality Rates Due to Aircraft Noise."* Presented to the Proceedings of Inter-Noise, August, Lueven, Belgium.

Miller, Arthur, Patricia Gurin, and Gerald Gurin. 1980. "Age Consciousness and Political Mobilization of Older Americans." *The Gerontologist* 20:691–700.

Osberg, J. Scott, Gayle E. McGinnes, Gerben DeJong, and Marymae L. Seward. 1987. "Life Satisfaction and Quality of Life Among Disabled Elderly Adults." *Journal of Gerontology* 42:228–30.

Pasco, Jean O. 1999. "Age Limit Could Mean New Hassles for New City." *The Los Angeles Times, Orange County Edition*, March 24, p. B3.

Pasco, Jean O. and Meg James. 2000. "El Toro Prospects Soar: Judge Voids Measure F." *The Los Angeles Times, Orange County Edition*, December 2, p. A1.

Pope, C. Arden, III, Michael J. Thun, Mohan M. Namboodiri, Douglas W. Dockery, Jon S. Evans, Frank E. Speizer, and Clark W. Health, Jr. 1995. "Particulate Air Pollution as a Predictor of Mortality in a Prospective Study of U. S. Adults." *American Journal of Respiratory and Critical Care Medicine* 151:669–74.

Pratt, Henry J. 1976. *The Gray Lobby*. Chicago: University of Chicago Press.

____. 1997. "Do the Elderly Really Have Political Clout?" Pp. 81–91 in *Controversial Issues in Aging*, edited by A. Scharlach and L. Kaye. Boston, MA: Allyn & Bacon.

Price, Matthew C. 1997. *Justice Between Generations: The Growing Power of the Elderly in America*. Westport, CT: Praeger.

Raina, Parminder, Toews D. Waltner, Brenda Bonnett, Christel Woodward, and Tom Abernathy. 1999. "Influence of Companion Animals on the Physical and Psychological Health of Older People: An Analysis of a One-Year Longitudinal Study. *Journal of American Geriatrics Society* 47:323–29.

Rhodebeck, Laurie A. 1993. "The Politics of Greed? Political Preferences Among the Elderly." *Journal of Politics* 55:342–64.

Rose, Arnold M. 1965. "Group Consciousness Among the Aging." Pp. 19–36 in *Older People and Their Social World*, edited by A. Rose and W. Peterson. Philadelphia, PA: Davis.

Rosenbaum, Walter A. and James W. Button. 1989. "Is There a Gray Peril? Retirement Politics in Florida." *The Gerontologist* 29:300–306.

____. 1992. "Perceptions of Intergenerational Conflict: The Politics of Young vs. Old." *Journal of Aging Studies* 6:385–96.

Smelser, Neil J. 1963. *Theory of Collective Behavior*. Glencoe, IL: Free Press.

Strate, John M., Charles J. Parrish, Charles D. Elder, and Coit Ford. 1989. "Life Span Civic Development and Voting Participation." *American Political Science Review* 83:443–64.

Street, Debra 1999. "Special Interests or Citizens' Tights? 'Senior Power,' Social Security, and Medicare." Pp. 109–30 in *Critical Gerontology: Perspectives From Political and Moral Economy*, edited by M. Minkler and C. L. Estes. New York: Baywood Publishing.

Streib, Gordon F., Edward Folts, and Anthony J. La Greca. 1985. "Autonomy, Power, and Decision-Making in Thirty-Six Retirement Communities." *The Gerontologist* 25:403–9.

Streib, Gordon F. and Clement J. Schneider. 1971. *Retirement in American Society*. Ithaca, NY: Cornell University Press.

Tessler, Ray and Jay Gottlieb. 1999. "New O. C. City Puts a Gleam on Governing." *Los Angeles Times, Orange County Edition*, March 4, p. A1.

U. S. Senate Committee on Aging. 1991. *Aging America: Trends and Projections*. Washington, DC: Government Printing Office.

Van Doorn. Oom. 1992. "Budget Priorities of the Nation." *Science*, December 11, pp. 31–40.

Walker, Cheryl. 1999. "Laguna Woods Mayor Resigns, Citing Colleqgues' Inexperience." *The Orange County Register*, July 22, p. A3.

Wallace, Steven P., John B. Williamson, Rita G. Lung, and Lawrence A. Powell. 1991. "A Lamb in Wolf's Clothing? The Reality of Senior Power and Social Policy.": Pp. 95–114 in *Critical Perspectives on Aging: The Political and Moral Economy of Growing Old*, edited by M. Minkler and C. L. Estes. Amityville, NY: Baywood Publishing.

Willon, Phil, and David Reyes. 2000. "Campaign 2000: County's Turnout Hits 20-Year High." *Los Angeles Times*, March 9, p. B1.

AUTHORS' NOTE: The authors presented a poster of the submitted study at the annual meeting of the Gerontological Society of America in Washington, D. C., in November 2000. The article was presented at the annual meeting of Western Political Science Association in Las Vegas, Nevada, in March 2001. The authors wish to express their appreciation to Laguna Woods Mayor Brenda Ross, Mayor Pro Tem Bert Hack, city manager Leslie Keane, and activists Helen Ensweiler and Betty Hohwiesner for their contribution to this article. Correspondence should be addressed to Ross Andel, Andrus Gerontology Center, University of Southern California, 3715 McClintock Avenue, Los Angeles, CA 90089–0191; telephone: (213) 740–2210; Fax: (213) 746–5994; e-mail: randel@use.edu.

Ross Andel, BA, is a doctoral student at the Leonard Davis School of Gerontology at the University of Southern California. His prior research interests include the study of motor learning and motor performance in Alzheimer's patients. His current research interests are senior political participation and cognitive aging. His publications appear in Journal of Clinical Geropsychology, Aging, Neuropsychology, and Cognition, *and the upcoming issue of* Journals of Gerontology: Psychological Sciences.

Phoebe S. Liebig, Ph.D., is an associate professor at the Leonard Davis School of Gerontology at the University of Southern California. Her research interests and publications focus on the politics and policy processes in aging and state-level policies and programs in housing and long-term care. A fellow of the Gerontological Society of America, her publications have appeared in such journals as Technology and Disability, Journal of Applied Gerontology, Housing Policy Debate, *and the* Journal of Aging and Social Policy.

From *Research on Aging*, January 2002, pp. 87-105. © 2002 by Research on Aging. Reprinted with permission of Sage Publications, Inc.

UNIT 8

Social Policies, Programs, and Services for Older Americans

Unit Selections

Key Points to Consider

- Why do most older persons not see the new Medicare prescription drug card as really solving the problem of high cost drugs?

- Why do many people believe the U.S. government should legalize the practice of importing drugs from foreign countries?

- Why does Pamela Herd believe that privatization of Social Security or Medicare would be most harmful to poor older persons?

- What are the advantages and disadvantages of a single payer system of universal health coverage?

- What does William Greider propose as a new retirement program to replace all those that are now having financial difficulties of being terminated?

Student Website

www.mhcls.com/online

Internet References

Further information regarding these websites may be found in this book's preface or online.

Administration on Aging
http://www.aoa.dhhs.gov
American Federation for Aging Research
http://www.afar.org/
American Geriatrics Society
http://www.americangeriatrics.org
Community Transportation Association of America
http://www.ctaa.org
Consumer Reports State Inspection Surveys
http://www.ConsumerReports.org
Medicare Consumer Information From the Health Care Finance Association
http://cms.hhs.gov/default.asp?fromhcfadotgov=true
National Institutes of Health
http://www.nih.gov
The United States Senate: Special Committee on Aging
http://www.senate.gov/~aging/

It is a political reality that older Americans will be able to obtain needed assistance from governmental programs only if they are perceived as politically powerful. Political involvement can range from holding and expressing political opinions, voting in elections, participating in voluntary associations to help elect a candidate or party, and holding political office.

Research indicates that older people are just as likely as any other age group to hold political opinions, are more likely than younger people to vote in an election, are about equally divided between Democrats and Republicans, and are more likely than young people to hold political office. Older people, however, have shown little inclination to vote as a bloc on issues affecting their welfare despite encouragement by senior activists, such as Maggie Kuhn and the leaders of the Gray Panthers, to do so.

Gerontologists have observed that a major factor contributing to the increased push for government services for the elderly has been the publicity on their plight generated by such groups as the National Council of Senior Citizens and the American Association of Retired Persons (AARP). The desire of adult children to shift the financial burden of aged parents from themselves onto the government has further contributed to the demand for services for the elderly. The resulting widespread support for such programs has almost guaranteed their passage in Congress.

Now, for the first time, there are groups emerging that oppose increases in spending for services for older Americans. Requesting generational equity, some politically active groups argue that the federal government is spending so much on older Americans that it is depriving younger age groups of needed services.

The articles in this section raise a number of problems and issues that result from an ever-larger number and percentage of the population living to age 65 and older. In "Have Seniors Been Dealt a Bad Hand? Medicare's Drug Discount Cards," the article

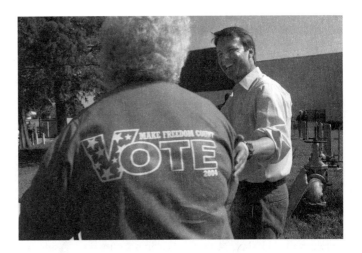

points out how much money older people would save by ordering drugs online from Canadian pharmacies rather than using the new Medicare drug prescription card program. In "Universalism Without the Targeting: Privatizing the Old-Age Welfare State," Pamela Herd points out how privatization would threaten the current redistribution of monies and services that Social Security and Medicare provide to maintain an adequate standard of living for the very poor.

In "Prescription for Change," Matt Leingang points out the advantages of a universal health-care system where the government would collect taxes and pay for everyone. William Greider in "Riding Into the Sunset" gives the economic problems of the current retirement funds and proposes a mandatory and universal saving system that he believes would be more durable than the current programs.

Have Seniors Been Dealt A Bad Hand?

MEDICARE'S DRUG DISCOUNT CARDS

When Medicare's drug discount cards were unveiled in May, 74-year-old Evelyn Levin considered enrolling in a plan. An interim measure until Medicare's full drug benefit begins in 2006, these cards would, in the words of the Bush administration, "give seniors the power to save on prescription drugs" and "demand the best prices." The only tangible benefit of the 2003 Medicare law seniors will see before November's elections, the White House and other supporters of the law are anxious to see the cards succeed.

The question is: Are seniors grateful for the cards or just confused and frustrated?

Evelyn and her husband, Seth, 70, together take six prescription medicines daily. For the past several years, this Manhattan couple has purchased their drugs online from a Canadian pharmacy. A web-savvy senior, Evelyn figured she would visit Medicare's website to research the cards. It was there she ran into her first problem. "I couldn't get through to the site because too many people were trying to access it at the same time and it was overloaded."

Medicare officials estimated 7 million hits to the website were made the first week the cards became available. Medicare's toll-free hotline, an option for seniors without Internet access, was also busy, logging 1.7 million calls in the first week, 10 times more than usual.

Choosing from the more than 70 Medicare-approved cards has generated widespread confusion among many seniors and their families. "When I was finally able to get through to the website I found

it very, very confusing," Evelyn remarked. Aside from the sheer number of choices, the cards do not lend themselves to simple comparisons. Each card offers different discounts, different drugs and different participating pharmacies.

"It took a lot of research and reading to get the information I needed to make the right choices for us," Evelyn said. "And after all that, I was furious by what I found. The card companies can change their discounts every week, but we would be locked into a card for a year! There may be a 15 percent discount one week and none the next. It's just not worth it."

Evelyn's complaints echo those commonly expressed by other seniors and advocates. As drug prices and discounts continue to fluctuate, confused seniors are struggling to determine which card will work best with their personal circumstances. A Harvard University study revealed average drug card savings would range around 17% off retail prices. However, those savings pale in comparison to the 40% discounts Levin finds in Canada. "I have an ulcer and for 100 pills it's $190 in Canada, compared to $360 in the United States—it's almost half the price," Evelyn explained. "Buying from Canada always saves me money and buying online couldn't be more simple. It's a no-brainer. For middle-class people like us, it ensures there's money for other things like food." Evelyn and Seth Levin are not the only ones to discover that the cards do not yield the same savings as retiree

Comparing Your Prescription Drug Discount Options

Ask prospective card sponsors these questions before joining a drug discount program

Cost of Drugs

1. How much will each drug I take cost under the program?
2. What other costs will I have?
  • Is there a monthly premium
  • Is there an annual enrollment fee?
  • Is there a deductible?
  • Is there a co-pay?
3. Are the costs of the program worth it?
4. How will I be able to find out about changes to the list of discounted drugs?

Access to Discounts

1. Will I be able to use the pharmacies I normally use?
2. Are discounts available by mail order?

If you are in a Medicare Private Plan (HMO or PPO)

1. How does the HMO's drug coverage coordinate with the program?

Service Area

1. Does the program work outside my state?
2. What happens if I travel outside my area?

---

health benefits, state drug assistance programs, or Canadian purchases.

As of June 1, the first day card discounts went into effect, only 2.8 million of Medicare's 35 million eligible beneficiaries had signed up for a card. Most, however, were automatically enrolled into the cards because they belong to a Medicare-managed care plan. Only about 400,000 actually chose to sign up. Medicare officials are hoping that 7.3 million beneficiaries will eventually sign up for a card.

There is little dispute, however, that the 7.2 million low-income beneficiaries who have no drug coverage and are eligible for the $600 credit should sign up for a card. The government will spend $4.6 million on outreach programs in urban and rural areas to enroll low-income seniors and persons

with disabilities, according to the Department of Health and Human Services. At least six states—Maine, Massachusetts, Michigan, New Jersey, Connecticut and New York—intend to automatically enroll low-income seniors who are already in state drug assistance programs into a Medicare-approved card plan. Some states have decided against automatic enrollment because the state drug program is already more generous than the discount cards.

As seniors try to make sense of the new Medicare reality, the cards portend the greater complexity that lies ahead. "The 2006 drug benefit promises even more daunting complexity," predicts Robert Hayes, president of the Medicare Rights Center, an independent organization that provides counseling services. "The administration and Congress

should create what the American people want and need: a prescription drug program that treats everyone equal, negotiates fair drug prices and provides reliable and comprehensive coverage."

Despite Medicare's offerings, Evelyn and Seth Levin are likely to continue doing what they've been doing all along: getting their drugs outside the U.S. "I'm not one to march or go to rallies," Evelyn said, "but I will march in protest if the government stops allowing seniors to buy their drugs from Canada. Once again, we are at the mercy of big business and the administration. We must all speak out against those who would make it difficult, and in some cases impossible, to pay for our needed medications."

From *Agewise*, Summer 2004, pp. 7-9. Copyright © 2004 by Alliance for Retired Americans, Washington, DC. Reprinted with permission.

LONG-TERM CARE
The Ticking Bomb

WITH THE POPULATION AGING, states are struggling to balance the relentless need for nursing home care, increased demands for home and community-based services and a way to fund it all. Further compounding the problem is another Medicaid population in need of expensive long-term care services: younger disabled adults unable to live independently without assistance.

Diagnosis
Long-term care threatens to bankrupt Medicaid and the states that pay for it. The best hope for a cure lies in cutting down on the need for institutional care.

The cost for long-term care for the elderly and disabled who qualify for Medicaid is enormous. Traditionally, the bulk of those services is provided by nursing homes, and increasingly, the greater proportion of people in those nursing homes are Medicaid patients. In the past few years, the federal-state Medicaid partnership has been the primary payment source for over 60 percent of all nursing home patients. The state share of that tab was $21 billion in 2002.

As the demand for non-institutional care grows, many state Medicaid programs have expanded home and community-based care. All totaled, the Medicaid program spent $16.4 billion in 2002 for home and community-based care; states paid about $8 billion of that bill.

That translates into a heavy load for each state. On average, long-term care eats up 35 percent of state Medicaid budgets. Among those above the average is North Dakota, where long-term care accounts for 60 percent of the state's Medicaid budget. Four other states that are also well above the average are Connecticut, Kansas, South Dakota and Wisconsin, where long-term care is more than 50 percent of Medicaid costs.

As fiscally challenging as long-term care expenditures are now, the pressure on states will intensify. The aging of the population is inexorable. One hundred years ago, only one in four Americans lived past 65. Today, three in four do, thanks in part to advances in medical science. Medical advances have also helped many younger people injured in accidents or afflicted with devastating illnesses recover, even though many of them remain physically disabled and unable to live independently or without assistance in basic personal care.

Given the fiscal and demographic pressures, it's not surprising that Mike Lewis, chief financial officer of the Alabama Medicaid Agency, wonders "how the system will sustain itself."

Case History

Before the 1970s, the elderly or disabled generally had one alternative to living with family, and that was to take up residence in a nursing home. A societal shift began about 30 years ago with a move to de-institutionalize the developmentally disabled. This was accompanied by an active independent-living movement on the part of people with physical disabilities and a similar push from advocates for the elderly to seek alternatives to nursing homes. "All three groups struggled against the cultural beliefs of the time, which were that if you had a disability, you were broken and somebody needed to fix you and that needed to be a health care worker," says Lee Bezanson, of Boston College.

The movement toward de-institutionalization got a big boost from a 1999 Supreme Court decision, *Olmstead v. L.C.* The court ruled that, based on the Americans with Disabilities Act, unjustified institutionalization is a form of discrimination. As long as an individual wanted transfer to the community and was judged to be qualified for community living, the state should work to move him to a less restrictive setting.

The court acknowledged that this might not be immediately possible if the move required "a fundamental alteration" of a state's programs—a sizable limitation that is being tested in courts around the country. Nonetheless, the ruling has been "a catalyst decision," says Sara Rosenbaum, chair of the Depart-

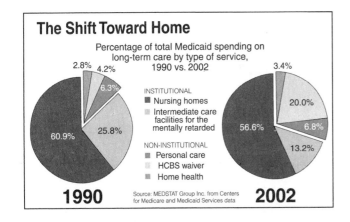

The Shift Toward Home

Percentage of total Medicaid spending on long-term care by type of service, 1990 vs. 2002

INSTITUTIONAL
- Nursing homes
- Intermediate care facilities for the mentally retarded

NON-INSTITUTIONAL
- Personal care
- HCBS waiver
- Home health

1990: 2.8%, 4.2%, 6.3%, 60.9%, 25.8%

2002: 3.4%, 20.0%, 6.8%, 13.2%, 56.6%

Source: MEDSTAT Group Inc. from Centers for Medicare and Medicaid Services data

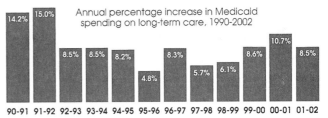

Budget Roller Coaster

Annual percentage increase in Medicaid spending on long-term care, 1990-2002

90-91: 14.2%, 91-92: 15.0%, 92-93: 8.5%, 93-94: 8.5%, 94-95: 8.2%, 95-96: 4.8%, 96-97: 8.3%, 97-98: 5.7%, 98-99: 6.1%, 99-00: 8.6%, 00-01: 10.7%, 01-02: 8.5%

Source: MEDSTAT Group Inc. from Centers for Medicare and Medicaid Services data

ment of Health Policy at George Washington University Medical Center. "The law didn't simply prohibit certain conduct," she says. "It imposed an affirmative requirement among states to start redirecting their public expenditures to get community integration to happen at a reasonable pace."

The federal government is pushing this prescription. Its Centers for Medicare and Medicaid Services, known as CMS, set up a resource network for states to share their experiences with alternative forms of services and by 2000 began awarding "real systems change grants." These provide seed money for states to experiment with fundamental alterations in the delivery of services. In 2001, President George W. Bush issued an executive order requiring federal agencies to "promote community living for persons with disabilities," and two years later the administration launched a five-year program called "Money Follows the Person." It enables an individual in an institution to take the money provided for his or her care in that setting and use it to live in the community instead.

As the demand for alternative-care options emerged, Medicaid began issuing waivers that permit the states to use federal matching funds to finance home or community-based care for patients who would otherwise qualify for nursing-home care. While the cost of that care cannot exceed that of care in a nursing home, Medicaid waivers provide substantial freedom for states to design their own systems.

In addition to those eligible for nursing home care, however, there are elderly and disabled people who qualify for Medicaid and require ongoing assistance, but require a lower level of assistance than a nursing home provides. All states offer home health services, largely medical in nature, but they are often very limited. About 30 states provide some level of personal care, which is not medical but includes help with basic personal activities: dressing, bathing, eating, using the bathroom, shopping or managing medicines. There also are state-financed services that can help prevent the need for more expensive institutional care.

Complications

Logic suggests that keeping Medicaid patients out of institutions and in their communities would drive down program

costs. In Arkansas, for example, the cost of caring for a person through home and community-based services available through the state's Elder Choices waiver program—homemaker services, a personal emergency response system, adult day care and a respite program for family caregivers—is a third as much as placing that person in a nursing home. In Vermont, it costs $25,000 a year to provide care to someone at home and $50,000 in a nursing home.

But the long-term care fiscal ledger is more complicated than that. Individuals who use non-institutional care are often a different patient base than those who enter nursing homes. An analysis by the University of Michigan found that 45 percent of state Medicaid patients receiving waiver-funded home-care services were at the lower end of the spectrum in terms of the acuity of their personal and health needs, whereas only 8 percent of nursing home residents were at that same level.

When Michigan expanded its Medicaid waiver for home care, the state went from paying for 2,000 days a year of home care to 3 million days a year. "But we didn't see a 3 million-day decline in nursing home use. It was flat," says Paul Reinhart, Michigan's Medicaid director. When the state put a lid on home-care enrollment, demand for nursing home placement did not, as one would expect, increase. "It's decoupled," Reinhart says. "Nursing home utilization doesn't decline unless there is some forceful front-end mechanism that really constrains enrollment in nursing homes."

Funny Figures

To control long-term care spending, states need to tamp down their nursing home bill, but lowering those costs isn't as simple as, say, capping nursing home enrollment for Medicaid patients. To start with, nursing home finances are similar to those of an airline. It costs a lot to fly a Boeing 747 from New York to Los Angeles, but the costs are about the same whether the plane is full of bi-coastal fliers or has only three people on board. The airline still needs fuel, pilots, flight attendants and, of course, the 747. The same applies to nursing homes. Cutting down on the population of any individual home doesn't save much money. The facility still has to spend a set amount of money—on utilities, on the mortgage, on the medical infrastructure—to keep operating, whether the home is full of patients or nearly empty.

As a result, simple reductions in nursing home populations don't substantially lower a nursing home's costs—or the price

The Long-Term Care Tab

Long-term care expenditures, and institutional vs. non-institutional care as percentage of spending FY2002

STATE	TOTAL LTC SPENDING FY 2002	% CHANGE 2001–02	INSTITUTIONAL CARE AS % TOTAL SPENDING	HOME CARE AS % TOTAL SPENDING
Alabama	$978,581,437	5.5%	77.0%	23.0%
Alaska	$198,817,419	27.1	43.9%	56.1%
Arizona*	$22,341,354	48.4	84.0%	16.0%
Arkansas	$704,103,233	8.8	74.7%	25.3%
California	$5,293,058,462	–1.6	64.4%	35.6%
Colorado	$845,928,300	10.1	48.6%	51.4%
Connecticut	$1,894,697,686	2.9	65.4%	34.6%
Delaware	$213,273,008	9.1	73.0%	27.0%
Florida	$2,941,546,297	11.1	74.3%	25.7%
Georgia	$1,269,886,217	15.5	74.5%	25.5%
Hawaii	$242,841,956	15.5	73.3%	26.7%
Idaho	$277,166,785	7.5	64.0%	36.0%
Illinois	$2,732,511,976	5.8	81.8%	18.2%
Indiana	$1,447,190,635	10.7	83.7%	16.3%
Iowa	$1,128,372,617	49.4	80.9%	19.1%
Kansas	$954,446,858	7.6	61.0%	39.0%
Kentucky	$996,229,926	6.5	71.6%	28.4%
Louisiana	$1,871,062,823	11.6	90.2%	9.8%
Maine	$438,813,760	6.8	56.2%	43.8%
Maryland	$1,146,893,390	8.1	71.2%	28.8%
Massachusetts	$2,496,135,688	3.5	64.8%	35.2%
Michigan	$2,389,481,098	0.2	75.7%	24.3%
Minnesota	$2,156,106,529	12.5	51.1%	48.9%
Mississippi	$717,479,703	11.1	87.4%	12.6%
Missouri	$1,954,434,032	16.5	72.9%	27.1%
Montana	$247,938,432	15.1	62.7%	37.3%
Nebraska	$630,758,950	9.0	69.6%	30.4%
Nevada	$187,693,295	15.7	73.4%	26.6%
New Hampshire	$465,133,927	29.8	65.4%	34.6%
New Jersey	$3,442,406,247	7.8	80.1%	19.9%
New Mexico	$491,324,098	19.7	38.2%	61.8%
New York	$14,445,209,022	6.7	62.8%	37.2%
North Carolina	$2,154,225,906	5.7	60.6%	39.4%
North Dakota	$284,396,238	13.4	80.6%	19.4%
Ohio	$4,109,314,347	12.8	83.5%	16.5%
Oklahoma	$881,771,565	8.7	63.8%	36.2%
Oregon**	$768,706,305	–28.2	27.1%	72.9%
Pennsylvania	$5,541,859,959	8.3	81.2%	18.8%
Rhode Island	$453,786,912	6.3	59.3%	40.7%
South Carolina	$864,374,865	9.6	65.4%	34.6%
South Dakota	$259,654,434	9.8	73.2%	26.8%
Tennessee	$1,418,262,915	18.0	84.4%	15.6%
Texas	$3,665,310,642	11.5	70.4%	29.6%
Utah	$258,915,418	7.6	58.2%	41.8%
Vermont	$212,155,946	11.3	44.2%	55.8%
Virginia	$1,250,230,746	23.8	73.1%	26.9%
Washington	$1,592,849,651	11.6	52.7%	47.3%
West Virginia	$577,800,830	8.8	62.1%	37.9%
Wisconsin	$2,193,324,965	21.0	70.4%	29.6%
Wyoming	$133,927,383	18.7	49.2%	50.8%

*Arizona has a statewide managed care system. These figures reflect only the very small fee-for-service population.
**Drop in spending is due to significant one-time costs in 2001.
Source: MEDSTAT Group Inc. from Centers for Medicare and Medicaid Services data

The Promise of Coverage

INSURANCE FOR LONG-TERM HEALTH CARE has yet to make it into the mainstream of financial planning. Most Americans carry health insurance that covers them, whatever their age may be, in case of a heart attack or the onset of diabetes—but not if they come down with Alzheimer's or suffer the aftereffects of disabling events that often occur with the onset of old age.

Medicare does not provide long-term care for the chronically debilitated, but Medicaid does. And that can be a problem. There is concern that, in an effort to make sure they have access to care, some elderly citizens are artificially impoverishing themselves to qualify for Medicaid. While it is illegal for someone to give away money for the purpose of making himself eligible for Medicaid, there are huge loopholes, and there are attorneys and financial planners who specialize in what is sometimes called "Medicaid estate planning." The effect of this, asserts Stephen A. Moses, president of the Center for Long-term Care Financing, "is that people with very substantial income and assets qualify routinely for Medicaid."

How routine and how substantial a problem this is for Medicaid is uncertain. But several states are trying to fight the problem and help plan for the financial burdens of long-term care by encouraging citizens—middle-aged and older—to invest in an alternative: long-term care insurance. Right now, under 10 percent of the elderly, and a smaller portion of middle-aged adults, have purchased private health insurance to cover their long-term care.

That said, the number of people buying long-term care insurance is increasing, and the policies themselves are much improved. More policies are now comprehensive and have a better balance of institutional and home-based coverage. States are also coming up with assistance. In 2002, about half the states offered some form of tax incentive for people who buy long-term care insurance. And some states, such as Minnesota and North Carolina, include long-term care insurance benefits for their own employees. "They get quality coverage for their constituency, and they serve as a role model for other employers," says Mark Meiners, associate director of the University of Maryland Center on Aging.

Four states have been particularly aggressive in pushing long-term care insurance. California, Connecticut, Indiana and New York started programs in the early 1990s that offered double protection for those who buy the insurance. Someone who purchases, say, $100,000 of insurance is able to shield $100,000 in personal assets. That means that after the $100,000 in insurance is used up, the shielded assets are not counted against eligibility requirements for Medicaid. Congress barred other states from instituting similar programs in 1993 but grandfathered these four in. The Bush administration has indicated an interest in revisiting this approach.

---

states have to pay for Medicaid patients living in the facility. For instance, when the number of patients in Kansas nursing homes dropped by 13 percent between 1996 and 2001, the per-person bill for Medicaid patients doubled. And in Idaho, when the nursing facility population declined by 7 percent during the same time period, the bill for the state's patients increased by 39 percent.

It's only when many beds in a nursing home are closed—or the facility is shut down altogether—that Medicaid can realize savings on its nursing home bills. But almost any state action to control nursing home costs—whether it's by limiting the number of beds that can be built or operated or other means—runs smack into powerful state-level nursing home lobbyists. They have proven themselves adept at pressuring legislatures to increase rates and keep up the count of nursing home beds. They've also been effective in fighting attempts to siphon off long-term care resources for other service options. One convincing argument for legislators, many of whom have a nursing home in their district: Nursing homes are good for local economies and provide jobs.

"The business interests in the nursing home sector are very powerful," says Barbara Edwards, Medicaid director in Ohio, where 83.5 percent of the state's Medicaid budget goes to institutional care. Nursing home reimbursement is set by statute, and the facilities are guaranteed rate adjustments. "Change is inevitable," she says, "but it will be a slow change becasue so much revenue is tied up in bricks and mortar."

In Louisiana last winter, the state's executive branch proposed diverting some nursing home residents into home and community programs—a potential blow to an industry in which 7,000 beds in the state are currently empty. The reason behind the proposal was simple. "The demand for nursing home care is declining. And yet we have this vast institutional network that we continue to support," says David Hood, secretary of the Louisiana Department of Health and Hospitals. Nonetheless, the proposal went nowhere, and the lobbyists' role in fighting it off was clear.

Remedies

Limiting Supply

Gaining control over the supply of nursing home beds is clearly one key to taming the cost of long-term care. States can use certificate-of-need programs to restrict the building or purchase of new medical facilities or equipment, nursing homes included. But many states have abandoned the certificate-of-need approach, and that limits their ability to cap nursing home supply. A case in point is Utah. After it eliminated certificates of need in the 1980s, a number of new nursing homes opened and occupancy rates slipped to 84 percent by the mid-1980s. In 1989, when the state placed a moratorium on accepting new nursing home providers for Medicaid, the old providers kept adding beds. Occupancy is now at 75 percent. "We are hugely over-bedded," says John Williams, the state's long-term care director.

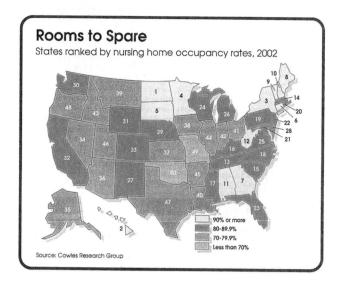

Rooms to Spare

States ranked by nursing home occupancy rates, 2002

90% or more
80-89.9%
70-79.9%
Less than 70%

Source: Cowles Research Group

Oregon and Vermont, on the other hand, have both been quite effective at controlling the growth of nursing homes through certificates of need. Oregon has used more than the blunt hammer of regulation. The state initially sweetened the pot with incentives for nursing home operators to develop alternative services, such as assisted-living facilities. These are apartment-like complexes that provide living quarters in individual apartments but also make available basic non-nursing services—personal care, meals, transportation and the like. This less expensive form of long-term care did get overbuilt, however, and there is now a moratorium on new construction. The state's success in shifting people away from nursing home care has resulted in low occupancy levels as well.

A critical element in developing Oregon's approach was the work legislators did on the state's Nurse Practice Act. In many states, such laws restrict the performance of a variety of patient-care tasks to nurses. Oregon embraced the concept of teaching and transferring skills to other individuals who could then perform them at lower cost. The newly trained personnel also helped address another issue, the shortage of nurses, particularly in the field of long-term care.

The changes dovetailed well with Oregon's overall attitude toward long-term care, which is to build a home and community services infrastructure for people who can afford to pay their own way as well as for those dependent on Medicaid.

Thanks to its tough line on limiting nursing home beds, Oregon was able to divert spending on nursing facilities to home and community care. Today, the state devotes a significantly higher proportion of its long-term care budget to home and community programs than any other state. In so doing, its overall long-term care costs are well below the national average: $604 per capita compared with the U.S. average of $996 per capita.

Vermont is on a similar course. As the state began to realize savings from limiting nursing home beds, it put the unspent money in a trust fund. That fund was then used to provide seed money to develop community programs. "We made smart investments," says Patrick Flood, commissioner of aging. "The

more you build the system, the more people can go to it, and the fewer people go to nursing homes." According to a 2002 AARP report, the percentage of long-term care dollars that Vermont spent in nursing homes dropped from 55.4 percent in 1996 to 44.1 percent in 2001. But it's still using nursing homes efficiently. The occupancy rate is 90.6 percent, compared to the U.S. average of 82.5 percent.

Leveling Care

Several states have been able to hold down long-term care costs by making sure that the nursing home option is reserved only for those whose needs cannot be met safely in less restrictive—and less expensive—ways. This is only possible, of course, if a wide range of alternatives is available. But the approach starts with, in effect, a system of triage.

Maine, for instance, created a uniform assessment system in 1995 that is carried out by an independent agency. The agency oversees admissions for both private- and public-pay nursing home stays.

Arizona has a particularly unusual system, one that has helped that state achieve an enviable record: Its nursing-home population is 1.1 percent of residents who are 65 or older—well below the U.S. average of 3.7 percent.

To accomplish this, the state starts with individual screening to see if an applicant for care qualifies for long-term services. Those who do are then assigned to a managed care organization that receives a pre-set payment for every individual under its care—a blended rate corresponding to nursing home costs and home-based costs that is generally similar for every individual for whom it provides care. The MCO—five of the seven that cater to the elderly and disabled long-term community are county run—helps its patients select the setting that's right for them, but there is a clear incentive to keep people in their homes as long as those services can be offered at less cost than a nursing home.

What's to stop managed care officials from overutilizing low-cost options? "If the program contractors don't ensure that they have the right amount and type of services for those people living in home and community-based settings, they will experience more acute care and more emergency room utilization later on," says Alan Schafer, program manager for Arizona's long-term care system. In Arizona's model, those cost increases will be born by the managed care organization, not shifted to some other group.

Arizona isn't just trusting to fiscal pain to assure that care is appropriate. The state has established a number of quality-assurance mechanisms to make sure that people are getting good services and that they are being placed in a program that provides the proper level of care.

Another creative but simple approach to determining who gets what kind of care is the way Vermont handles its waiting list for home and community-based services. Instead of admitting people on a first-come, first-served basis, the state sets priorities: Those in the greatest need—the ones most likely to end up in a nursing home if they have to wait for services—are pushed to the front of the list.

In an effort to expand on that idea, Vermont is currently asking CMS to approve a waiver that will allow the state to divide the people who qualify for long-term care into two groups: a higher need group and a lower need group. Those with the most acute needs would have a choice: They would be entitled to either home and community-based care or nursing home care, depending on what would be the most appropriate level of care for them. After that population is taken care of, the money that remains would be spent on those in the lower-need group.

Cash and Counseling

The approach that may have the greatest promise for national overhaul of long-term care is called "Cash and Counseling." Since 1996, it has been jointly funded by the Robert Wood Johnson Foundation and the federal government.

The idea is to give people who need long-term care—the frail elderly, the disabled—the choice of using cash to purchase the personal care, equipment, remodeling or other services that they need to keep them living at home safely. Instead of using an agency, the recipients (or a responsible family member on their behalf) are put in charge of hiring and firing employees and arranging for care by the individuals they choose.

To help people make their plans and choices, a counselor or consultant helps them establish a budget that will meet their needs. The adviser also stays in contact with each client to make sure that all is going well. A bookkeeping service is offered for people who want help in administrative and financial tasks, such as paying employment taxes.

The program has been implemented in Arkansas, Florida and New Jersey, with a total of 6,700 individuals. Results are being closely watched.

The first set of evaluations centered on Arkansas, since it was the first to get the program up and running. Arkansas won an A for its efforts. There were no instances of fraud or abuse—one of the big fears officials have when control shifts from a bureaucracy to an individual. Since 1998, when the program started, only four people out of the 3,000 who have enrolled were shifted out of the program because of problems in the way they were handling their own services.

The differences Cash and Counseling makes are clear. When outcomes for those in a control group in the old system were compared to those in the new program, the disparities were "gigantic," according to Kevin J. Mahoney, national program director for Cash and Counseling Demonstration and Evaluation. In Arkansas, there was a 20-point difference in the levels of customer satisfaction. What's more, people who had control over their own employees had equal or fewer health problems, and there was a major reduction in unmet needs.

The program also appeared to provide a solution to the long-standing problem of worker shortages and to providing help in difficult-to-reach rural areas. Since participants were able to hire neighbors or even family members to help them, they had a much easier time finding people to work at difficult hours, such as early morning or weekends. "Access improved markedly," says Mahoney.

This approach was such a notable success in Florida that the legislature unanimously passed a bill making consumer-directed care a permanent option in state programs. In May 2002, CMS came out with model "independence-plus waivers," which provide a template for states to set up programs that are similar to Cash and Counseling. Meanwhile, the Robert Wood Johnson Foundation and its federal government partner are expanding their specific Cash and Counseling program to an additional 10 states.

Prognosis

Regardless of the remedies states try, long-term care is going to grow more expensive. Simple demographics, coupled with advances in medical care, dictate that. The number of elderly people residing alone without living children or siblings is expected to reach 1.2 million in 2020—up from about 600,000 just a decade ago. Some of them will qualify for public programs, and the number of younger people available to pay that bill is declining as a percentage of the population.

The quality of services in nursing homes and in the community is improving—even as those improvements boost costs. And that is likely to continue, as will the pressure for states to deliver more and better services. The power of older Americans as a voting and lobbying group is well known to politicians, and their concerns are not easily ignored.

So, are the states stuck with an inexorably growing budget item for long-term care? Possibly, although state associations are working on the issue. The National Governors Association has argued for a shift in funding responsibilities to the feds for years, but the emphasis is now greater than before. The new chair of the NGA, Idaho Governor Dirk Kempthorne, has announced that making changes in the long-term care system in this country is his number one initiative.

A greater reason for guarded optimism lies in state efforts to encourage citizens to take individual responsibility—expressed, for example, by bolstering families' capacity to take care of one another and by encouraging more affluent citizens to buy insurance to cover long-term care costs.

What appears to be missing from the equation is appropriate education of the American people about the horrific financial burdens that await them. Just as many self-interested Americans finally realized that they could not have a comfortable retirement based exclusively on Social Security income, states would be well advised to encourage a similar awakening regarding long-term care. Only 15 percent of Americans polled by AARP were able to make a remotely accurate guess as to the cost of long-term care; most were totally confused about whether Medicare would pay for their long-term needs. As an AARP report concludes, Americans "know less about long-term care than they think—and than they should."

Universalism Without the Targeting
Privatizing the Old-Age Welfare State

Pamela Herd, PhD[1]

Decades of conservative attempts to scale back Social Security and Medicare, by limiting the program's universality through means testing and drastic benefit cuts, have failed. Thus, after numerous unsuccessful attempts at dismantling the U.S.'s universal old-age welfare state, or even meaningfully restraining its growth, conservative critics have developed a new approach. They are wrapping promarket "privatization" policy proposals in the popular universal framework of Social Security and Medicare. What is fundamentally different about privatization is that it embraces (or at least acquiesces to) key aspects of universalism, including broad-based eligibility and benefits that "maintain accustomed standards of living," which leave universal programs with rock-hard public support. Proponents argue privatization will "save" these programs. What distinguishes this approach from past retrenchment efforts is that promarket privatization policies, while supporting key universal tenets, will retrench Social Security's and Medicare's redistributive facets. Instead of limiting the most popular features of universalism, privatization proposals limit the redistributive elements of our large social insurance programs.

Social Security and Medicare are the United States' most popular social welfare policies. Despite decades of conservative attempts to scale them back, our universal old-age welfare state remains the bedrock of American social policy. Attempts to limit the programs' universality through means testing and drastic benefit cuts have failed. Moreover, Social Security and Medicare have almost exclusively expanded their breadth and depth since their inceptions.

Thus, after numerous unsuccessful attempts at dismantling the U.S.'s universal old-age welfare state, or even meaningfully restraining its growth, conservative critics have developed a new approach. They are wrapping promarket "privatization" policy proposals in the popular universal framework of Social Security and Medicare. As President Bush argues, he wants to institute individual accounts to save Social Security. What is fundamentally different about privatization as a reform goal is that it embraces (or at least acquiesces to) key aspects of universalism, including broad-based eligibility and benefits that "maintain ac-

customed standards of living," which leave universal programs with rock-hard public support (Korpi, 1983; Korpi & Palme, 1998).

Privatizing Social Security and Medicare would not change universal eligibility, unlike means testing reforms or proposals to make contributions to both programs voluntary. And in regards to benefits, a common refrain from privatization proponents runs along these lines: "Such an enormous financial gap (referring to Medicare and Social Security's current fiscal problems) cannot be closed by raising taxes and cutting benefits, which would greatly harm working people and retirees. The only solution is to reform the system by taking advantage of the efficiencies, incentives, competition, and productivity of the private sector" (Ferraro, 1998). Basically, privatizing will address the program's fiscal problems with a limited, and in some cases, positive impact on benefits. The validity of these claims are addressed in this article. Nonetheless, true or not, the key claim with this new reform approach is the promise to maintain key features of universal policies, particularly broad-based eligibility and generous benefits, which keeps middle-class Americans happy and the program popular.

But while privatization proponents promise a generous and robust old-age welfare state, privatization will retrench the redistributive aspects of both Social Security and Medicare. Ironically, past less popular retrenchment efforts, including means testing and even benefit cuts, did not directly challenge the redistributive nature of these programs.

The Political Strength of Universal Programs

Throughout the world, universal programs, like Social Security and Medicare, are consistently the most popular social welfare policies. Basically, when all citizens contribute to and benefit from a social policy it engenders enormous amounts of public support and loyalty for those policies. The evidence for this is overwhelming (Korpi & Palme, 1998). Any cuts or retrenchment to these programs must pass the muster of middle-class voters who benefit from them, and politicians are loathe to risk negative reactions from such a large voting block.

[1]LBJ School of Public Affairs, University of Texas, Austin.

Any approach that would have significantly and negatively impacted the Social Security benefits of middle-class Americans, thereby undermining the program's universal principles, has gained no traction. Conservative politicians in the United States have faced voters' wrath in the past when they have attempted to do just that. Republican nominee Barry Goldwater's suggestion that participation in Social Security be made "voluntary" became a symbol of his "radical conservativism" (Derthick, 1979, p. 187) and contributed to his landslide loss to Lyndon Johnson in the 1964 election. Throughout the 1980s and into the 1990s proposals to means test Social Security benefits fell on deaf ears. Reagan was attacked in the 1980s for proposals to reduce Social Security benefits. Examples like these led to Social Security's nickname as the "Third Rail" of politics. Thus, during the past 50 years, most changes to Social Security have expanded the number of beneficiaries and the size of those benefits.

Medicare, created in 1965 compared to Social Security's inception in 1935, has a similar, albeit a much shorter, political history. Most changes to the program have expanded, as opposed to retrenched, benefits. The most recent of which was the inclusion of a prescription drug benefit. And programmatic reforms that would undermine its universal principles have been met with significant resistance. One of the prime examples of this is the 1988 Medicare Catastrophic Coverage Act, which while expanding benefits, would have instituted significantly higher charges for higher income beneficiaries. The Act was unpopular with seniors, and it was repealed in 1989 (Rice, Desmond, & Gabel, 1990).

What connects all these past reform efforts is that they did not explicitly challenge Social Security's and Medicare's redistributive features. Instead, they tried to limit the programs' universality through means testing or significantly limit the depth of that universality by advocating large benefit cuts. Means testing, in theory, is actually more redistributive. And benefit cuts, though they would be hardest for the poorest, would not alter the programs' redistributive structures. Of course, though, the long-term concern with means testing or dramatic benefit cuts is that they would *eventually* destroy our most successful redistributive social policies by undermining the programs' popularity among the general public; means testing and drastically cutting benefits would hamper middle-class benefits and thus their support for the old-age welfare state.

This is not to say, however, that small benefit cuts, means testing, and decreasing eligibility ages have not happened or that they are no longer being proposed. Universalism has been "stretched" (Kingson, 1994). Social Security's eligibility age rose from 65 to 67, and higher income beneficiaries now have their benefits taxed. In the next few years, high-income Medicare beneficiaries will pay higher premiums, and changes in 1997 entailed that beneficiaries would pay more for their benefits. Further, proposals to privatize have been accompanied by proposals to reduce benefits to offset Social Security's long-term fiscal problems. But these potential benefit cuts are a separate policy issue from privatization. Moreover, advocates argue that necessary benefits cuts due to Social Security's fiscal problems will be smaller because of privatization.

Ultimately, what makes privatization different from past retrenchment efforts is that it embraces key aspects of universalism to generate public support for reforms while attacking these programs' redistributive features that have for so long been protected within the programs' popular universal frameworks. That said, I am not arguing that privatization will have no negative impact on universality. The extent to which universal programs inspire social solidarity and mutual obligation would likely be harmed by a reform that fosters the individualistic, rather than collective, aspects of Social Security. Moreover, privatization would likely weaken important insurance aspects of the program, particularly disability and spousal and survivor benefits. That said, Social Security has always fostered an individualistic spirit by clearly linking individual retirement worker benefits, and to a lesser extent disability benefits, with individual earnings. In the end, most privatization proponents claim privatization will maintain the aspects of universalism that keep programs popular—broad-based eligibility and generous benefits.

The Growing Popularity of Privatization

Unlike past retrenchment efforts, the idea of privatization is gaining traction among the public. Support for privatizing Social Security varies from 50% to 70% depending on the question wording, though the support is far greater among younger than older Americans. Contrastingly, public support for past retrenchment efforts is far weaker. The percentage of individuals approving means testing Social Security benefits comes in at about 40%, while reducing benefits comes in at 35% (Public Agenda, 2004). Even in the most recent polls where support for President Bush's partial privatization plan has fallen, the majority of Americans (56%) support diverting a portion of their payroll tax into an individual account, whereas support for means testing benefit cuts is much lower (Social Polling Report, 2005).

Support for privatizing Medicare is even more striking. To fix Medicare's fiscal problems, almost 8 in 10 Americans support allowing seniors to choose among many private health plans with a fixed monetary contribution from the government (Employee Benefit Research Institute [EBRI], 2001). Comparatively, 54% support increasing Medicare premiums for those with incomes above $50,000, while 27% favor increasing the age of eligibility (EBRI).

The following two sections, which explore Social Security and Medicare separately, answer these two questions. First, why is privatization more popular than past reform or retrenchment efforts? Specifically, how is this reform agenda being sold? Second, how does this reform agenda line up with the conservative agenda and what are the impacts of this on the redistributive elements of Social Security and Medicare?

Social Security

Most Social Security privatization proposals entail shifting about 2%–4% of the 12.4% payroll tax (split between employers and employees) into individual accounts that Americans would invest in the stock market. That 2%–4% would now be a contribution to an individual account. The key reason for the popularity of these reform proposals, compared to past reform approaches, is that they do not undermine the principles of universalism that have kept the program popular. These reforms promise the maintenance of relatively generous benefits and universal eligibility. In fact, proponents argue that privatizing Social Security will "save" it from bankruptcy and limit the need for large benefit cuts to fix its fiscal problems (President's Commission to Strengthen Social Security, 2001).

While I will examine these claims momentarily, what is critical to point out is that a major reason why privatization has been a relatively popular reform idea is because politicians and policy advocates no longer talk about eliminating or downsizing the program. Instead, privatization is framed as a way to save Social Security. Yet, this is a reform that can still meet a common conservative principle: limited government intervention. Specifically, privatization would give individuals more control over their payroll taxes, and the government would have a lesser ability to redistribute. Privatizations falls in line with past retrenchment efforts, means testing and benefit cuts, because it shifts individual contributions back toward individuals who would bear the risks and rewards of controlling these resources.

Part of the public support for privatization is because proponents argue it will help save a bankrupt social policy. But is it really bankrupt? Many have shown how the "crisis" is severely overstated (Quadagno, 1996). The Social Security trustees estimate that the program's 75-year shortfall could be fixed by a 1.9% increase in payroll tax (shared between employers and employees), which hasn't been raised since 1983, while the Congressional Budget Office (CBO, 2004a) estimates a 1% increase. Another way to lend some proportion to the issue is that while President Bush has specifically argued Social Security is financially unsustainable in its current form, the money spent on the recent tax cut would have completely offset the 75-year shortfall. Finally, the projections that show a deficit are based on all kinds of assumptions about fertility, mortality, immigration, and the economy. For those in their 20s, the analogous forecast is predicting what their children, who are not born yet, will be doing in retirement. (Herd & Kingson, 2005)

Further, would privatization "save" Social Security? The argument to prefund the system is theoretically appealing. There would be no fiscal problem if each individual was funding their own retirement. But when theory hits the ground, the possibility that creating individual accounts will financially save Social Security is not even a remote certainty (Diamond & Orszag, 2002). First and foremost it would cost around 2 trillion dollars to switch the system over. Current beneficiaries need their benefits as future individual account holders shift their payroll taxes towards those accounts. Thus, there is a need for additional revenue.

And though proponents argue privatization would increase peoples' benefit, this claim is questionable. The privatization proposal that came from the President's Commission to Strengthen Social Security made benefit comparisons between the current and proposed system based on current projected benefit levels reduced by 30% to account for the shortfall (Diamond & Orszag, 2002). Then, using this baseline, they claimed privatization would increase Social Security benefits when, in fact, benefits would be substantially reduced to address the shortfall. Aside from the shortfall issue, administrative costs and the ability of individuals to invest wisely call into question whether individual accounts can produce the strong return proponents of privatization hope for (CBO, 2004a).

How Privatizing Undermines Redistribution

The effort to privatize Social Security has its roots in neoliberalism, which argues against most government intervention. The basic theory is that income is best left in the hands of individuals, as opposed to the government. The notion of redistribution, shifting resources from wealthier to poorer Americans, runs contrary to this sentiment. And this is precisely why opponents of government intervention dislike Social Security. While it is questionable that privatizing Social Security will "save" it, there is little doubt it will have a significant and negative impact on the program's progressiveness. So how does creating individual accounts, or privatizing Social Security, undermine the program's progressiveness? Privatization limits the program's ability to redistribute.

While Social Security's universal structure has engendered wide public support among middle class Americans, it has also been enormously successful at protecting some of the poorest Americans. In 1970, before the largest expansion of Social Security benefits with the automatic cost of living increases, about 1 in 4 elderly persons lived below the poverty line. In 2003, just 1 in 10 elderly persons lived below the poverty line (Census Bureau, 2004). Comparatively, the poverty rate for children rose and remained stagnant for working-age adults.

Social Security protects poor Americans because, as Theda Skocpol (1991) argues, it "targets within universalism." Poor Americans benefit from the re-distributive benefit formula. Simply, low-income workers have a higher percentage of their lifetime earnings replaced by their benefits than do high-income workers. It is these beneficiaries who are most vulnerable to poverty. Not including Social Security benefits in individuals' incomes raises the poverty rate from 10% to almost 50% (Porter, Larin, & Primus, 1999).

Targeting, however, is done under the cover of universalism. Unlike means tested programs, like the eliminated Aid to Families with Dependent Children (AFDC), which are constantly retrenched because they lack broad support, universal programs like Social Security maintain popular support because everyone contributes to and benefits from the program.

The shift toward individual accounts would restrain Social Security's ability to redistribute resources. The high-income replacement rates that low-income workers receive may be threatened by privatization. Quite simply, the more payroll taxes are diverted to individual accounts, the less the government will be able to redistribute those resources. Of course, women, Blacks, and Hispanics would be particularly hard hit given their relatively low earnings. Compared to the White man's dollar, women still earn just 70 cents, Black women earn just 63 cents, Hispanic women earn 53 cents, and Black and Hispanic men earn 60 cents (National Committee on Pay Equity, 2004).

One of the most enlightening studies of privatization was done in the county of Galveston, Texas (Wilson, 1999). On January 1, 1982, the county opted out of Social Security and developed a privatized system. The study found that those with higher earnings had higher benefits under this plan than they would have under the Social Security system. Contrastingly, low earners had lower benefits under the plan than they would have under Social Security. Their initial benefit was about 4% lower. But because Social Security institutes cost of living increases to offset inflation, the difference grows over time. So after 15 years, their benefit would be 63% of what it would have been under Social Security. More moderate earners would have a higher initial benefit, but after 15 years their benefit would be 91% of their original benefit and after 20 years it would be just 78%. Contrastingly, the highest earners would have an initial benefit 177% of their Social Security benefit. After 20 years it would be equivalent to what their Social Security would have been. Overall, they would have obtained a substantial gain through a private contribution system.

There are numerous reasons other than restricting redistribution as to why disadvantaged groups do not fare well. There is concern about peoples' ability to make good investment decisions (Williamson & Rix, 1999). Others point out the relatively high administrative costs for small accounts (CBO, 2004b). Women, who live 7 years longer than men on average, will not gain as much from individual benefits more directly linked with overall contributions; Social Security does not penalize women for their longer life spans (Williamson & Rix). And of course the smaller one's income in retirement the less able one is to absorb large changes in income that would likely occur if it was heavily tied to the stock market (Herd & Kingson, 2005).

A final salient concern is how those benefiting from the insurance portion of the program, particularly disabled workers and survivors, would fare given money would be shifted out of the insurance portion of the program and into private accounts. The basic insurance benefit would thus be around one third lower for survivors and disabled beneficiaries (Diamond & Orszag, 2002). Survivors, however, could inherit whatever savings had built up in the deceased worker's account, which would be highly dependent on the age he or she died at. The size of disabled workers' accounts would be highly dependent on the age at which they became disabled. Generally, the individual account, particularly for disabled workers, would not have accrued enough value, leading to lower benefits overall than under the current system.

Medicare

Currently, older Medicare beneficiaries pay the same premiums, deductibles, and co-payments to their primary health insurance provider: the federal government. A small percentage of beneficiaries are covered by HMOs. But regardless of whether beneficiaries participate in fee-for-service or an HMO, individuals are guaranteed a set of covered services (benefits) regardless of cost. It is a defined benefit. Moreover, all those individuals are placed in the same "pool" to determine the cost of premiums. The most common privatization proposal for Medicare would basically entail providing older Americans with a voucher with which they would buy their health insurance coverage from a host of private insurance providers, who would offer an array of different plans with varying copayments and services, in addition to traditional Medicare. In essence, the system would shift toward a defined contribution approach, where a contribution, as opposed to a certain level of benefits, is guaranteed. Unlike in the current system (a defined benefit) where the government contributes more toward sicker and generally poorer beneficiaries, everyone would receive the exact same monetary voucher benefit (a defined contribution). How this amount is determined will depend upon policy details. A pure defined contribution would pay, for example, $500 toward a premium. Another variation, however, premium support, would set the amount at a percentage, say 90%, of the average premium amount. Another key difference is that older Americans would no longer be in the same insurance pool. The result is that premiums and benefits would vary widely.

The reason privatizing Medicare is a more popular reform than limiting eligibility through significant means testing or raising the program's eligibility age is because, similar to privatizing Social Security, privatizing Medicare is being sold as the way to save this universal program. Some privatization proponents argue it would protect Medicare from fiscal ruin and improve its benefits without requiring increases to the eligibility age, benefit cuts, or significant means testing (Bush, 2004). Other proponents, however, are more pragmatic and acknowledge benefits cuts will be necessary (Pauly, 2004). While I will examine these claims momentarily, it is critical to note that privatization is being sold in such a way that does not challenge the basic aspects of universalism that make Medicare popular. Everyone contributes and everyone would continue benefiting; the size of the beneficiary pool would not be decreased due to an increased age of eligibility or significant means testing. What would change is the extent to which Medicare subsidizes the sickest, and generally the poorest, beneficiaries.

Much like the claims made by proponents of privatizing Social Security, there is no evidence that privatizing Medicare will improve its fiscal problems. Medicare's dilemma is far more serious than Social Security's. Currently, Medicare comprises 2.7% of gross domestic product (GDP). By 2030 it will comprise 7% of GDP (MedPAC, 2004). But what is often ignored is that Medicare's fiscal problems are rooted in the larger problems of the U.S. health care system. Overall, health care spending is expected to rise from 15.3% of GDP to 25% of GDP from 2004 to 2030 (MedPAC). The only country in the industrialized world without the government as the primary health insurer for its citizens and residents is also consistently the most expensive system in the world.

Proposals to privatize would severely limit the government's role as the primary health insurer to all older Americans and expand the private sector's role. But Medicare has been far more effective at controlling health care costs than the private sector has been (Boccuti & Moon, 2003). From 1972 to 2002, average annual cost increases have been 9.6% in Medicare compared to 11.1% in the private sector. There are two reasons for the government's success at holding prices down. First, the large pool of beneficiaries (almost all older Americans) makes it easy to negotiate low prices with health care providers and suppliers. Second, it has much lower administrative costs: 3% compared to the private sector's 12.8% (Davis, 2004).

The goal of privatizing Medicare is to reduce the government's current role as the primary health insurer for almost older Americans. Proponents argue that older Americans should be able to "decide what kind of health plans they want, the kinds of benefits packages they want, the medical treatments and procedures they want, and the premiums, co-payments, deductibles, and coinsurance they are willing to pay" (Lemieux, 2003; Moffit, 2004). More choice will lead to more competition and further reduce prices. Ultimately, proponents argue that the increased competition that results from privatizing Medicare is a way to "save" and improve Medicare without resorting to benefit cuts or tax increases.

But there is no evidence that increased competition will reduce costs (Moon & Herd, 2002; Rice & Desmond, 2002). First, the larger number of companies, and consequently different health plans, involved will increase administrative costs. Second, for competition to reduce costs, elderly people would have to switch plans on an almost yearly basis, but there is significant evidence that older adults will not switch plans (Buchmueller, 2000). Third, it will be very difficult for seniors to sort out which plans will give them the most for their money. It is difficult to compare plan benefits and costs because plans vary so widely within and between health insurance companies.

How Privatization Will Undermine Redistribution Within Medicare

How does Medicare redistribute? The redistributive nature of Medicare is less obvious than Social Security's. But the key progressive feature of Medicare is that, regardless of how sick or poor, individuals are guaranteed access to the same basic coverage at the same costs as wealthier and healthier individuals. This is most certainly not the case for younger Americans who may not be able to access health insurance or often have to pay considerably more for it depending on their employment status, health status, and where they live.

The key to understanding Medicare's success is understanding what older people's health insurance dilemmas were before Medicare. Before Medicare was enacted in 1965 about three quarters of older Americans had inadequate health insurance coverage, and half had no coverage whatsoever (Century Foundation, 2001). Wealthier older Americans were the only ones able to afford health insurance. Moreover, buying health insurance as individuals in the market left them with few protections. The sickest older Americans could be charged exorbitant premiums making the coverage unaffordable. Now all older

Americans are guaranteed affordable health insurance. Their Medicare premiums are not effected by how sick they are or where they live. And most polls show approval ratings for the program at almost 90% among the elderly people who rely on it (Public Agenda, 2004).

Again, the long-term goal of privatization supporters is to dramatically reduce the role of Medicare fee-for-service or rather limit the government's current role as the primary health insurance provider for older Americans. Though the government does contract out Medicare's administrative responsibility to private companies, ultimately the government determines what services beneficiaries receive and how much they have to pay. Under a defined contribution approach, the government plan—Medicare fee-for-service—would just be one of hundreds of primary health insurance plans with varying premiums and services covered.

The problem for poorer and sicker beneficiaries is that these changes are likely to increase their health care costs. Multiple insurance pools make it much harder to spread and redistribute the costs of health care from the sickest and poorest beneficiaries to the healthiest and wealthiest. In the current system, everyone is in the same insurance pool so costs are spread evenly; the more pools, the harder to evenly spread costs. The problem is that HMOs are skilled at attracting the healthiest individuals who bring the highest profits. Studies show that sicker individuals end up concentrated in certain plans when people have multiple options. With a defined contribution approach, the sickest and most expensive beneficiaries would be concentrated in fee-for-service Medicare. Sick and expensive beneficiaries concentrated in one plan drives up costs, leaving these vulnerable beneficiaries with extraordinarily high premiums, deductibles, and copayments (Moon & Herd, 2002; Rice & Desmond, 2002).

Unlike with Social Security, partial privatization of Medicare has already begun. And these experiments demonstrate the problems with privatization for sicker and poorer Americans. The main example is the participation of HMOs in Medicare. Millions of older Americans have participated in an HMO as opposed to traditional Medicare fee-for-service. Beneficiary premiums remained the same, but for years those elders in HMOs, who are the healthiest and wealthiest, received better benefits than the average participant in Medicare fee-for-service. The government was overpaying the HMOs. But as soon as the reimbursements were corrected, HMOs began dropping Medicare coverage. In 1998, 17% of beneficiaries participated in an HMO; by 2004 that had fallen to 11% (Kaiser Family Foundation, 2004a). In 2002, Congress significantly increased reimbursements to HMOs to further encourage their participation. Currently, the government pays an extra $552 per enrollee in Medicare HMOs as compared to fee-for-service, even though the sickest and poorest beneficiaries are in Medicare fee-for-service (Cooper, Nicholas, & Biles, 2004).

The second piece of privatization in Medicare is the new prescription drug bill, whereby private insurers, as opposed to the government, will provide coverage (Kaiser Family Foundation, 2004b). The benefit premium will vary depending on where beneficiaries live and what kind of plan they choose. Beneficiaries already in HMOs will simply receive their coverage through them. Beneficiaries who want to remain in Medicare fee-for-service (who are sicker and poorer beneficiaries) will have to buy an additional policy from a private insurer, which is on top of whatever Medigap coverage they currently have. There is concern that Medicare fee-for-service participants will have to pay more for less coverage due to the stand-alone nature of the coverage. The overall incentive is to push more individuals into HMOs and away from fee-for-service Medicare.

Conclusion

Neither privatizing Social Security nor privatizing Medicare explicitly threatens two basic universal principles that keep these programs popular: broad-based eligibility and relatively generous benefits for the middle class. While additional policy changes to deal with these programs' fiscal problems could threaten either of these principles, proponents argue that privatization will help offset the impact of any benefit cuts. This is likely a key explanation as to why these reforms have received far more public support than past attempts at retrenching Social Security and Medicare. Instead of attacking Social Security and Medicare as draining and wasteful programs that should be limited, proponents argue privatization will "save" these programs.

What privatization does clearly limit is the redistribution that occurs within these programs. The magnitude of the impact on redistribution, however, will depend on policy details. A few recent proposals for Medicare and Social Security have tried to limit the impact of reform on poor beneficiaries (see Pauly, 2004). That said, the basic premise of these proposals is to more tightly link individual contributions with individual benefits, which reduces the potential for redistribution. Given Social Security's and Medicare's success at securing the incomes and protecting the health of elderly Americans, we need to pay close attention to the ramifications of privatization on the beneficiaries who need these programs the most.

References

Boccuti, C., & Moon, M. (2003). Comparing Medicare and private insurers. *Health Affairs, 22,* 230–237.

Buchmueller, T. C. (2000). The health plan choice of retirees under managed competition. *Health Services Research, 35,* 949–957.

Bush, G. W. (2004). *Framework to modernize and improve Medicare fact sheet.* Retrieved September 15, 2004, from http://www.whitehouse.gov/news/releases/2003/03/20030304-1.html

Census Bureau. (2004). *Income, poverty, and health insurance coverage in the United States: 2003.* Retrieved September 10, 2004, from http://www.census.gov/prod/2004pubs/p60-226.pdf

Century Foundation. (2001). *Medicare reform.* Retrieved September 10, 2004, from http://www.medicarewatch.org

Congressional Budget Office. (2004a). *The outlook for Social Security.* Retrieved January 15, 2005, from http://www.cbo.gov/showdoc.cfm?index=5530&sequence=0

Congressional Budget Office. (2004b). *Administrative costs of private accounts in Social Security.* Retrieved January 15, 2005, from http://www.cbo.gov/showdoc.cfm?index=5277 &sequence=0

Cooper, N., Nicholas, L., & Biles, B. (2004). *The cost of privatization.* New York: Commonwealth Fund.

Davis, K. (2004). Making health care affordable for all Americans. Testimony before the Senate Committee on Health, Education, Labor, and Pensions, January 28, 2004. Retrieved January 15, 2005, from http://www.cmwf.org/usr_doc/davis_senatehelptestimony_714.pdf

Derthick, M. (1979). *Policymaking for Social Security.* Washington, DC: Brookings Institution.

Diamond, P., & Orszag, P. (2002). *Reducing benefits and subsidizing individual accounts.* New York: The Century Fund.

Employee Benefit Research Institute (EBRI). (2001). *Medicare awareness, satisfaction, confidence, and reform.* Retrieved September 10, 2004, from http://www.ebri.org/facts/0701fact.pdf

Ferrara, P. (1998). *The next step for Medicare reform.* Policy analysis no. 305. Washington, DC: CATO Institute.

Herd, P., & Kingson, E. (2005). Selling Social Security. In R. Hudson (Ed.), *The future of age-based public policy* (pp. 183–204). Baltimore, MD: Johns Hopkins University Press.

Kaiser Family Foundation. (2004a). *Medicare fact sheet: Medicare Advantage, March 2004.* Retrieved January 15, 2005, from http://www.kff.org

Kaiser Family Foundation. (2004b). *Summaries of the Medicare Modernization Act of 2003.* New York: Author.

Kingson, E. (1994). Testing the boundaries of universality. *The Gerontologist, 34,* 736–742.

Korpi, W. (1983). *The Democratic class struggle.* London: Routledge.

Korpi, W., & Palme, J. (1998). The paradox of redistribution and strategies of equality. *American Sociological Review, 63,* 661-687.

Lemieux, J. (2003). *Explaining premium support.* Retrieved September 1, 2004, from http://www.centrists.org

MedPac. (2004). *A data book: Health care spending and the Medicare program.* Medicare Payment Advisory Commission. Retrieved September 1, 2004, from http://www.medpac.gov/publications/congressional_reports/Jun04DataBookSec6.pdf

Moffit, R. (2004). What federal workers are doing today that you can't. Webmemo #604. Washington, DC: The Heritage Foundation.

Moon, M., & Herd, P. (2002). *A place at the table.* New York: The Century Foundation.

National Committee on Pay Equity. (2004). Fact sheet on gender pay gap. Retrieved September 3, 2004, from http://www.pay-equity.org/info.html

Pauly, M. (2004). Means testing in Medicare. *Health Affairs,* web exclusive, W4 (549).

Porter, K., Larin, K., & Primus, W. (1999). *Social security and poverty among the elderly.* Washington, DC: Center on Budget and Policy Priorities.

President's Commission to Strengthen Social Security. (2001). *Strengthening Social Security and creating personal wealth for all Americans.* Retrieved September 4, 2004, from http://www.css.gov

Public Agenda. (2004). *Opinion polling on Medicare.* Retrieved Month, day, year, from http://www.publicagenda.org/issues/major_proposals_detail.cfm ?issue_type=ss&list=1

Quadagno, J. (1996). Social Security and the myth of the entitlement crisis. *The Gerontologist, 36,* 391–399.

Rice, T., & Desmond, K. (2002). *An analysis of reforming Medicare through a premium support plan.* New York: Henry J. Kaiser Foundation.

Rice, T., Desmond, K., & Gabel, J. (1990). The Medicare Catastrophic Coverage Act. *Health Affairs, 9,* 75–87.

Skocpol, T. (1991). Targeting within universalism. In C. Jencks & P. E. Peterson (Eds.), *The urban underclass*, (pp. 411–436). Washington, DC: The Brookings Institution.

Polling Report. (2005). Title of report. Retrieved April 3, 2005, from `http://www.pollingreport.com`

Williamson, J., & Rix, S. (1999). Social Security reform: Implications for women. Boston College, Boston, MA. Retrieved September 1, 2004, from `http://www.bc.edu/centers/crr/papers/wp_1999-07.pdf`

Wilson, T. (1999). Opting out: The Galveston plan and Social Security. PRC WP 99–22, Wharton School, University of Pennsylvania, Philadelphia.

Address correspondence to **Pamela Herd,** *LBJ School of Public Affairs, University of Texas, Austin, PO Box Y, Austin, TX 78713-8925. E-mail: pherd@mail.utexas.edu*

Prescription for change

Lobbying under way for single-paper system

Matt Leingang

A push for universal health coverage is being rekindled in some states by the soaring cost of health care and the lack of political support in Washington for federal changes.

Advocates of a single-payer system—where the government would collect taxes and cover everyone, similar to programs in Canada and across Europe—have introduced bills in at least 18 state legislatures. Some are symbolic gestures, but heated debate is taking place in California and Vermont.

> **"There's no other solution out there. The system we have now is immoral, it's foundering and it's on its last legs."**
>
> David Pavlick, Cleveland

In Ohio, doctors, union officials and religious leaders are gathering signatures to get a single-payer health system placed on a ballot next year.

"The level of misery with private insurers is rising, and that's why we're seeing this increased activity," said Larry Levitt, vice president of the California-based Kaiser Family Foundation, which analyzes health care issues. "But whether one state can succeed, I don't know."

Not since Oregon in 2002 has a state voted on a single-payer health system. Voters there soundly rejected it, as did Californians in 1994. Both times, the proposals came under fierce assault from the medical, insurance and pharmaceutical industries.

However, Oregon supporters are aiming for another ballot measure in 2008, and a bill in California would have the government pay for health care in a state where 7 million people are uninsured.

Across the nation, the number of uninsured is 45 million and rising, and 16 million lack enough insurance to cover all their medical bills.

Premiums for employer-sponsored health plans rose an average of 11.2 percent in 2004, the fourth consecutive year of double-digit growth, according to the Kaiser Family Foundation. Companies are raising employee fees for health care, increasing co-payments and decreasing benefits.

Mainstream medical groups, including the American Medical Association, oppose single-payer systems. The AMA fears they would stifle the development of new medical technology and create longer waits for patient care should government budgets become strapped for money.

Advocates dismiss those arguments as scare tactics.

"There's no other solution out there," said David Pavlick, a member of the United Auto Workers in Cleveland, which has endorsed the Ohio campaign. "The system we have now is immoral, it's foundering and it's on its last legs."

A single-payer system would be financed through a mix of payroll tax increases and new taxes on personal income. The new taxes would take the place of insurance premiums that many people currently pay for health coverage, and there would be no out-of-pocket expenses.

States would use their leverage to negotiate lower prices for prescription drugs and other health services. Hospitals and doctors' offices would be relieved of the hassles and expense of dealing with multiple health insurers.

RIDING INTO THE SUNSET
The Geezer Threat

WILLIAM GREIDER

In 1900 Americans on average lived for only 49 years and most working people died still on the job. For those who lived long enough, the average "retirement" age was 85. By 1935, when Social Security was enacted, life expectancy had risen to 61 years. Now it is 77 years—nearly a generation more—and still rising. Children born today have a fifty-fifty chance of living to 100. This inheritance from the last century—the great gift of longer life—surely represents one of the country's most meaningful accomplishments.

Yet the achievement has been transformed into a monumental problem by contemporary politics and narrow-minded accounting. "The nation faces a severe economic threat from the aging of its population combined with escalating health costs," a *Washington Post* editorial warned. Others put it more harshly. "Greedy geezers" are robbing from the young, bankrupting the government. Painful solutions must be taken to avoid financial ruin. Or so we are told.

A much happier conviction is expressed by Robert Fogel, a Nobel Prize-winning economist at the University of Chicago and a septuagenarian himself. America, he reminds us, is a very wealthy nation. The expanding longevity is not a financial burden but an enormous and underdeveloped asset. If US per capita income continues to grow at a rate of 1.5 percent a year, the country will have plenty of money to finance comfortable retirements and high-quality healthcare for all citizens, including those at the bottom of the wage ladder. When politicians talk about raising the Social Security retirement age to 70 in order to "save" the system, they are headed backward and against the tide of human aspirations. The average retirement age, Fogel observes, has been falling in recent decades by personal choice and is now around 63. Given proper financing arrangements, he expects the retirement age will eventually fall to as low as 55—allowing everyone to enjoy more leisure years and to explore the many dimensions of "spiritual development" or "self-realization," as John Dewey called it.

"What then is the virtue of increasing spending on retirement and health rather than goods?" Fogel asked in his latest book, *The Fourth Great Awakening and the Future of Egalitarianism* (2000). "It is the virtue of providing consumers in rich countries with what they want most." What people want is time—more time to enjoy life and learning, to focus on the virtuous aspects of one's nature, to pursue social projects free of economic necessity, to engage their curiosity and self-knowledge or their political values. The great inequity in modern life, as Fogel provocatively puts it, is the "maldistribution of spiritual resources," that is, the economic insecurity that prevents people from exploring life's larger questions. Everyone could attain a fair share of liberating security, he asserts, if government undertook strategic interventions in their behalf.

Fogel's perspective is generally ignored by other economists, but sociologists and psychologists recognize his point in the changing behavior of retirees. The elderly are redefining leisure, finding "fun" in myriad activities that lend deeper meaning to their lives. An informal shadow university has grown up around the nation in which older people are both the students and the teachers. They do "volunteer vacationing" and "foster grandparenting." They rehab old houses for the needy, serve as self-appointed environmental watchdogs or act as ombudsmen for neglected groups like indigent children or nursing-home patients. They dig into political issues with an informed tenacity that often withers politicians. In civic engagement, they are becoming counselors, critics, caregivers and mentors equipped with special advantages—the time and freedom to act, the knowledge and understanding gained only from the experience of living.

When the "largest generation" reaches retirement a few years from now, the baby boomers will doubtless alter the contours of society again, perhaps more profoundly than in their youth. Theodore Roszak, the historian who chronicled *The Making of a Counter Culture* thirty-six years ago, thinks boomers taking up caregiving and mentoring roles will inspire another wave of humanistic social values (perhaps expressed more maturely this time around). "More than merely surviving we will find ourselves gifted with the wits, the political savvy and the sheer weight of numbers to become a major force for change," Roszak wrote in *America the Wise* (1998). "With us, history shifts its rhythm. It draws back from the frenzied pursuit of marketing novelties and technological turnover and assumes the measured pace of humane and sustainable values. We may live to see wisdom become a distinct possibility and compassion the reigning social ethic." The "retired," he predicts, will seek to become reintegrated with the working society and claim a larger role in its affairs. Some elderly may reclaim the ancient role of respected "elders" who keep alive society's deeper truths and remind succeeding generations of their obligations to the nation's longer term. None of these possibilities are likely to unfold, however, if the promise of economic security for retirement is eviscerated in the meantime.

Fogel's optimism sounds eccentric amid the gloom and doom of the Social Security debate and the more threatening deterioration under way in private pensions and personal savings. Fogel skips over the snarled facts of current politics. He thinks big-picture and long-term. He won the Nobel Prize by producing unorthodox economic history that traced the deeper shifts in demographics and living conditions across generations, even centuries. His thinking is especially provocative because the conclusions collide with both left and right assumptions. Fogel is a secular Democrat, yet he extols the conservative evangelical awakening as a valuable social force. He sounds alternately conservative and liberal on economic issues, yet he thinks government should engineer a vast redistribution of financial wealth, from top to bottom, to insure equitable pensions for all.

Fogel's solution is a new national pension system alongside Social Security—a universal "provident fund" that requires all workers to save a significant portion of their wage incomes every year to provide for their future. He proposes a savings rate of 14.7 percent (though taking Social Security benefits and taxes into account, a lower rate would suffice for a start). The contributions would be mandatory but set aside as true personal savings, not as a government tax. The accumulating nest eggs would belong to the individual workers and become a portable pension that goes with them if they change jobs, but the wealth would be invested for them through a broadly diversified pension fund. Employers would no longer be in charge (though they could still contribute to worker savings to attract employees). The government or independent private institutions would manage the money, investing conservatively in stocks, bonds and other income-generating assets while allowing workers only limited, generalized choices on their investment preferences.

Fogel's vision of expanding leisure and greater human fulfillment is actually receding at the moment. The time for big ideas is now.

The concept resembles the forced savings plans adopted in some Asian and Latin American countries, but Fogel's favorite prototype is American: TIAA-CREF, the pension system that exists for nearly all college professors (a nonprofit institution founded in 1917 by Andrew Carnegie). Another model could be the government's own Thrift Savings Plan, which manages savings wealth for federal employees. Lifelong healthcare, Fogel adds, could be guaranteed for all by setting aside another 9.8 percent from current incomes. "If you take the typical academic, we all have TIAA-CREF," he explains. "The universities require of us that we invest anywhere from 12.5 to 17.5 percent of our salaries in a pension fund—mandatory—but it's

all in my name. I can leave it to whomever I want. It has entered my sense of well-being for many years. The fund has earned about 10 percent a year since the 1960s, so retirement is not a burden to the university."

Obviously, people with low or even moderate incomes could not afford such savings rates, and even diligent savings from their low wages would not be enough to pay for either retirement or healthcare. Fogel has a straightforward solution: Tax the affluent to pay for the needy. A tax rate of 2 or 3 percent, applied progressively to families in the top half of income distribution, could finance the "provident fund" for those who can't pay for themselves. "This is a problem, not of inadequate national resources, but of inequity," he observes.

Fogel's big thinking—a system of compulsory savings, with the federal government taking charge—sounds way too radical for this right-wing era, and probably even most Democrats would shy away from the concept. But keep Fogel's solution in mind as we examine the sorry condition of retirement security. The current political debate is not even focused on the right "crisis," much less on genuine solutions. It is not Social Security that's financially threatened but healthcare and the other two pillars of retirement security—employer-run pension plans and the private savings of families. Many millions of baby boomers realize as they approach the "golden years" that they can't afford to retire at all, much less retire early. They will keep working because they lack the wherewithal to stop. Retiring for them would mean a drastic fall in their standard of living. Fogel's vision of expanding leisure and greater human fulfillment is actually receding at the moment. The time for big ideas is now.

Grasshoppers and Ants

When George W. Bush launched Social Security reform with his promise of new personalized savings accounts for everyone, he did not seem to grasp that most Americans already have such accounts. During the past generation tax-exempt 401(k) and IRA accounts—the individualized "defined contribution" approach—became the principal pension plan for working people, displacing the traditional company pension provided by employers who assume the risks and promise a "defined benefit" to workers at retirement. The do-it-yourself version of pensions is a flop, as many Americans have painfully learned. When older employees look at their monthly balance statements, they are more likely to experience fear than Bush's romanticized thrill of individual risk-taking.

Picking stocks for themselves has left many employees, perhaps as many as 40-45 percent, without an adequate nest egg for retirement. When Bush explains further that he intends to divert trillions from Social Security to finance his "ownership society," it makes people even more nervous. Social Security pays very modest average benefits—roughly equivalent to the federal minimum wage—but it is the last safety net. For nearly half of the private-sector workforce, it is the only safety net. The far more threatening problem is elsewhere—shrinking pensions, collapsed personal savings and soaring costs for health insurance.

The bleak reality is reflected in those 401(k) account balances. Of the 48 million families who hold one or more of the accounts, the median value of their savings is $27,000 (which means half of all families have less than $27,000). Among older workers on the brink of retiring (55 to 64 years old) who have personal accounts, the median value is $55,000. That's only enough to buy an annuity that would pay $398 a month, far short of middle-class living standards. What's strange and disturbing about their low accumulations is that these older workers have been investing during the best of times—the "super bull market" of soaring stock prices that lasted nearly twenty years. The Congressional Research Service summarized the sobering results: Median pension savings "would not by themselves provide an income in retirement that most people in the United States would find to be adequate."

This grand experiment was launched nearly twenty-five years ago by Ronald Reagan, but with very little public debate because the pension changes were obscured by more immediate controversies—Reagan's regressive tax cuts and massive budget deficits. His Treasury under secretary explained the reasoning: "The evidence of the past suggests that people do not behave like grasshoppers. They are much more like ants." For lots of reasons, most Americans turned out not to be like the proverbial ants, storing food for winter. People either misjudged their future need for savings or couldn't afford to put much aside or bet wrong in the stock market and got wiped out. But corporate managements turned out to be the true grasshoppers, living for the moment and ignoring the future. Companies took advantage of the 401(k) innovation to escape their traditional responsibility to employees. They dumped old defined-benefit pension plans and adopted the new version, which requires much smaller employer contributions and thereby reduces labor costs dramatically. Good for the bottom line, bad for the country's future.

"The whole thinking was: Let's relieve the employers of this burden and empower individuals," explains Karen Ferguson, longtime director of the Pension Rights Center in Washington. "The problem is, it has failed—and failed miserably—and no one wants to say that."

Pension protection is actually shrinking, despite the proliferation of 401(k) accounts and the alleged prosperity of the 1980s and '90s. In the private sector, fewer employees participate in pension plans of any kind now than twenty years ago, down from 51 percent to 46 percent (the defined-benefit company pensions that once covered 53 percent now protect only 34 percent). The value of pension wealth, meanwhile, fell by 17 percent for workers in the middle and below, mainly because their voluntary savings were weak or nonexistent, yet soared for those at the top—"an upsurge in pension wealth inequality," economist Edward Wolff of New York University observed.

In sum, pensions became less valuable. And fewer families have one. That helps explain why Bush's plan encountered popular resistance. In these circumstances, whacking Social Security benefits or raising the retirement age does not sound like "reform." But neither political party has yet summoned the nerve to acknowledge the implications of the failed experiment or to propose serious solutions.

The most threatening problem is not Social Security; it is shrinking pensions, collapsed personal savings and soaring health costs.

The circumstances look even more ominous—the very opposite of Professor Fogel's sunny vision—because personal savings also collapsed during the long, slow-motion weakening of pensions. Given the stagnating wages for hourly workers and easier access to credit, families typically managed to stay afloat by working more jobs and by borrowing more. Saving for the future was not an available option for many. In 1982 personal savings peaked at $480 billion, then began an epic decline. Last year the national total in personal savings was only $103 billion—down nearly 80 percent from twenty-five years ago. As Eugene Steuerle of the Urban Institute points out, the federal government now spends more money on tax subsidies to encourage the individual forms of pension savings—$115 billion last year—than Americans actually save.

The one potential bright spot in this story might be real estate—the family wealth that accumulates gradually through home ownership and the rising market value of houses. Given the current housing boom and runaway prices in the hotter urban markets, many families might salvage retirement plans by selling their homes and moving to less expensive dwellings. The trouble is, families have been living off that wealth—borrowing, almost dollar for dollar, against the rising price of their homes through equity-credit lines or refinanced mortgages. From 1999 through 2003, the value of family homes rose by a spectacular $3.3 trillion, but families' actual equity in those properties changed little because mortgage borrowing rose nearly as fast.

Thus, people financed routine consumption by borrowing against their long-term assets—that's real grasshopper behavior. And the situation could turn very ugly if the housing bubble pops and home prices fall. People will find themselves stuck paying off a mountain of debt on homes that are suddenly worth less than the mortgages. They will not only need to keep working; they might also be filing for bankruptcy.

'Just as wealth and income are being redistributed to the wealthy, so is leisure.' —economist Teresa Ghilarducci

How could this have happened in such a wealthy nation—especially during an era when stock prices were rising explosively? The basic explanations are familiar: rising inequality and reactionary economic policies, launched first by Reagan, then elaborated by Bush II and resisted only faintheartedly by Democrats. The corporate "social contract" was discarded; regressive tax-cutting rewarded capital and the well-to-do; numerous other measures fractured the broad middle class. The wages of hourly workers—80 percent of the private-sector workforce—have been essentially unchanged in terms of real purchasing power for three decades (no one in politics wants to talk about that, either). The political system continues to defer to the needs of corporations despite the torrent of financial scandals and extreme greed displayed by egomaniacal CEOs. All these factors contributed to the erosion of retirement security. Economist Teresa Ghilarducci, a pension authority at Notre Dame, remarks, "Just as wealth and income are being redistributed to the wealthy, so is leisure."

In fact, Ghilarducci argues, allowing the pension system to deteriorate serves a long-term interest of business: avoiding future labor shortages when the baby-boom generation moves into retirement. "All this retirement policy is really a labor policy," she asserts. "It's motivated by these experts who say, Hey, wait, we're going to need to do what we can to encourage people to work longer. A whole range of economists and elite opinion makers is talking about a labor shortage where, God forbid, wages would increase. That's what they're worried about—making sure there isn't a corporate profit squeeze, that skill shortages and upward wage pressures are checked."

This development is already lengthening working lives, she finds. The average retirement age, rather than gradually declining toward 55, as Fogel foresees, has turned around in the past few years and is slowly increasing. "I'm not against older people working if they want to," Ghilarducci says. "I'm against policies that force them back into the workforce because they've lost their pensions or their healthcare costs have gone up."

One need not question the sincerity of the right's ideological convictions to see that their policy initiatives are also designed to benefit important political patrons. With the transition to 401(k) accounts, corporate employers were major winners. Ghilarducci's examination of 700 companies over nearly two decades found that their annual pension contributions dropped by one third—from $2,140 to $1,404 per employee—as they shifted from defined-benefit pensions to the less expensive defined-contribution model. Not surprisingly, the traditional company pension began to disappear or shrink as large industrial companies hacked away at the uncompetitive costs. The number of younger workers with the traditional form of pension is much smaller and falling fast.

Wall Street banks and brokerages were big winners too, since they began competing for the millions of new "investors" with their individual stock accounts. This enormous influx of customers helped fuel the long stock-market boom and encouraged the exaggerated promises made by both corporations and financial firms. The overall economy was probably damaged too, because mutual funds competed for customers by going after rapid, short-term gains rather than focusing on the long-term investments financed by patient capital. When the stock-market illusions burst in 2000, the meltdown evaporated lots of retirement accounts too, especially for those innocent risk-takers who had bet their savings on NASDAQ's high-flying tech stocks.

The most damning fact about the 401(k) experiment is that it has failed to fulfill the original purpose: boosting savings for ordinary Americans. Academic studies have confirmed that the personal accounts produced "very little net savings" or "statistically insignificant" gains. While every worker could participate in theory, the practical reality is that only the more affluent families could afford to take full advantage of the 401(k) tax break—sheltering their annual 401(k) contributions from income taxes. But typically they did so simply by moving money from other conventional savings accounts into the tax-exempt kind.

More affluent Americans thus reduced their income taxes, but their net savings did not actually increase. For two decades, the federal government has been heavily subsidizing "savings" by the people who needed no inducement because they were already saving. Think of it as welfare for the virtuously well-to-do. A rational government would phase out such a misconceived program. Bush is instead proposing to make the contradictions worse by adding still other tax-exempt savings vehicles designed to benefit the affluent.

The old system of defined-benefit pensions had many strengths by comparison, but it was never a solution to the national problem either. Even at their peak, the traditional corporate pensions left out half of the workforce. Larger companies, especially in unionized industrial sectors, provided strong benefits for their employees, responding to labor's bargaining demands and to attract well-qualified people. But the millions of very small firms, where more Americans work, almost never offered pensions. The burden either seemed too costly or too complicated to administer. Generally, their workers are the folks who depend solely on Social Security.

The corporate pensions are also not portable (a problem the individual accounts were supposed to solve). And pension law gives corporate managers ample latitude to game their pension funds to enhance the company's bottom line. Stories of elderly retirees stranded by their old employers are now commonplace: broken promises on healthcare and other benefits that go unpunished. Instead of accumulating larger surpluses during the good times, the corporations often did the opposite, leaving their pension funds severely underfunded for the bad times, when shortfalls couldn't be overcome. Employees have no representatives to speak for them in the decision-making. If a corporate pension fund goes belly up, its liabilities are dumped on the government's insurance agency, which is getting strapped itself.

A logical and achievable solution exists to correct this mess. Government should create a new hybrid pension that combines the best aspects of defined-benefit and defined-contribution versions—one that requires all workers to save for the future and no longer relies on the "good will" of employers. Given modern employment patterns, workers do need a portable pension that stays with them, job to job. But their voluntary savings are simply too small and erratic—too vulnerable to manipulation by financial brokers—to produce secure results in the stock-market casino. Either they get lured into wild gambles or they park their savings in mutual funds that gouge them with inflated fees and commissions while catering to the corporations that are the funds' largest customers (this conflict of interest between large and small customers is endemic to the US financial system; guess who loses). The employees' money will produce far more reliable accumulations if it is invested for them by professionals at a major independent pension fund that works only for them.

The fundamental truth (well understood among experts) is that individualized accounts can never match the investment returns of a large common fund, broadly diversified and soundly managed, because the pension fund is able to average its results over a very long time span, thirty years or more. A few wise guys might beat the casino odds, but the broad herd of small investors will always be captive to the random luck of bad timing and their own ignorance. The right wing's celebration of individual risk-taking in financial markets is like inviting sheep to the slaughter.

The super bull market is over. Its gorgeous returns will not return for many years, maybe many decades. But a very large, diversified pension fund—managed solely in the interests of its contributors—provides the vehicle for "shared luck." It can smooth out the ups and downs among all participants, young and old, lucky and unlucky. It can invest for long-term economic development rather than chase stock-market fads. Good returns for retirees, good results for the economy.

These are the very qualities Professor Fogel envisions. They describe trustworthy pension systems, like TIAA-CREF, which reliably serves many thousands of individual employees (teachers and professors) who are scattered across many different employers (schools and universities). The present reform debate is not thinking this way. Collective action is out of fashion, especially if the government is involved. Significant reform would require institution-building. The transition would pose many technical difficulties. "There are obstacles, but I don't think that's the problem," Ghilarducci says. "The obstacle is imagination."

Pro-Life Pension Reform

The Pension Rights Center just conducted a year-long "conversation on coverage" that pulled together experts from business and labor, the insurance industry, Wall Street finance, academia, AARP and other interested sectors. The workshop sessions produced a long list of worthy ideas for patching up the broken system, but that was the problem: The proposals basically involved incremental tinkering with the status quo, not universal, mandatory solutions. To get all these diverse interests to join the conversation, Karen Ferguson confides, the center had to stipulate that "mandatory" would not be discussed.

"The bottom line is that the companies always have the upper hand, even though they've gotten huge subsidies and tax benefits," she explains. "The system is voluntary, so companies can always opt out." Indeed, the politics of pension reform is usually a discussion about what new favors and concessions should be granted to employers to get them to do the "right thing" for their employees. This political logic led to the current failure. "Voluntary" is a loser, as the past twenty years amply demonstrated, because it gives companies controlling leverage over what is possible. And even well-intentioned executives will always have to choose between the company's self-interest and its employees (guess who usually loses). Only the government

has the reach and power to design and oversee a pension system that truly serves all. During the past generation, most corporations discarded their obligations under the old social contract. It seems only fair they should forfeit political control too.

A universal savings system that covers everyone because it is mandatory could prove to be as durable (and popular) as Social Security.

Plausible plans in addition to Fogel's do exist that offer genuine solutions. A universal savings system that covers everyone because it is mandatory could prove to be as durable (and popular) as Social Security. It balances equity by subsidizing the savings of lower-income workers. It creates authentic individual ownership and incentives to save more for the future, consume less in the present. It operates free of Wall Street profiteers and under government supervision, adhering to well-established principles of sound investing. Employers could be discouraged from further abandoning their obligations by penalties in the tax code. Many other nations, large and small and far less wealthy, have created such systems. Americans would need to craft their own distinctive version.

One promising example, designed by economist Christian Weller for the Economic Policy Institute, proposes a modest savings rate of 3 percent of wages, but combined with the existing Social Security benefits, it would approach the level of retirement security envisioned by Fogel. The government would contribute substantial savings for low earners and also match additional contributions made by the workers or their employers. Weller estimates this would cost around $48 billion a year—less than half the federal tax subsidy now devoted to all pension plans. Weller's design is robustly equitable, scaled to help the bottom rungs most and top income earners least. Combined with Social Security, low earners (wages of $24,000 or less) would enjoy a pension that replaces 83 percent of their peak working wages. Average earners would get 60 percent replacement, high earners only 48 percent. This makes sense, because higher-income families have much greater opportunity to augment pensions with other sources of income and savings. The working poor do not.

Essentially, Weller has updated and expanded a mandatory savings plan that was proposed nearly twenty-five years ago—a last gasp from the Carter Administration. Reagan's election and laissez-faire politics snuffed the idea. While still modest in scale, Weller's design represents a meaningful start toward Fogel's larger vision of a 15 percent savings rate. Since the Social Security tax now collects 12.6 percent of wages jointly from workers and employers, it is not plausible at this point to add another 15 percent to labor costs for pension savings. However, as the new pension system matures and public confidence is established, a gradual transition can be pursued that adds little by little to the personal savings rate, offset by equivalent reductions in the payroll tax for Social Security—thus yielding greater savings and lower taxes. Both government systems would continue in place, one as the fundamental safety net of social insurance, the other as the universal, expanding pillar for comfortable retirement.

Ghilarducci thinks much of the accumulating wealth could be stored and invested by large private pension funds, organized by unions or other groups for workers at multiple employers (much like TIAA-CREF's role for universities). A successful existing model is the unified pension systems for the building and construction trades. Co-managed by unions and companies, they encourage industry and labor to collaborate on joint training and other productivity-enhancing endeavors that can raise the quality of work and wages.

While most politicians don't dare embrace a "mandatory" solution—not yet, anyway—it is not self-evident that ordinary Americans would reject one, if properly educated about the alternatives. Most people are conflicted. They know they need to save more—retirement is a very meaningful investment for them—but it's very hard to accomplish, given the competing pressures. They like the concept of personal accounts but are also aware of their vulnerability as amateur investors. In her conversations with union presidents, Ghilarducci finds they are more in favor of an "add on" national pension than raising the payroll tax for Social Security. "You can sell workers if their name is on it," she concludes. "If you had a system that says you must contribute 3 percent of wages to your mandatory savings account, you would actually have two-thirds of the workers grateful that they are being forced to save. You wouldn't get that if they were forced to pay another 3 percent in taxes into Social Security."

The retirement question—choices of mandatory or voluntary, universal or incremental—embodies a classic dilemma often facing liberal politics. Do reformers pursue the larger, more provocative approach that invites greater resistance but would fundamentally solve the problem? Or do they opt for smaller, safer measures that have a better chance of adoption and will demonstrate good intentions, if not a genuine remedy for society? For several decades, it seems obvious, most Democrats have chosen the side of caution: thinking small, offering symbolic gestures, avoiding fights over fundamental solutions. One can see where this strategy has gotten the party. The gestures are no longer taken seriously, since they don't lead anywhere. The public no longer associates Democrats with big ideas or principled commitments to authentic reform. We await incautious politicians with the courage to pursue their unfashionable convictions.

Index

Index

Test Your Knowledge Form

We encourage you to photocopy and use this page as a tool to assess how the articles in *Annual Editions* expand on the information in your textbook. By reflecting on the articles you will gain enhanced text information. You can also access this useful form on a product's book support Web site at *http://www.mhcls.com/online/*.

NAME:

DATE:

TITLE AND NUMBER OF ARTICLE:

BRIEFLY STATE THE MAIN IDEA OF THIS ARTICLE:

LIST THREE IMPORTANT FACTS THAT THE AUTHOR USES TO SUPPORT THE MAIN IDEA:

WHAT INFORMATION OR IDEAS DISCUSSED IN THIS ARTICLE ARE ALSO DISCUSSED IN YOUR TEXTBOOK OR OTHER READINGS THAT YOU HAVE DONE? LIST THE TEXTBOOK CHAPTERS AND PAGE NUMBERS:

LIST ANY EXAMPLES OF BIAS OR FAULTY REASONING THAT YOU FOUND IN THE ARTICLE:

LIST ANY NEW TERMS/CONCEPTS THAT WERE DISCUSSED IN THE ARTICLE, AND WRITE A SHORT DEFINITION:

We Want Your Advice

ANNUAL EDITIONS revisions depend on two major opinion sources: one is our Advisory Board, listed in the front of this volume, which works with us in scanning the thousands of articles published in the public press each year; the other is you—the person actually using the book. Please help us and the users of the next edition by completing the prepaid article rating form on this page and returning it to us. Thank you for your help!

ANNUAL EDITIONS: Aging 06/07

ARTICLE RATING FORM

Here is an opportunity for you to have direct input into the next revision of this volume.
We would like you to rate each of the articles listed below, using the following scale:

1. **Excellent: should definitely be retained**
2. **Above average: should probably be retained**
3. **Below average: should probably be deleted**
4. **Poor: should definitely be deleted**

Your ratings will play a vital part in the next revision.
Please mail this prepaid form to us as soon as possible.
Thanks for your help!

RATING	ARTICLE
	1. Elderly Americans
	2. The Economic Conundrum of an Aging Population
	3. A Study for the Ages
	4. Puzzle of the Century
	5. The Demographic Drivers of Aging
	6. Will You Live to Be 100?
	7. The Coming Death Shortage: Why the Longevity Boom Will Make Us Sorry To Be Alive
	8. Women's Sexuality as They Age: The More Things Change, the More They Stay the Same
	9. Successful Aging
	10. The Do or Die Decade
	11. We Can Control How We Age
	12. Society Fears the Aging Process
	13. Ageism in America
	14. The Activation of Aging Stereotypes in Younger and Older Adults
	15. The Under-Reported Impact of Age Discrimination and Its Threat to Business Vitality
	16. Primary Care for Elderly People: Why Do Doctors Find It So Hard?
	17. Breakthrough
	18. Will You Still Need Me When I'm...84? More Couples Divorce After Decades
	19. The Disappearing Mind

RATING	ARTICLE
	20. Alzheimer's Disease as a "Trip Back in Time"
	21. How to Survive the First Year
	22. Reshaping Retirement: Scenarios and Options
	23. Old. Smart. Productive.
	24. Work, Retirement, and Well-Being
	25. Work/Retirement Choices and Lifestyle Patterns of Older Americans
	26. More Hospice Patients Forgoing Sustenance
	27. Expectancy of Spousal Death and Adjustment to Conjugal Bereavement
	28. Start the Conversation
	29. Trends in Causes of Death Among the Elderly
	30. (Not) the Same Old Story
	31. A Home for the Rest of Your Life
	32. Assisted Living: How Much Assistance Can You Really Count On?
	33. The City of Laguna Woods: A Case of Senior Power in Local Politics
	34. Have Seniors Been Dealt a Bad Hand? Medicare's Drug Discount Cards
	35. Long-Term Care: The Ticking Bomb
	36. Universalism Without the Targeting: Privatizing the Old-Age Welfare State
	37. Prescription for Change
	38. Riding Into the Sunset

(Continued on next page)

BUSINESS REPLY MAIL
FIRST CLASS MAIL PERMIT NO. 551 DUBUQUE IA

POSTAGE WILL BE PAID BY ADDRESEE

McGraw-Hill Contemporary Learning Series
2460 KERPER BLVD
DUBUQUE, IA 52001-9902

Ihlhmlhllllmllhmmllllhlhlhlllhmhlhhll

ABOUT YOU

Name   Date

Are you a teacher? ❒   A student? ❒
Your school's name

Department

Address   City   State   Zip

School telephone #

YOUR COMMENTS ARE IMPORTANT TO US!

Please fill in the following information:
For which course did you use this book?

Did you use a text with this ANNUAL EDITION?   ❒   yes ❒   no
What was the title of the text?

What are your general reactions to the *Annual Editions* concept?

Have you read any pertinent articles recently that you think should be included in the next edition? Explain.

Are there any articles that you feel should be replaced in the next edition? Why?

Are there any World Wide Web sites that you feel should be included in the next edition? Please annotate.

May we contact you for editorial input?   ❒   yes ❒   no
May we quote your comments?   ❒   yes ❒   no